A Thinker's Guide
to Ultrasonic Imaging

A Thinker's Guide
to Ultrasonic Imaging

Raymond L. Powis, Ph.D.

Wendy J. Powis, D.M.U. *(Australia)*

Urban & Schwarzenberg
Baltimore—Munich

Urban & Schwarzenberg, Inc.
7 E. Redwood Street
Baltimore, Maryland 21202
USA

Urban & Schwarzenberg
Landwehrstrasse 61
D-8000 München 2
West Germany

Printed in the United States of America

10   9   8   7   6   5   4   3

Library of Congress Cataloging in Publication Data

Powis, Raymond L.
  A thinker's guide to ultrasonic imaging.

Includes index.
  1. Diagnosis, Ultrasonic. I. Powis, Wendy J.
II. Title.
RC78.7.U4P68   1984   616.07'543   83-21704
ISBN 0-8067-1581-2

Compositor: Automated Graphic Systems
Printer: Automated Graphic Systems/Maple Press Company
Manuscript editor: Molly Ruzicka
Indexer: Author
Production and design: John Cronin and Norman Och

ISBN 0-8067-1581-2 Baltimore

ISBN 3-541-71581-2 Munich

THIS BOOK IS

Dedicated to Every Sonographer

WHO HAS EVER LOOKED AT AN ULTRASONIC IMAGE
AND WONDERED WHAT WAS GOING ON.

Contents

PART ONE
Inner Workings of the Sonograph

PART TWO

Extracting Information
from the Images

How to Use This Book

A quick look through the book will show that it is divided into two major sections. The first section addresses the physical and electronic events in sonography. This section is a detailed description of the science underlying diagnostic ultrasound.

Within this first section, the division of chapters is not along technology lines but highlights the steps that lead to the ultrasound display. Thus, chapters 1 and 2 on waves and signal processing are the starting point for someone new to ultrasound. The remaining chapters can be read in any order. As much as possible, each chapter in this section stands alone, with references to other chapters for more detailed reading. Several figures and concepts are repeated in each chapter so the reader does not have to jump around the book to completely follow the discussion.

The second section of the book is intimately connected with the information in the first section. The second section points the reader's attention to the many connections between the clinical utility of a sonograph and the underlying science. In sum, the second section demonstrates why ultrasound science is valuable to a sonographer. Consequently, many of the ideas in this section are predicated on knowing facts from the first section. A reader just learning about ultrasound will find this section more difficult to completely understand without the core ideas detailed in the first section. As in the first section, the chapters have no special order and a reader can safely follow the pulls of curiosity or need.

In total, the book is neither a clinical text nor a rigorous science text. It is, instead, a book on building a mental model of ultrasound, a way of thinking, that may eventually give the excellent clinical and physics texts now available added dimension and meaning.

Preface

Nineteen seventy-eight was a windfall year for us. Although we had been working 12,000 miles apart, on separate continents, in different cultures, and each of us with different educational backgrounds, we quickly discovered at our first meeting that we had been using a common set of words to teach ultrasound in Australia and the United States. In our classes, solutions to ultrasound problems and an understanding of events had been achieved by an approach we had called "thinking through the problem." But we had soon found that to be an effective educational tool, "thinking things through" required that users have access to a set of fundamental facts that would integrate both the informal and documented observations that we and others had made. Searches of the available literature on ultrasonic imaging on two continents had provided the facts, but seldom in a form we could use to teach others or that others could use to teach themselves. So, we each started to collect and transcribe into usable form the principles of ultrasound science. This book, then, is the result of our separate and combined efforts to provide users with a "thoughtful" approach to ultrasound.

A Thinker's Guide to Ultrasonic Imaging is directed to every individual who holds a transducer in hand and must make and interpret the visual results. In terms of difficulty, this book is designed as an intermediate step—midway between a rudimentary text and an advanced treatment—in the continuing education of both sonographer and sonologist. Although each chapter addresses a separate area of interest and can be read alone, each chapter is connected to the others by frequent cross references. Often the same ideas are repeated in later chapters, a reflection not of a lack of things to write about, but of the importance of certain key ideas to the mechanical and electrical events of diagnostic ultrasound.

The acid test for any text is the number of new and productive avenues of thought it generates in its readers. A successful text is a conduit to bigger and better things and seldom an end in itself. Writing this book has been a condensing force for us, bringing together ideas that would have remained uncorrected without the effort. We hope it does the same for its readers.

Raymond L. Powis
Wendy J. Powis (Aldous)

Acknowledgments

Writing a book is a lonely business most of the time. And the singular effort of writing could make an author believe that the final result is singularly his. We have no such illusions about this book. Without the assistance and support of many different people, companies, and institutions, this book would never have come to be.

We would like to especially thank Christopher Merritt, M.D. and Melissa Foreman, R.D.M.S. at the Ochsner Foundation Hospital, New Orleans, Louisiana. Dr. Merritt and Ms. Foreman kindly opened their facilities to us and provided assistance in gathering many of the real time images and nearly all of the B-scan images for this book.

We also extend thanks to the companies who provided aid without hesitation to our requests: Advanced Technology Labs (ATL), Bellevue, Washington for generously providing their facilities to make the quality assurance real time images; Radiation Measurements, Inc. (RMI), Middleton, Wisconsin for providing the tissue equivalent phantoms used in making the quality assurance images; and Technicare Ultrasound Division, Englewood, Colorado, for making special efforts to secure otherwise unavailable pictures.

So many people have helped us put parts of this book together, it is hard to name them all. We extend personal thanks to: Norman Rantanen, D.V.M., who provided positive criticism for many of the chapters; Ann McClary, International Marketing Manager at Technicare, who personally provided photos; and Chuck Wood, Ph.D. of Biomedical Illustrations, Bellevue, Washington for drawing a few of the more difficult art pieces.

We would like to extend a special thanks to the publisher, who kept faith through numerous delays and rewrites.

And lastly, we would like to thank the sonographers and sonologists in Australia and America who have shared their experiences and ideas with us. Their knowledge lives in the pages of this book.

PART ONE

Inner Workings of the Sonograph

Chapter 1

Waves and Wave Analysis

The world abounds with waves. Waves appear on the surface of water when it is disturbed, they roll over a flag or banner in the wind, they move outward from us when we speak. Some waves are visible, like those on a water surface, while others are invisible, like the electromagnetic waves in the radio spectrum or the sound waves that travel through air. Despite their diverse forms, qualities, and quantities, all waves contain nearly the same properties. Thus, by studying a limited number of wave types, it is possible to begin to generalize our thinking for all waves.

Of all the available waves, this book focuses on only two: *electromagnetic* waves and *mechanical* waves. Electromagnetic waves arise from the movement of charged particles such as electrons. As their name implies, electromagnetic waves are made of both electrical and magnetic components. If the frequency of these waves is high enough, we can see them; such waves represent the visible portion of the electromagnetic spectrum. Today, scientists know a great deal about the physical properties of light, information that helps to explain the second form of waves that concerns us, the mechanical waves. Of the mechanical waves, this text centers on two types, the longitudinal waves and the transverse waves. Once again, however, the apparent difference between these waves is deceiving, for they both exhibit nearly identical properties. The more-familiar transverse wave is used here to study the less-familiar longitudinal wave. We begin with a description of wave anatomy.

Wave Anatomy

Mechanical waves are initiated as a physical displacement of material particles away from a rest position, with the displacement moving from its starting point as in Figure 1-1. As the mechanical wave travels, it interacts with the carrying medium, sometimes altering the wave or medium as it moves. If a displacement is repeated at regular intervals, a long series of waves forms, the waves moving away from the source in a regular fashion. The displacement can be across or along the direction of travel: If across the direction of travel, the wave is called *transverse;*

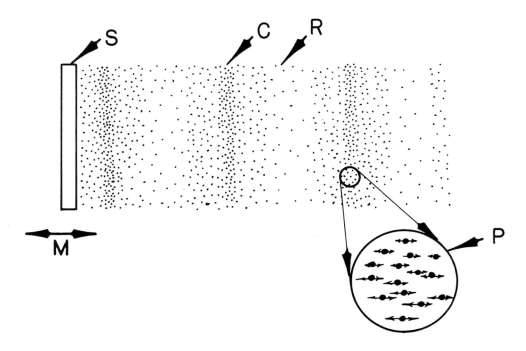

1-1   Formation of longitudinal waves. The vibratory motion *M* of the source *S* forms compressions *C* and rarefactions *R*. Particle motion *P* is along the same direction as the source motion *M*.

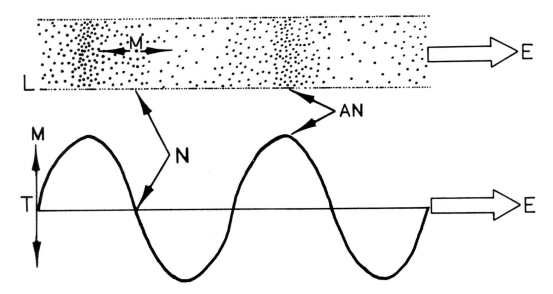

1-2   The connection between longitudinal and transverse waves. For the longitudinal wave *L,* the motion *M* is along the same direction as the energy flow *E*. For the transverse wave *T,* motion *M* is transverse to the direction of energy flow *E*. In both waves there are regions where the displacement is either minimum, called nodes, or *N,* or maximum, called antinodes, *AN*.

if along the direction of travel, the wave is called *longitudinal*. Both waves, however, have a common set of events, as shown in Figure 1-2, even though they carry different names.

As the displacements move away from the source, they take on a pattern that forms the final waves. To better visualize this pattern, consider the surface waves on a body of water. A basin filled with water that is disturbed at the surface forms a set of waves that moves away from the disturbance as concentric waves, and appears to us as a set of concentric circles. If we mentally cut through the surface of the water while this is happening, as in Figure 1-3, we can see the transverse waves in cross section, an exercise that helps to visualize wave anatomy and events.

Figure 1-3 shows that the surface of the water is displaced both upward and downward as the wave passes. The peaks of this displacement, both up and down, are called *antinodes*. At the same time, the portions of the wave that do not represent any surface displacement are called *nodes*. As shown in Figure 1-2, nodes and antinodes are primary markers to reference events within the wave itself.

Unless we are able to monitor the instant that a wave cycle starts, it is hard to know where a wave starts or stops. A cycle of activity can be traced, but the absolute timing of events is unknown. In order to provide some reference points, we will focus here on a single segment of one cycle. A cycle extends from one node past the next to the third node. This period of time includes a set of nonrepeated events. The distance traversed by a single cycle is called the *wavelength*, represented by the Greek letter *lambda* (λ). Stated another way, the wavelength represents the distance from one event to the repetition of that event; thus, the wavelength can extend from any part of the wave to the next repetition of that event, including from one antinode past the next to the third antinode.

The time it takes to form a cycle is called the period, represented by *T*. *T* can be calculated by dividing a single second by the number of cycles that occurs in each second, which is frequency. Thus:

$$T = 1/f \qquad (1.1)$$

where f is the number of cycles that occurs in one second. The unit used to describe cycles per second is the hertz. Thus, a wave vibrating at 10 cycles per second has a frequency of 10 Hz; if vibrating at 1,000 cycles per second it has a frequency of a kilohertz (kHz); and if vibrating at 1,000,000 cycles per second it has a frequency of a megahertz (MHz). These are the basic labels applied to the wave and wave components.

Let us look again at the formation of waves on a water's surface. The surface disturbance created a set of waves that moved away from the source point symmetrically and at a constant velocity. This wave velocity is called the *propagation velocity* and represents the rate at which the mechanical wave can be coupled from one region of the water surface to another. How fast this happens depends in part upon the spacing of particles that compose the propagating medium.

In general, gases carry mechanical waves more slowly than do fluids, which, in turn, carry waves more slowly than do solids. These characteristics provide clues to the varying distances between the molecules or particles that make up the wave-

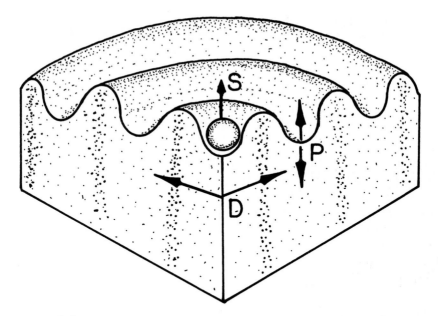

1-3   A systematic connection between surface and longitudinal waves. A source *S* disturbs the surface of a fluid, forming surface waves that result in particle displacement *P* and corresponding density and pressure changes *D* below the surface.

carrying medium. If the propagation velocity is high, the distance between nodes or antinodes within the material is larger than in a material with a lower propagation velocity. If the frequency is increased, the spacing between nodes decreases, shortening the wavelength. Thus, a fundamental relationship between the velocity of propagation, the wavelength, and frequency may be expressed in the equation:

$$V = F \lambda, \tag{1.2}$$

where V is the velocity of propagation in units of length per unit time, F is the frequency in hertz, and λ is the wavelength in units of length. In most materials, the velocity of propagation for a mechanical wave is nearly constant, regardless of frequency, which is nearly the same for ultrasound. Thus, as the frequency increases, the wavelength decreases. And by knowing the velocity of propagation and the frequency, the wavelength can be easily calculated from equation 1.2.

If a wave lasts for only a few cycles, it is called a finite wave train. Indeed, no real limit exists on the number of waves that can constitute a wave train, except that the number is finite. If the source makes waves continuously, the wave train can become very long and can be considered an infinite wave train. Sometimes, if the wave train is short and part of a larger set of wave events, it is called a wavelet.

Waves represent the transport of energy away from an energy source. As a result, waves are usually traveling from one region to another. At times, however, waves can be standing, or at least appear to be standing. Such waves are often the sum of several traveling waves that together form a standing wave. This process of adding waves together is covered in more detail later in the chapter.

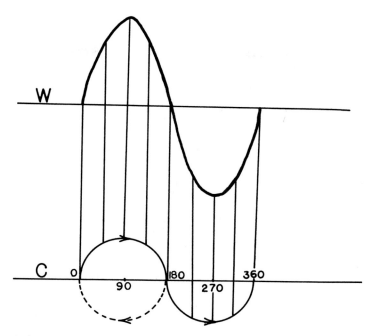

1-4 Expressing timing and phase for a sine wave using degrees. Because a sine wave is cyclic, each segment of the wave cycle can be expressed in degrees. The first half of the cycle spans 180°, and the second half of the cycle spans 180° to 360°, as if a particle were moving around a circle (dotted line).

Most waves are repetitive, that is, they exhibit a sequence of events that represents a single cycle that is repeated. The times comprised by events within a single cycle are called *phases,* as shown in Figure 1-4. A phase can reference any event from the start to the finish of a wave cycle. Typically, events are marked by their appearance in the cycle, according to which the time within a cycle is expressed by angular degrees. The use of degrees stems from the practice of considering a cycle as a trip around a circle, with the entire trip representing 360°. Thus, the cycle begins at 0°, one-quarter of a cycle is 90°, a half cycle is 180°, three-quarters of a cycle is 270°, and, of course, full circle is 360°. Given this division of the cycle, timing changes within one cycle can be expressed in terms of phase changes. For example, if a wave is suddenly advanced by one-quarter of a cycle, it has been shifted in phase by 90°. Alternately, if a wave is suddenly delayed a quarter of a cycle, it has been shifted back in phase by 90°.

However, expressing the relative timing of events between waves would be difficult if frequency or amplitude (see below) were the only means of doing so. If two waves coincide on a one-to-one basis, where each node and antinode match, the two waves are said to be alike in both phase and frequency. On the other hand, two waves can have the same frequency but not the same phase. By relating the landmarks of one wave to the other, for example, comparing nodes or antinodes in a cycle, the amount of phase difference can be expressed in degrees, and waves will add together as a function of amplitude, frequency, and phase, in which phase plays a dominant role.

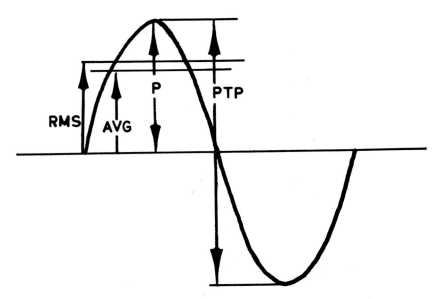

1-5   Peak and average values for a sine wave. The total swing in the wave is the peak-to-peak value *PTP*. The greatest displacement in either direction is the peak value *P*. The *RMS* average is calculated by taking the square *R*oot of the *M*ean value *S*quared. The mean value is the first moment of the wave, *AVG*.

As a mechanical wave progresses through its formation, the particles of the carrying medium experience a displacement away from the normal resting position. The relative size of this displacement is called the *wave amplitude.* By tracing events within a cycle it can be seen that the amplitude constantly changes. Thus, when speaking of amplitude, it is necessary to specify where in the cycle the amplitude is being considered. Wave amplitude usually means the peak amplitude, representing the maximum displacement that occurs during the wave cycle, as shown in Figure 1-5. A related parameter is the peak-to-peak value, the distance from the largest upward displacement to the largest downward displacement. These values are used to evaluate such things as the amount of energy present in the wave and how disruptive the wave is to the material carrying it.

The discussion so far has defined events only around waves in two dimensions, such as a transverse wave traveling on a line within the plane of this page. That concept can now be extended to include three-dimensional waves, such as those on the surface of water. Disturbing the water's surface generates a set of concentric traveling waves that moves outward from the disturbance over the water's surface. Moving the source or disturbance into the volume of water causes a set of concentric spherical waves that moves out from the source at a constant velocity. Each spherical surface is formed by connecting all the components of the waves that have a common phase, as in Figure 1-6. The curved surface so created is called a wave front. In this case, the wave fronts are curved into spheres. As the waves continue to travel, they form an increasingly larger radius of curvature to the point that when a small portion of the wave front is examined, it appears flat, forming what is called a plane wave front.

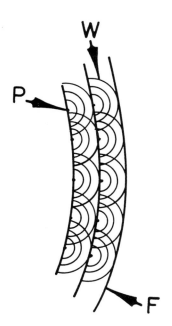

1-6 Christian Huygens's principle for advancing waves. For an advancing wave front moving through a homogeneous medium, each point on a wave front *P* acts like a point source of waves *W*. The new wave front *F* can be formed by connecting together all the wave positions at the same point in time.

Once the wave front is formed, the front advances at a fixed velocity that is determined by the material the wave is traveling through. We can determine the direction a wave front will advance by drawing small arrows everywhere perpendicular to the surface of the wave front. These small arrows symbolize rays, with each ray composed of a wavelet. By always connecting together the common phase points in the waves, the shape of the advancing wave front can be determined.

We now have a wave, generated by a source, with a known frequency and propagation velocity that determines the wavelength within the carrying medium. We can gauge the amplitude of the wave by measuring the amount of displacement that occurs when the wave passes a given point. And by connecting together the common phase points, we can determine the shape of the wave front. Given these definitions and parameters, we are ready to look at some properties of various waves and at wave interactions.

Wave Properties

The previous section referred to the transverse wave to explain various aspects of wave anatomy. Next, we will examine the longitudinal wave in more detail.

Unlike the transverse wave, the longitudinal wave is formed by the movement of material particles along the direction the energy is traveling. This results in regions where the molecules of the medium are compressed closely together (called *compressions*), and other regions where the molecules are pulled apart (called *rarefactions*). The compressions form regions of higher-than-normal density, and the rarefactions form regions of lower-than-normal density. The ability to form these compressions and rarefactions is limited by the relative elasticity of the carrying medium. In addition, the rate at which these regions form determines how well the wave can move through the material. All these facets of material-wave interaction are factors in the production and propagation of ultrasound in tissue.

The ability to squeeze molecules of a material closer together is called *compressibility,* and is determined by how close the molecules are already. Molecules that are widely separated, as in a gas, can be easily compressed. On the other hand, the molecules of a metal are already tightly packed and resist further compression. Fluids are somewhere between these two extremes of compressibility. In terms of wave action, it follows therefore that longitudinal waves are easy to form in air but difficult to form in metals, with water once again somewhere in between. In general, as the density of a material increases, the ability to form compressional waves decreases.

The longitudinal wave is a mechanical wave and needs a material that can couple the energy from one region of space to another. Again, this is a function of how closely together the molecules are arranged and of how well they are connected with intermolecular forces. The ability to couple energy is witnessed in the propagation velocity of a material. If a material has a high propagation velocity, the ability to form longitudinal waves decreases, because the energy moves along before the compressional process is complete. Low propagation velocities, on the other hand, encourage longitudinal wave formation because the energy moves slowly enough to form compressions.

The compressibility of a material as a function of density and wave propagation velocity within that same material can promote or impede the formation of compressional waves, or for that matter, any mechanical wave. A parameter has been invented to evaluate how well mechanical waves can be formed in a material. Called the material characteristic impedance, it expresses the amount of impedence a material raises to compressional wave formation. It is the product of the material density and propagation velocity and appears as:

$$Z = pc, \tag{1.3}$$

where Z is the characteristic impedance, p is the material density, and c is the velocity of propagation. In ultrasound, Z is known as the acoustic impedance.

According to this model, the material carrying the wave is not considered to be removing energy from the wave. However, the geometry of the propagation still imposes a decrease in wave amplitude as the wave front advances from the source. This is easily understood by examining a point source of waves located inside a body of water. The waves, and therefore the wave fronts formed from the source, have a finite amount of energy contained in each. As the wave front increases its distance from the point source, the wave front enlarges its surface area proportional to the radius squared. Thus, the wave-front geometry spreads the wave energy over a larger and larger area, decreasing the amount of energy contained in any unit wave front area, as shown in Figure 1-7. In the process, the wave front experiences a decrease in intensity.

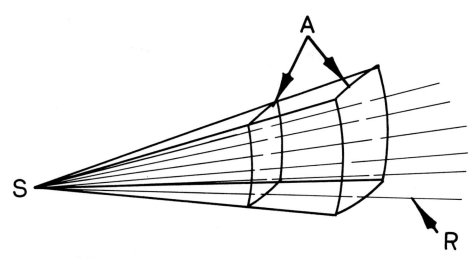

1-7 Geometric spread of waves from a point source. As a wave front *A* expands from a point source *S,* corresponding points on the wave front travel along straight lines to form rays *R*. As the distance from the source increases, the rays become farther apart, and the wave energy per unit area decreases.

But what is intensity? To understand this concept, look again at the decreasing energy per unit area on a growing, spherical wave front. Consider a small area perpendicular to the direction of energy flow. Energy is passing through this area as a function of time, and energy per unit time is power, expressed in watts. Dividing power by the small sample area gives watts per unit area, or the units of intensity. Thus, intensity is a measure of the amount of energy passing through a unit area per unit time. In ultrasound, the units are W/m^2 or mW/cm^2. To return to the example, the unit area moves outward with the advancing wave front; the amount of energy passing through it decreases, thereby decreasing the intensity.

The wave-front geometry, however, is not the only source of energy loss from an expanding front. The material carrying the waves can also remove energy. The process can be thought of as a randomization of the normally organized motion of particles forming compressional waves. Since random motion is really heat, the energy contained in a wave converts to heat in the carrying medium. This type of energy loss is called *absorption,* and represents a steady energy loss from the advancing wave front.

Our model so far has considered only one source of waves. When several sources are present, the space surrounding them receives waves from all the sources. In any one volume of space, a series of traveling waves from each source may be passing through. As the waves travel through, they add together in a process called *superposition*. At the same time, each wave continues its own existence, unmodified by the presence of the other waves. Yet, the motion of the medium particles at any point in space is a sum of all the motions imparted by all the waves at that instant. This ability to add together without losing individual identity is common to nearly all waves, both mechanical and electromagnetic. Superposition is difficult to see and measure with acoustical waves, but not with light waves. Thus, many

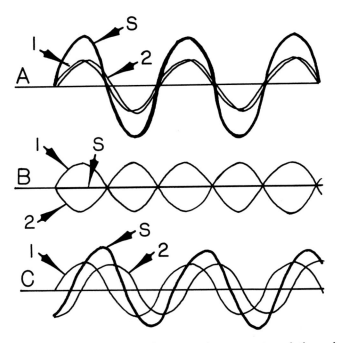

1-8 The superposition of waves. As waves travel through space, they can maintain their individuality and still add together to form a complex wave. If waves 1 and 2 are in phase, they sum together to form a larger resultant wave *S*, as in Part A. If the waves are out of phase 180°, the sum is zero, as in Part B. If the two waves are out of phase less than 180°, they sum together to form a lower amplitude wave than A with a phase different from either component wave, as in Part C.

of the models used to describe the superposition of acoustic waves were determined and predicated on observations of light interactions.

To better understand some wave interactions and the superposition process, a two-dimensional model is utilized here. Consider just two waves traveling past a common point. If the two waves are identical, with the same amplitude, phase, and frequency, they will add together to form a resulting wave that is the sum of the two individuals, as shown in Figure 1-8. Because the waves are in phase, the summation is simple: the new wave has twice the amplitude of the components, the same frequency, and the same phase. If, however, the phase of one wave is slipped 90°, the sum will produce a new wave shifted in phase 45°, with the same frequency, but a new peak value about 1.4 times larger than either component. If the phase is shifted 90° farther, the total phase shift is 180°, and the sum of the two waves is zero. Thus, if the waves have the same frequency and amplitude, but not the same phase, the resulting wave can change all the way from twice the original amplitude to zero. Yet, despite the various amplitudes, the waves still have not lost their individuality, but pass through the region of space unaltered.

Waves that are sufficiently in phase to form a new wave larger in amplitude than the components are said to constructively interfere with one another. If the summary wave has an amplitude less than its components, the components are said to

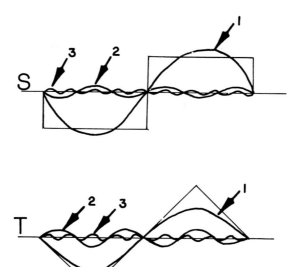

1-9   The summation of simple waves to form complex waves. Complex wave forms, such as square waves *S* and triangular waves *T* can be formed by adding together simpler component waves such as *1, 2,* and *3*. Each wave component has a different amplitude, phase, and frequency.

destructively interfere with one another. If the component waves differ in frequency and amplitude, they will form regions of constructive and destructive interference with one another. In the case of light, this interference results in a visible light pattern that can be measured.

The superposition of waves works so long as the elastic limit of the material carrying the waves is not exceeded. Beyond this limit, the waves do not add, and recognizable interference patterns do not arise. A good example of this process is the inability of waves that make up the surf to add with the wind-driven waves on top. As might be expected, very high-intensity mechanical waves will not add with smaller mechanical waves traveling through the same space.

The superposition properties of waves permit complex waves to be formed from the interaction of several waves that vary in amplitude, phase, and frequency. For example, human speech is a complex mix of different waves, a fact that can be appreciated when the waves are seen on an oscilloscope. Various analytical techniques, however, show that the individual wave elements still exist and can be separated out. They have not lost their individual identities just because the final form is complex.

If the phase relationship among waves is steady, the resulting wave will appear to stand in place, despite the traveling wave components. A good example of added traveling waves that produce a standing wave is the vibration of a tethered rope or string. The standing wave that appears on the vibrating string is composed of traveling waves moving along the string from end reflections, and a full wave vibration on the string will look like a fuzzy figure eight.

If a complex wave can be made by adding together a set of simpler waves with varying amplitude, phase, and frequency, and each of these waves does not lose identity, then complex waves might by analyzed by extracting wave components. The mathematical concept of this process was first introduced by Jean Baptiste Fourier in the early 19th century. In this process, a complex wave is analyzed by applying mathematical techniques that extract each of the simpler component waves. These waves are called Fourier components, and represent a set of simple sine waves of varying amplitude, phase, and frequency that, when added back together, produce the original complex wave. An example is shown in Figure 1-9. Several digital devices can perform this analytical process quickly and are discussed in Chapter 8.

One result of using a Fourier analysis technique is the opportunity to observe the relationship between the shape of a complex wave and its frequency components. For example, as the rate of rise or fall of a complex wave increases, the frequency components increase both in number and frequency. If we consider a simple vibrating body, the frequencies present in the resulting wave will be determined by the shape of the vibrating process, including the rise and fall in amplitude associated with starting and stopping the vibration. One way of changing the shape of a vibrational sequence is to rapidly remove energy from the vibration process. The result is called a damped vibration, which forms an envelope of waves, with a shape that introduces frequencies other than the measured center frequency of the vibration. These additional frequency components are an outgrowth of the shape of the resulting wave train, and the components will change by changing the shape of the envelope.

Damping is only one way in which the shape of a traveling wave can be altered. If the medium carrying the mechanical wave has different velocities of propagation for different frequencies, the shape of a traveling wave can be modified as it moves along. This change in shape accordingly changes the frequency components of the traveling wave. This process is called *dispersion,* in which the medium carrying a mechanical wave can change the wave shape. Many materials are dispersive. For example, waves on the surface of water will become broader as they move out from a disturbance, because lower frequencies travel faster in water than higher frequencies.

To this point, this chapter has considered the waves traveling only through a uniform, or homogeneous material. When the medium is not uniform, that is, heterogeneous, waves may not be propagated with equal facility in all directions. If the medium is a mixture of materials with varying densities and velocities of propogation, then another process occurs called *reflection.* Reflection takes place at interfaces where two materials of different wave-carrying capabilities meet, and can involve changes in material density or propagation velocity. At the interface, a portion of the incident wave energy is reflected back.

A string model can be used to illustrate some of the events surrounding reflection. Figure 1-10 shows a string made of two parts, one with a weight per unit length of D_1, and the other with a weight per unit length of D_2. The string is also very long, in order to remove any end reflections in the model. When a train of waves travels along the string from segment D_1 to D_2, a portion of the incident wave energy is

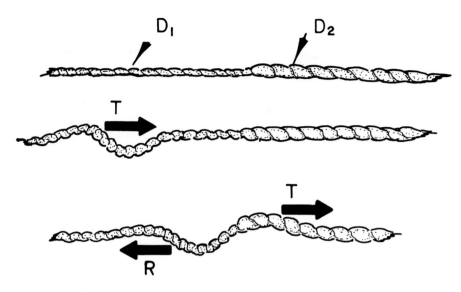

1-10 Reflection on a string. As a transverse wave *T* travels down a string with an abrupt change in density from D_1 to D_2, where D_2 is larger, the wave loses a portion of its energy at the change in density as a reflection *R*. The reflection moves back toward the source while the remainder of the incident wave *T* continues down the string.

reflected back along D_1 at the transition between D_1 and D_2. Thus, at the transition, the wave train is separated into two components, one continuing in the original direction along D_2, and a reflected component moving in the opposite direction along D_1. The sum of the energy in the reflected and traveling wave is equal to the energy in the incident wave. When the phase of the two wave components is compared to the incident wave, the traveling wave in segment D_2 will be in phase, but the reflected wave may or may not be, depending upon the density transition at the D_1–D_2 interface. For example, if D_1 is greater than D_2, the reflected wave will be in phase with the incident wave; but if D_2 is greater than D_1, the reflected wave is shifted in phase 180°, that is, it is inverted.

Earlier in the chapter, acoustic impedance was described as a function of material density. In the string model, the two segments of string had different densities, which corresponds to different characteristic impedances for the two string segments. A fundamental ultrasonic relationship may thus be demonstrated. If a mechanical wave moves from a high to a low acoustic impedance, the reflected wave will not have a phase shift. But if a mechanical wave moves from a low acoustic impedance to a high acoustic impedance, the reflected wave will have a phase shift of 180°.

Although it is tempting to generalize from the string to waves in the tissue, the various interfaces in tissue have neither the same size nor the same shape as those on the string. Lacking any other easy reference, however, the wavelength of a wave train serves well, and reflection processes can be separated according to reflector size relative to the wavelength.

As stated, when a traveling mechanical wave encounters a change in acoustic impedance, a portion of incident wave reflects back. If the interface is laterally large relative to the wavelength, the reflection will be governed by the same rules that apply to light reflection at a mirrored surface. Such reflection is called *specular reflection,* in which the angle of reflection is equal to the angle of incidence (Figure 1-11). On the other hand, the amount of energy reflected is determined by the magnitude of the characteristic impedance change, which is expressed through the interface pressure reflectivity. The reflectivity equation is as follows:

$$R = (Z_1 - Z_2)/(Z_1 + Z_2) \tag{1.4}$$

where Z_n is the characteristic impedance for each of the materials as numbered, always going from material 1 to material 2. If the transition is from a low impedance to a higher impedance, the sign of R is negative, indicating a phase shift of 180°, that is, the reflected wave is inverted. If the transition is from a high impedance to a low impedance, the sign of R is positive, indicating no shift in phase at reflection. Within this simple equation resides information on the amount of pressure (amplitude) reflection, or reflectivity, expressed as a fraction, and the phase of the reflected wave.

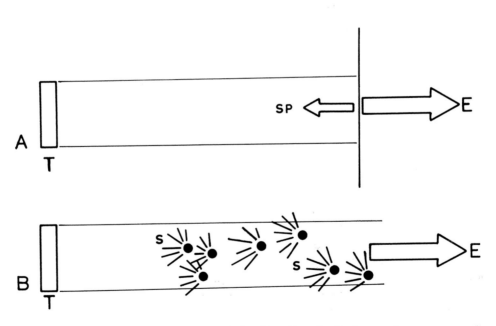

1-11 Longitudinal wave reflections. Longitudinal waves traveling through a medium can experience two forms of reflection. As the waves move from the source *T,* they can experience a mirror-like reflection called a specular reflection *SP,* as in part A. Alternately, the wave can intercept small scattering bodies *S* that intercept a portion of the wave energy and scatter it in all directions, with only a portion of the scattered energy returning to the wave source *T.*

The same reflection process can be considered in terms of the intensity reflectivity, as well. *R* represents the pressure reflectivity and, therefore, a reflection-amplitude ratio between the reflected pressure and the incident pressure. Normally, energy is proportional to the square of amplitude. The same is true here. The intensity reflectivity is expressed as the square of the pressure reflectivity, *R*. Thus:

$$\propto = R^2 \tag{1.5}$$

where $\propto$ is the intensity reflectivity and *R* is the pressure reflectivity.

Still, most biological materials do not have interfaces that are all larger than the ultrasound wavelength. Lateral dimensions of interfaces are often equal to or much smaller than the incident wavelength. For interfaces with dimensions less than one wavelength, a new set of reflecting events called scattering takes over. As the name implies, the scattering process simply takes a portion of all the incoming energy and redirects that portion in all directions. As before, the ability to be a scatterer depends upon a change in characteristic impedance. Just how evenly the energy depends upon the size of any scattering body. Furthermore, the distance apart that the scatterers are spaced and the degree of regularity in their spacing will alter the characteristics of the scattering process. Because these wave properties apply to the interaction of X rays and molecules in crystals, scattering information from X rays can provide intimate information on the organization (separation and regularity) of a crystalline material. Similarly, the regularity and separation of the scattering bodies in tissue will affect scattering processes, forming a speckle pattern that permits separation of one organ from another and one sort of tissue from another.

With the exception of scattering, we have considered an incident wave as continuing on in a straight line after crossing an interface. Given the proper conditions, however, the incident waves will be bent at the interface, but in a predictable manner. If the change in characteristic impedance comes in part or totally from a change in propagation velocity, a ray crossing the interface at an angle will be bent. This process is called refraction. The amount of bending is predicted by an equation that relates the angle of refraction to the relative change in propagation velocity across the interface. The equation is called Snell's law, and appears as:

$$(\text{Sin } i)/(\text{Sin } r) = (V_1/V_2), \tag{1.6}$$

where *i* is the incident angle between a perpendicular to the surface and the incident ray, *r* is the refraction angle between the emerging ray and a perpendicular to the surface, and V_n is the propagation velocity in each medium.

We can now identify many of the mechanisms that contribute to energy loss from a wave as the wave travels through a heterogeneous material. These mechanisms include the geometry of the expanding wave front; the absorption of energy and conversion to heat; and the scattering of incident energy away from the normal propagation path. Each of these processes can be considered an example of *attenuation,* a term used to describe the process of energy loss from a wave for any reason. Depending upon the materials the wave happens to be traveling through, attenuation is a function of frequency. This is also true for ultrasound in tissue.

Up to now, propagation and attenuation have been discussed in general terms, using wave fronts generated by some mechanical wave source. We have also been dealing with the complete wave front. But another set of events occurs when only a portion of a wave front is permitted to travel on. These events, which are grouped under the general label, *diffraction,* are described below.

Waves and Diffraction

Once a wave front is formed and propagating, the ability of segments in the front to interact with one another is limited. On the other hand, when discrete portions of a wave front are brought together, new interactions occur that can produce interference patterns. Called diffraction, the process involves the addition of several wave fronts to form a common interference pattern. The different wave fronts

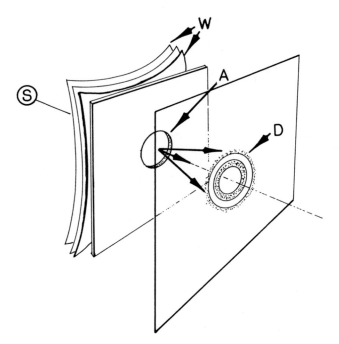

1-12 Forming a Fresnel diffraction pattern. Fresnel diffraction occurs when wave fronts *W*, from a point source of waves *S*, encounter an aperture *A*, that is close to the source. Close to the source, the wave fronts are not planar, causing a complex diffraction pattern *D* on a plane surface beyond the aperture. The interaction between wave front and aperture is difficult to describe mathematically because the curved and complex wave fronts formed as the incident waves pass through the aperture.

are produced by letting a single wave front pass through an aperture. In this particular application of wave science, light is one of the best models, and most of the predictions about diffraction come from the study of light. Because surface mechanical waves are still waves, a few simple experiments with mechanical waves on the surface of water can show relationships like those presented in light.

Consider a circular aperture formed in the face of an infinite plane, with light waves reaching the aperture from a point source a short distance behind the aperture, as in Figure 1-12. The waves that enter the aperture are not planar because they are still so close to the source. At the plane, the waves interact with the aperture and are thus bent, causing a complicated pattern of rays to emerge from the aperture. The pattern of light reaching a viewing plane a short distance from the aperture is so complicated, in fact, that no well-developed means of mathematically predicting the pattern is possible. The resulting light pattern on the viewing plane will not replicate the geometry of the aperture. The light pattern on the viewing surface is called a Fresnel diffraction pattern, named after the physicist and mathematician who studied this form of diffraction in the 19th century. Principle characteristics of this Fresnel diffraction are the nonparallel rays that make up the light rays reaching the aperture and the complicated wave fronts formed after the aperture.

A better geometry may be used to permit a more predictable interaction between light and aperture. Events become easier to handle when light enters the aperture as parallel rays, and the wave fronts are planar. One way of doing this is to move the wave source farther from the aperture, so that the wave fronts are more planar when they reach the opening. Another method is to leave the source close to the aperture but apply a lens to the rays coming out of the aperture that makes them appear to have been parallel through the aperture. The focal point of the lens is set so that the wave fronts reaching the viewing plane are themselves planar. This application of a lens to the Fresnel diffraction setting is called Fraunhofer diffraction, the hallmark of which is the planar waves that reach the viewing plane (Figure 1-13).

The plane waves permit the process to be modeled with considerable accuracy. For a circular aperture, for example, a circular disc of light is formed from the light emerging from the aperture. This disc of emerging light subtends a half angle predicted by the equation:

$$\text{Sin } a = 1.22\, \lambda\, /D, \tag{1.7}$$

where a is the half angle in degrees, λ is the wavelength, and D is the diameter of the aperture [1]. Beyond the center disc are rings of light with decreasing intensity, spaced at regular and predictable intervals. The drop in intensity away from the center disc is very sharp, with 85% of the light contained in the center disc. It turns out that mechanical waves with apertures and a similar geometry will produce a distribution of wave energy like this light experiment.

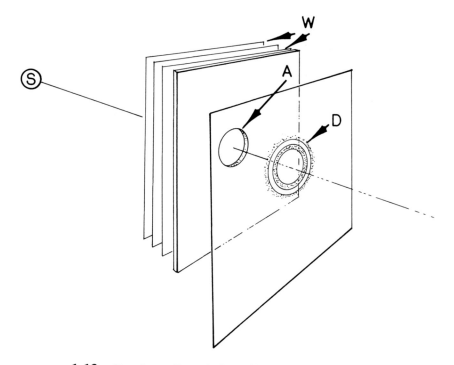

1-13   Forming a Fraunhofer diffraction pattern. Fraunhofer diffraction occurs when wave fronts W, from a point source of waves S, encounter an aperture relatively far from the source. At longer distances from the source, the wave fronts are planar as they encounter the aperture, causing a simple and well-described diffraction pattern D on a plane surface beyond the aperture.

The size of the disc formed by Fraunhofer diffraction can be predicted by considering basic optics and the geometry of the image formation. A classic treatment of the problem shows the radius of the disc to be:

$$r = 1.22\ \lambda\ F/D, \tag{1.8}$$

where r is the radius of the light disc, λ is the wavelength of the light, and D is the diameter of the aperture (when using a lens, the lens and aperture have the same diameter) [1]. Mechanical waves will adhere to these predictions of performance with surprising regularity. As a result, these equations and others like them are used to predict the behavior of ultrasonic waves in focusing, diffraction, and scattering processes.

Until now, we have considered only one source of waves and one aperture. When the number of apertures increases, the problem becomes more complex and requires the application of more stringent geometric limitations to adequately describe events. Again, light is used to model the observations of all waves.

Using a common source of light and two apertures (called Young's experiment [1]), the diffraction pattern becomes an intricate set of light intensities. With the addition of more apertures, the whole apparatus becomes what is called a diffraction grating. The resulting light patterns formed by constructive and destructive interference are wavelength dependent. A diffraction grating, then, can be used to divide white light into its frequency components. In mechanical waves, the diffraction pattern still mimics the events in light, and the same equations will apply. The diffraction grating forms off-center-axis lobes called grating lobes. These events will play a central role later in our discussion of multielement transducers in ultrasound.

Having outlined a model of waves and wave events, we can now look at the science of ultrasound.

Conclusion

Underlying the events associated with ultrasonic waves is the relationship ultrasound carries with all waves. Thus, an examination of the basic rules governing the behavior of waves in general yields information about the mechanical waves of ultrasound in particular. For example, the frequency and velocity of propagation determine wave length for both transverse and longitudinal waves. An expanding ultrasonic wave front will follow Huygen's principles, and like all waves, ultrasonic waves will add together in a simple fashion if the waves are working within the elastic limits of the propagating medium. In addition, ultrasonic waves can be reflected and refracted like transverse waves on a rope and light at an air-water interface. With a firm foundation of wave science, ultrasound in the body is much easier to understand.

References

1. Frank, N.H. 1950. Introduction to electricity and optics. 2nd ed. New York: McGraw-Hill Book Co.

Chapter 2

The B-Scanner Unclothed

It is difficult not to be impressed with the results of a skilled person working with a high-technology tool. Ask such a skilled user what accounts for the quality of his or her product, and the reply is likely to be that it begins with the quality of the tool. Equally important, however, is an understanding of the tool—what it is designed to do, how it is designed to do it, and how to extract from the tool the maximum utility. In the end, the tool and the guiding mind become one, and the tool becomes a physical extension of the user's mind. This is the ideal interaction between the sonographer and sonograph. In the hands of the sonographer, the sonograph becomes an acoustical eye to peer into the body's interior.

On the other hand, peering into the interior of the typical B-scanner yields little about the machine's ultimate performance capabilities. Within the machine perhaps half a million events and operations occur, some in a programmed sequence, others simultaneously in different parts of the machine. Yet, at first glance what we see between the tiers of circuit boards are ribbons of wire, and mounted in large numbers on each board are small, black, insect-looking devices. This is obviously not the level at which to gain maximum understanding about how to use the sonograph as an imaging tool.

Any approach to educating a practitioner about the sonograph must aim to provide some predictive power about how the machine will function under different conditions. Such predictive power can come only by understanding the signal-shaping events on the path from first ultrasound production to final display. Events such as conversion from one energy form to another, nonlinear amplification, detection schemes that remove specific information, and changing a signal from analog to digital are all elements in the formulation of a signal-flow diagram. Such a diagram lends structure to our understanding of the sonographic events that can influence the final display of tissue interfaces inside the body. Knowledge of the diagram is crucial in order to realize the full potential of the machine as an imaging tool.

Using the Echo-Ranging Process

The echo-ranging process initially seems far too simple to be a reliable source of image information. But, when echo ranging is performed in a fixed sequence and the results integrated, a two-dimensional image emerges. We will use a small model to trace the sequence of events.

Consider a transducer or energy source that is continuous with a medium that can carry the energy. The first assumption is that the propagation velocity for the energy through the medium is constant, regardless of frequency or direction of travel. With this assumption, the range of an echo source from the energy source can be calculated by plugging values into the well-known relationship:

$$d = vt, \tag{2.1}$$

where d is distance, v is the velocity of propagation, and t is the lapse time from the initial burst of energy to the return of an echo. In its present form, equation 2.1 calculates the total traveled distance, both to and from the echo source. The clock used to count time need not be a standard clock. For ultrasound, it is the moving beam of a cathode ray tube (CRT).

Events begin by starting the clock, that is, the movement of the CRT electron beam, simultaneously with transducer excitation, as shown in Figure 2-1. Time on

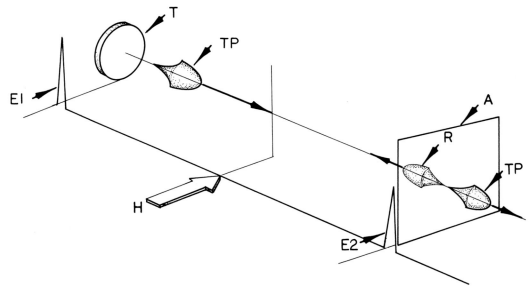

2-1   The echo-ranging process. The transducer T sends out a transmitted pulse TP, which travels at a fixed velocity. The display electron beam moves at one-half the propagation velocity. Transmitting the pulse of ultrasound forms the echo signal $E1$. When TP reaches the interface A, a portion of the energy reflects to form R, which begins to travel back to the transducer. The display electron beam is now at the half-way point H. As R travels back, the display electron beam continues to move until R reaches the transducer to form the echo signal $E2$. This relationship makes the range of $E2$ equal to the range of A.

the CRT clock is indicated by position on the CRT just as hands on a wall clock are used to show time. An initial requirement is to establish a one-to-one correspondence between distances on the CRT and distances within the medium. By moving the electron beam vertically to indicate the presence of an echo signal, the clock display shows not only the starting point, or time zero, but also the arrival of an echo back to the transducer. If the Y-axis movement is proportional to the echo strength, the information displayed on the CRT will be echo range and amplitude.

For any echo to be registered by the system, the echo must reach the transducer. This requires that the energy travel to an echo source within the medium, and that the echo travel back to the transducer. The lapse time between time zero and the arrival of an echo, then, is the time taken to traverse the distance to the echo source, produce an echo, and traverse the distance back to the transducer. By moving the electron beam at one-half the propagation velocity within the medium, a one-to-one relationship results between the signal position on the CRT face and the echo-source range within the medium.

The entire transmit-receive cycle is as follows: 1) At time zero, the transducer emits a burst of energy and the CRT clock starts to move the beam; 2) The beam moves at one-half the medium propagation velocity (in the time that it takes the energy to reach an echo source 10 cm from the transducer, the CRT beam will move 5 cm); 3) The echo is formed, and then must travel back to the transducer to be detected and displayed; 4) During the journey back to the transducer, the CRT clock moves another 5cm; and 5) The echo energy reaches the transducer, and the event appears on the CRT at a distance from the start of the CRT sweep equal to the echo-source range from the transducer in the medium. Echo strengths and echo ranges can now be accurately portrayed on the display, provided the ultrasonic wave propagation velocity is known.

Often a smaller CRT is a more efficient display, but a one-to-one correspondence will not fit on the small display. Putting the trace on a smaller display poses no problem if the units of distance are marked on the screen. The units will come from knowing the propagation velocity within the medium.

We can make the model more specific by using the average soft-tissue velocity for ultrasound, which is 1,540 m/s. At this velocity, it takes 6.5×10^{-6}s, or 6.5 μs, to traverse 1 cm of tissue. The display lapse time, however, includes time both out and back, so the total travel time for 1 cm of tissue takes $2 \times 6.5 \times 10^{-6}$s, or 13×10^{-6}s. By using an internal electronic clock that produces a small "pip" on the CRT trace for each 13-μs interval, an electronic ruler appears on the display, starting a time zero and continuing over the whole display trace, as shown in Figure 2-2. Now the CRT electron beam can move any velocity across the screen to count time, so long as the 13-μs clock puts distance markers on the display. To display very short distances, this 13-μs interval can be further divided into segments representing 1mm or 2mm each. This 13-μs clock is discussed later in connection with its use for depth markers in the two-dimensional image.

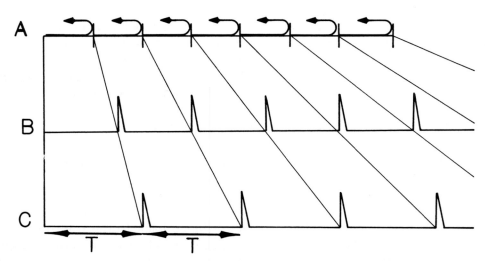

2-2 Scaling distance on the display. An array of echo sources in the tissue A produces a set of echo signals separated by 13 μs. Sweeping the display electron beam faster than one-half the tissue velocity produces echo signals physically farther apart on the display than in the tissue, B and C, but the echo signals are still the same time apart, T. By changing the display sweep speed, the display can scale the echo signals and make the image larger or smaller than life.

Clearly, what is placed on the display screen is not distance at all, but time. This fact helps explain some of the distinctive artifacts in ultrasound and covered in Chapter 18.

With echo ranging as a back drop, we can focus on the machine organization needed to do echo ranging.

Organization of an Echo-Ranging Device

An echo-ranging device depends upon the coordinated transmission of energy and counting time. It involves sending out a burst, or pulse, of energy and waiting for an echo to return. As a result, the words *echo-ranging device* and *pulse-echo device* will be used interchangeably here to describe system organization.

An ultrasonic echo-ranging device needs a transducer to make and receive ultrasound; a transmitter to excite the transducer into making ultrasound; a receiver to amplify and shape the signal that will represent the echo; a display to permit the operator to see the returning signal; and a central synchronizer, or timer, to assure that all of the above elements act in concert. These elements are shown in Figure 2-3. Naturally, an accurate measure of time is central to the coordination of events and interpretation of results.

While at first keeping the display simple, the sonographer sees the starting pulse that represents the zero time on the display, as well as the signals indicating returning echoes and the timing markers that represent units of distance into the

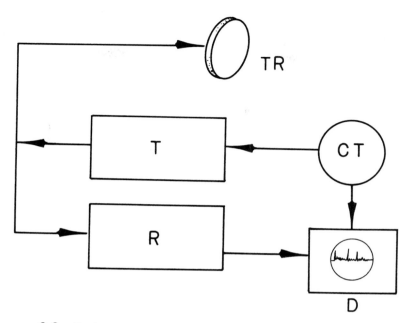

2-3   Basic organization of an echo-ranging device. The transducer *TR* makes and receives ultrasound. The transmitter *T* excites the transducer into vibration, and the receiver *R* shapes and detects the echo signal for display *D*. The display and the transmitter must be coordinated by a central timer *CT*.

tissue. The central timer simultaneously tells the CRT to start the trace and the transmitter to excite the transducer into vibration. In more complicated configurations, the central timer takes on more responsibilities and often is linked with other equipment that is very time-sensitive, such as a scan converter.

The display on our simple machine is a CRT with no memory. Consequently, a single pulse-listen cycle cannot be seen. To handle this problem, the sonograph goes through many pulse-listen cycles every second to refresh the display. The number of pulse-listen cycles per second is called the *pulse repetition rate* (PRR), or *pulse repetition frequency* (PRF). But the PRF does more than make the display easy to see; it also sets the maximum distance that the system can see from the transducer, called here the field of view.

In many sonographs, the PRF is set to a value that allows the largest desired field of view. At smaller depths, the receiver is turned on during the time of the display depth, then turned off during unneeded periods. The result is a steady PRF, irrespective of depth. As an example, a PRF of 1,000 Hz means that during each pulse-listen cycle, the receiver could be listening for 1/1,000th of a second, or 0.001 s. The number of centimeters traversed by ultrasound in this time period can be determined by dividing the time interval by 13×10^{-6} s. The result is 76.8 cm, which means that echoes arising as far as 76 cm from the transducer could be displayed. Special applications of ultrasound will later require higher PRFs than in this example. At the same time, higher PRFs limit the effective field of view. All these limits exist simply because of a finite propagation velocity for ultrasound.

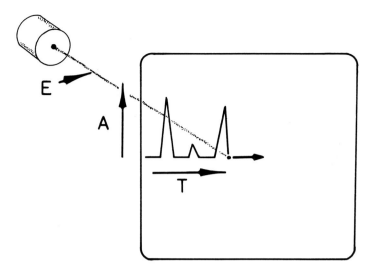

2-4 Forming the A-mode display. Forming an A-mode display with a cathode ray tube requires moving the electron beam *E* to form the A-mode signals. Moving vertically shows signal amplitude *A,* and moving horizontally shows the signal position in time *T.*

In this simple system, the information displayed about an echo includes echo amplitude and echo range (Figure 2-4). Such a display form is called A-mode, for amplitude-modulated display. (Other display forms are introduced later in this chapter.) In the right circumstances, an A-mode display can be very informative. While other forms of display have similar information, none is as quantifiable as an A-mode display.

Using the basic echo-ranging design shown in Figure 2-3 as a guide, a few of the function boxes need further explanation. All current echo-ranging machines, no matter how complicated, rely on the basic relationships just described; future machines will be equally dependent upon them. With these fundamentals in mind, our expanded discussion begins with the transducer.

Transducer

Transducers are treated in detail in Chapter 3. Several essential points must be made here in order to properly place the transducer into the B-scanner organization.

The first step is to remove the word *probe* from our vocabulary. Transducers change one form of energy into another and thus should be called transducers or crystals, rather than probes, to reflect accurately their properties and functions. *Probe* must now be recognized as a quaint term used during the early period of ultrasound when events in imaging were poorly understood.

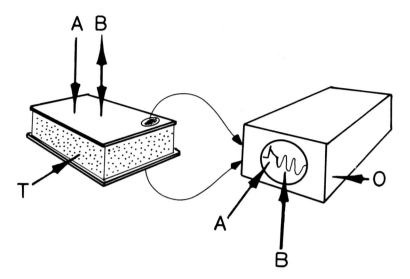

2-5 Piezoelectric transduction of pressure. Applying external pressure to a transducing material *T* changes the mechanical energy into electrical energy. A sustained pressure *A* will cause a voltage that steadily decays. A rhythmic pressure *B* causes a rhythmic voltage *B*, on the oscilloscope *O*.

Ultrasonic transduction involves converting mechanical energy into electrical energy and vice versa, all of which depends upon the physical organization of the transducer molecules. The transducer is made of a material called a ferroelectric, which has piezoelectric properties. Piezoelectric (pressure electric) means that the material responds to an applied external pressure by making an internal electric field. This field appears on the surface of the transducer. Piezoelectric transducers also transduce in the opposite direction, where applying an external electric field to the material causes it to change shape. In both energy conversions, the response of the transducer can follow the changes in the stress, whether the stress is mechanical or electrical. Thus, a rhythmic pressure applied to a transducer will produce a following rhythmic output voltage (Figure 2-5). Conversely, a rhythmic voltage applied to the transducer will produce a rhythmic motion following the voltage.

The transducer, however, needs to vibrate at its natural resonant frequency in order for it to produce ultrasonic waves easily. To do this, the transducer receives a large amount of electrical energy in a short period of time, which starts a physical vibration as if the transducer were struck by a small hammer. The electrical stimulation is typically a short electrical pulse with a maximum value of several hundred volts. The applied electrical pulse causes the material to change shape; then the stress is rapidly removed (Figure 2-6). After being displaced from its resting state, the transducer tries to return, and in so doing, sets up a vibration of the transducer surfaces. The frequency of this vibration is determined by the physical dimensions of the transducer. In this fashion, the electrical energy is stored for a short time in the ferroelectric, and then is quickly released as a mechanical, ultrasonic wave.

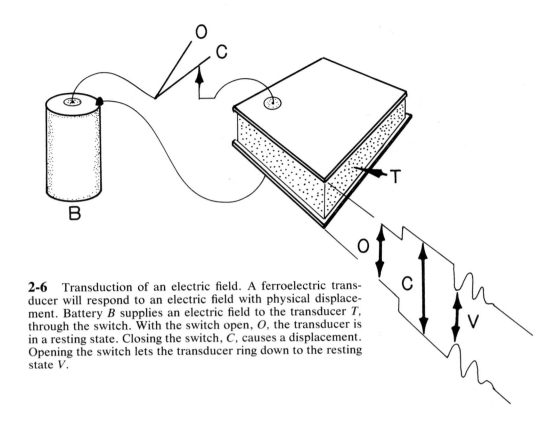

2-6 Transduction of an electric field. A ferroelectric transducer will respond to an electric field with physical displacement. Battery *B* supplies an electric field to the transducer *T*, through the switch. With the switch open, *O*, the transducer is in a resting state. Closing the switch, *C*, causes a displacement. Opening the switch lets the transducer ring down to the resting state *V*.

The mechanical waves set up both inside and outside the transducer are *compressional*, or *longitudinal*, waves. The particles carrying the waves move along the direction of energy travel. As these waves are formed and radiated away, the transducer loses energy, and the amplitude of the mechanical vibration decreases. How long the transducer vibrates (or rings) after excitation is a function of how fast the vibrational energy is removed from the transducer. A functional transducer is designed to make the time to ring down to its resting state as short as possible. The transducer vibration forms an envelope of ultrasonic waves, defined by the starting and stopping time for transducer vibration. This vibrational pattern appears in the return echo, and the resulting envelope is used to represent an echo in the sonograph, all the way to the final display. The size of the envelope determines, in part, the resolution of the system.

The returning echo, which is a compressional wave, applies a rhythmic squeeze to the transducer at the same frequency as the returning echo. An oscillating pressure applied to a transducer produces an oscillating output voltage, with the amplitude of the voltage proportional to the strength of the squeeze. Should the frequency of the returning echo be changed from the transmitted frequency, the output voltage from the transducer will have the new frequency. Furthermore, any shift in the phase of the echo will also appear in the electrical output. Thus, the returning ultrasound wave carries the following information: 1) The time of arrival, which can be translated into range or distance; 2) The amplitude of the

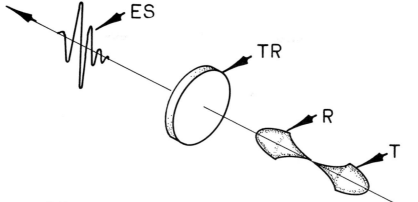

2-7   The role of the transducer. The transducer *TR* makes ultrasound *T* and receives reflected ultrasound *R*. The transducer converts the mechanical energy of the reflected wave into an electrical signal *ES*, with a phase, frequency, and amplitude proportional to the reflected wave *R*.

echo, which can be transcribed into relative signal strength; 3) The frequency of the echo, which can be related to echo-source velocity; and 4) The phase shifts that result from different reflecting conditions. During imaging, the echo amplitude and time of arrival are used to form the image. In Doppler applications of ultrasound, the phase and frequency information are used to form a Doppler "image." Of all the information possible in a returning echo, only about 3% is utilized for imaging, and hardly more with Doppler. The remaining information is more difficult to extract and represents an area for future ultrasound development.

The transducer provides an interface between body and machine, between ultrasound and electronics (Figure 2-7). Ultrasound occurs inside the body, with events such as propagation, reflection, and refraction. Outside the body are the electronics, with their own intricate internal organization and events that shape and place the signal representing the echo on display. The section following takes a look at events occurring inside the machine.

Transmitter

To make ultrasound, the transducer must be excited into vibration. The portion of the machine that handles this task is the transmitter.

The transmitter delivers an electromechanical kick that starts the transducer vibrating. The kick is a short electrical pulse applied across the crystal that is produced within the transmitter circuit by a high-voltage source that is rapidly gated to the transducer, then just as rapidly turned off. The peak pulse voltage can range from 60 V to as large as 400 V. In some early machines, the voltage was much higher still, sometimes reaching 1,000 V or more [1]. The amount of ultra-

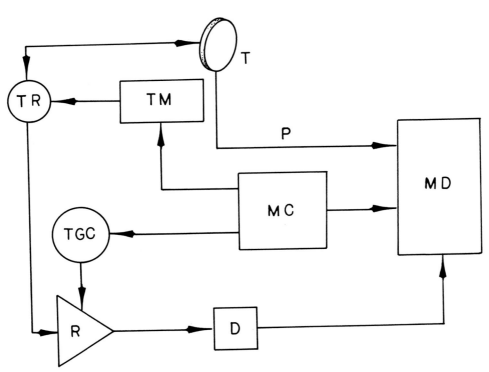

2-8 Organization of an imaging sonograph. *T* is the transducer; *P* is the information on the transducer position in space; and *TR* is the transmit-receive switch. *TM* is the transmitter, which excites the transducer into vibration. The received echo signal is amplified by the receiver *R*, detected by *D*, and sent to the memory and display *MD*. The master controller *MC* sends control signals to the transmitter, the display, and the time-gain compensation curve generator *TGC*.

sound energy transmitted by the transducer is in part a function of the transmitter peak voltage; thus, changing the transmitter voltage with a front panel control changes the whole system's response. Despite its function, this output control is often named something else, such as "gain" or "damping." The pulse is typically 1μs to 2μs long, which matches the ring-down time in many transducers. In turn, the ring-down time for a transducer is determined by the transducer design and by how rapidly energy is removed from the vibration. Despite the seemingly simple cause and effect relationship between the transmitter and transducer, influences on the relationship can be subtle.

Besides being a physically vibrating object, the transducer is also a bulk electronic component in the transmitter circuit (Figure 2-8). The transducer acts as if it were composed of electronic components such as capacitors, inductors (coils), and resistors. As a result, the transducer's response to an applied voltage depends upon more than just amplitude. For example, the phase relationship between the applied current and voltage will change the transducer's response. To help shape these relationships in the transducer, other components are often added to the transducer, such as capacitors or inductors, to set the phase relationship for better transducer excitation. In addition, part of the energy in a transducer vibration is electrical; thus, the electrical impedance seen by the transducer during vibration will influence both starting and stopping the vibration. Along with shaping the phase relationships for the transmitting electrical energy, the transducer must see the correct electrical impedance to vibrate properly.

All of these characteristics are designed into the transmitter and receiver circuits by each manufacturer, and each design is different. As a result, using a transducer designed for one brand of sonograph on another can often result in poor images. The transmitter and transducer must be matched in order to work in concert and to help ensure image quality.

Although the transducer receives rather large voltages for transmitting, the voltages produced by echoes are much smaller. In addition, most systems use the same transducer for both transmitting and receiving. This places the transmitter and receiver on a common line to the transducer, which represents a voltage-handling problem for the system. The engineering solution is a circuit called the transmit-receive switch, discussed next.

Transmit-Receive Switch

As stated, although the transmitter delivers several hundred volts to the transducer, this same voltage should not be delivered to the receiver, which has difficulty managing voltages even as large as 1 V. A 1-V input signal can easily saturate a contemporary ultrasound receiver. The need, then, is to deliver the transmitter voltages to the transducer and not the receiver, yet permit the small echo-signals to reach the receiver input. This division of signals is accomplished with a *transmit-receive,* or TR, switch.

The TR switch sits at the input to the receiver, rejecting the large transmitter voltages but passing the much-smaller echo-signals. Because of its strategic position at the receiver input, the TR switch sets the range of signals presented to the receiver for amplification. The upper edge of this range is usually in the neighborhood of 1 V. The lower edge is defined by the small-signal characteristics of the TR switch design. This signal range is called the input dynamic range, and ideally might span 1 V down to 1 μV (120 dB). Variations in circuit components and normal differences in manufacture can decrease this value to around 80 dB. Typical values are around 100 dB. Interestingly, this dynamic range has a major influence on the effective tissue-imaging depth; this area is examined in detail in Chapter 9.

When TR switches fail and the high transmitter voltages reach the front end of the receiver, the first radio frequency amplifier is nearly always fatally injured. This is a dramatic failure. On the other hand, the TR switch can become a very low-resistance path, decreasing the transmitter voltage to such a small level that little ultrasound energy leaves the transducer. This can be a much more subtle change, which might appear first as a growing need to run very high system-gain for normal penetration. In either case the sonograph will need immediate attention.

With the ultrasonic echo transduced into a voltage, the next link in the signal path is the receiver radio frequency amplifier.

Radio Frequency Amplifier

As the echoes reach the transducer, the output from the transducer is a set of oscillating voltages with a central frequency close to the transmitted ultrasound. A 2.25-MHz transducer will, for example, have an electrical output oscillating at close to 2.25 MHz, which is clearly in the radio frequency (rf) spectrum. Logically, the first amplifier in the receiver is an rf amplifier with a passband large enough to handle not only the central operating frequencies of the various transducers used with the machine, but also the additional frequencies produced by a highly damped transducer. A passband spanning 1 MHz to 10 MHz is a range chosen by many manufacturers.

Along with a large frequency range, the transducer electrical output, as noted earlier, also has a wide amplitude range. The signals arriving at the rf amplifier input can have a dynamic range extending from 80 dB to 120 dB for normal operation. In other words, the amplitude variations can range from 10,000 up to 1,000,000 to 1. This places severe constraints on the first amplifier design.

Such a large range of signal levels comes from two sources: 1) The normal variation in reflectivity among the tissue acoustical interfaces, and 2) The frequency-dependent, tissue attenuation. The largest signals will come from the specular reflectors close to the transducer; the smallest signals will come from the most-distant scatters.

Although a typical rf amplifier can handle such a signal amplitude range at the input, it cannot accommodate the corresponding output using linear amplification. A good rf amplifier design can handle a 50-dB dynamic range linearly, but not much beyond that [2, 3]. One method of extending the capability of the rf amplifier is to amplify nonlinearly, for example, as a logarithmic amplifier. In this technique, the output from the amplifier is proportional to the logarithm of the input voltage. The result can be an input signal range of 90 dB to 100 dB, and an output with signals unevenly compressed closely together, spanning 40 dB to 50 dB in range.

Another solution to this dynamic-range problem is to use an amplifier design with a voltage-controlled gain. Changing the control voltage to the amplifier will change the amount of gain through the amplifier. Thus, control voltages can be set so that signals from interfaces close to the transducer are amplified less than the signals from more distant targets. If the change in amplifier gain increases at the same rate as the signal strength falls off due to losses in beam intensity, the only signal variations left are those due to variations in echogenicity among the echo sources (Figure 2-9). These signals can vary 40 dB to 50 dB, ranges easily handled by a good rf amplifier design.

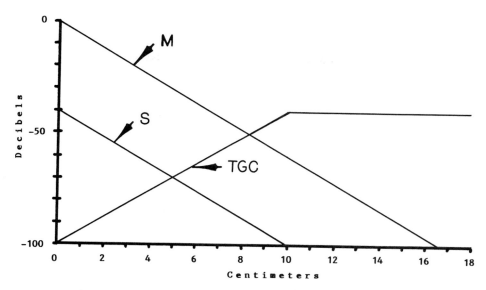

2-9 Matching TGC to the attenuation rate. Both the maximum signals *M* and smallest signals *S* are attenuated at the same rate. TGC is set so that all the tissue signals are represented as deeply as possible, increasing gain at the same rate as the tissue attenuates.

The controlled change in gain used to compensate for falling signal strength is called *time-gain compensation,* or TGC. It has other names as well, such as depth-gain compensation (DGC), and swept gain. Except for a few systems with automatic TGC, this gain function is set by the sonographer using front panel controls. Extracting image data accurately will depend upon TGC set up (the rules for which are discussed in more detail in Chapter 13).

Along with compressing the input dynamic range handled by the machine, the rf amplifier can also set the noise level within the machine, determining the ultimate signal-to-noise ratio. This fact imposes a need for low internal noise on the amplifier, and much design effort has gone into keeping this amplifier quiet. Modern solid-state amplifiers used in the communications industry are a good choice here. The most common amplifier used at this system input is the field effect transistor or FET. Quiet, linear amplifier designs are now available for this circuit, providing the required sensitivity and high signal-to-noise ratio of the modern sonograph [2].

Trying to reduce system noise can produce an amplifier placement problem in which the amplifier position within the sonograph can measurably affect noise levels. For example, using a long set of cables between the transducer mounted on the scan arm and an amplifier housed within the sonograph main frame can couple significant outside electromagnetic noise into the sonograph. To handle this problem, some manufacturers moved the first rf amplifier into the arm or into a connector between the transducer and the arm. Moving the amplifier so close to the transducer means that the noise sources that can affect the sonograph performance are kept low relative to the signal levels. This design, however, does not diminish the need for power sources that are free of electrical noise. Still, properly positioned amplifiers can effectively increase the sensitivity of a machine, improving both its useful dynamic range and effective penetration.

By the time the signal arrives at the sonograph display, it will grow in amplitude 30 dB to 90 dB. This amount of amplification will increase the signal amplitudes 30 to 32,000 times. Any system noise that might be present is also amplified along with the signals. This fact underscores again the need to keep the operating environment for any sonograph as free as possible of electromagnetic noise. Simple devices such as pagers, handie-talkies used by security personnel, diathermy, elevators, and X-ray machines can all generate great amounts of noise that can enter the rf amplifier and undergo the same amplification as signals from the transducer.

Unshielded transducers can pick up local radio and television stations that are close enough to generate effective electric fields in the scanning area. Any effort to produce an electromagnetically clean environment for the sonograph will be rewarded by scans free of signals that do not represent tissue-ultrasound interactions but bursts of noise.

The discussion following describes typical parameters cited often by manufacturers to characterize the static B-scanner; many of these parameters relate to the performance of the rf amplifier.

Because of a need to change transducers according to the clinical task and the frequency components in the highly damped transducer ringing process, the rf amplifier must have a wide passband. The limits on these frequencies are often stated in the receiver passband specifications. For example, a passband of 1.5 MHz to 7.5 MHz means that the amplifier can amplify the signals within these bounds in a nearly equal manner, in other words, differing not more than 3 dB. The amplifier will amplify a 1.5-MHz signal or a 7.5-MHz signal 3 dB less than frequencies between these two limits, and variations in gain for any frequencies in-between will not exceed 1.5 dB. A 7.5-MHz transducer operating on a sonograph with such a passband will have decreased performance, and a 10-MHz transducer will likely not work at all. Although many of the newer sonographs can handle these higher frequencies, most of the older machines cannot. The first limitation in considering any sonograph design is the passband of the rf amplifier.

Like other aspects of the rf amplifier, the passband depends upon the components that make up the amplifier circuit. As a result, the amplifier passband can change with temperature or age. Textural information that depends upon the total frequency content of the transducer will be affected first. The dot size and texture will alter along with the ability of the rf amplifier to handle the frequencies present. And experience indicates that a decreasing passband will decrease overall image quality.

The range of signal amplitudes an amplifier can accept at its input or output is called the signal dynamic range and should be specified as input or output. Such a signal range can be achieved by either rejecting or cutting off signals below a certain level—a process called signal supression—or compressing a larger range of signals to a narrower one [4]. These two processes, although described as "setting the dynamic range," are actually quite different (Figure 2-10).

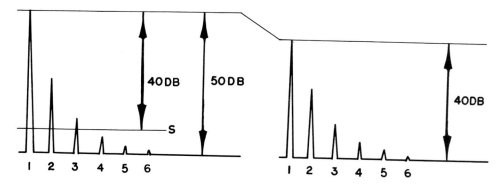

2-10 Compression versus suppression of echo signals. Video-signal processing can either compress or suppress to the video-signal dynamic range. During compression, which takes all the signals and brings them closer together, none of the signals is lost. Suppression S rejects signals below 40 dB; thus signals 4, 5, and 6 would not appear on the display.

If we first consider the input signals to the receiver and assume that such mechanisms as TGC and compression are not at work, then the input dynamic range of the receiver is equal to the output from the transducer, that is, about 90 dB to 120 dB (Figure 2-11). The specifications given by the manufacturer, however, are considerably lower, with typical values of 30 dB to 45 dB. These smaller numbers do not represent signal input, but, rather, the output dynamic range after TGC, compressions, and other events in the signal stream. They represent the signal dynamic range put into the display. Because many displays have dynamic ranges hardly beyond 30 dB and only a few have ranges with 40 dB, some signal compression is needed to fit the signals that arrive at a display into the display's dynamic range.

Whether at the input or output of a system, dynamic range is the ratio of the largest, nonsaturating signal that can be amplified, compared to the smallest signal just above the system noise. Thus, a dynamic range of 40 dB, for example, means that the largest signal that can be amplified without saturation within a system will be 100 times larger than the smallest. To understand this, we simply need to know if the dynamic range is an input- or an output-dynamic range. As an input-dynamic range, 40 dB is very poor; as an output-dynamic range, it is quite good.

The lower dynamic range limit is set by the noise floor of the system. When the noise increases and approaches the maximum signals, the signal range that can be handled by a sonograph might not be changed, but the range of discernable signals will be. Along with the overall system response, the output-dynamic range will affect the depth of useful imaging. Thus, a dynamic range that has been decreased because of noise will also decrease the useful imaging depth.

The presence of noise brings up another parameter, the signal-to-noise ratio, or SNR. This ratio changes with the various signal levels and a fixed noise level, but becomes important when examining the smaller echo signals. Effective penetration will cease when the SNR is unity. Many systems are designed to use rejecting

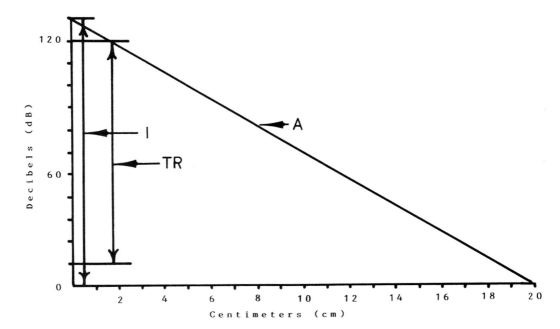

2-11.   Limiting the input dynamic range with a transmit-receive switch. The range of echo-signals out of a transducer can exceed 120dB, I. Transmit-receive switches, however, have a limited range, TR, which sets the maximum and minimum signals that can enter the sonograph. Y axis is signal level in dB; X-axis is distance in cm for maximum signal A.

diodes in a circuit that removes signals below a level just above the noise floor. This design keeps noise out of the image but also removes low-level echo signals that could be separated from the noise by sophisticated filtering.

Internal noise is hard to characterize without any real reference to place it against. As a result, system noise is often referred to the input, that is, the noise is expressed as an input voltage in microvolts that would produce a signal of that level within the system. Typical noise figures are in the 2-μV to 10-μV range for most current sonographs in good condition. In several well-designed systems, these noise figures are reaching the theoretical limits of design. Further noise reduction requires processes such as special narrow passband amplifiers or special averaging techniques that separate stationary from random signals.

With an rf signal amplified to a usable level, the system then detects or demodulates the signal.

Detector

The signals delivered to the detector contain four pieces of information: amplitude, phase, frequency, and time of arrival. For an imaging ultrasound device, two of these data will be used—amplitude and time of arrival (distance); the rest is

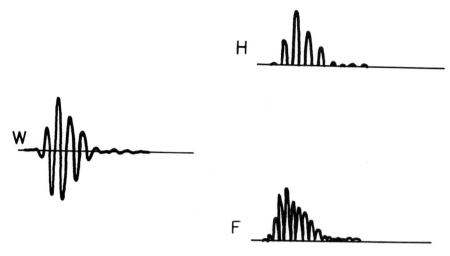

2-12 Half-wave versus full-wave detection. Detection requires rectifying and filtering the radio frequency echo signal *W*. Half-wave detection *H* realizes only one-half of the echo signal contributing to the video signal. Full-wave detection *F* uses all of the wave *W* to make the video echo-signal.

discarded. In contrast, pulsed-Doppler will use phase, frequency, and time of arrival, discarding signal amplitude.

The process of extracting amplitude information from a returning signal is called amplitude detection. In this process, the amplified rf signals are rectified and filtered to remove the rf (Figure 2-12). Rectification is a technique of turning rf alternating current into rf pulsating direct current. The effect is to take the oscillating rf and cut it in half. If it is full-wave rectification, the bottom half of the envelope is folded up on the top, producing a pulsating DC signal at twice the rf frequency. The pulsations are often then removed by filtering, and only the envelope of the rf signal remains. This is the same rectification and filtering as used in amplitude modulation (AM) transistor radios to detect the radio signals. Much of the detection technology from the communications industry is applied here.

Rectification depends upon the devices used to transform alternating current to direct current. These devices are usually diodes, designed to handle the high-frequency content of the rf signal shape, as well as the rf itself. The detector can "leak" the higher frequencies through the diodes by capacitance within the diodes, leading to a loss of both the envelope waveform and the direct-current qualities of the rectified signals. Such malformations of the video signal can gradually but markedly destroy the gray-scale qualities of a sonograph.

The voltage-current relationship in a detector must be linear in order to permit proper transfer of the rf envelope without distortion. Often a detector circuit will have nonlinearities in the low-voltage range, which pull the smaller signals farther apart than they were when entering the detector [4]. The result is an expansion of the signal range that must be corrected, usually by a compressing video stage after the detector.

The signal range out of an amplitude detector can be as large as 60 dB to 70 dB. A compressing video amplifier after the detector can reset the signals into a 30-dB to 45-dB range, depending upon the design of the particular machine. This is the dynamic range usually stated by the manufacturer to describe machine performance.

Signal compression need not be limited to the video stage. It can also occur in the rf stage, coupling amplifier compression with TGC compression. Some designs use an even-greater amount of compression at the rf level, and in such cases, the TGC is often applied at the video level rather than at the rf level. This design should theoretically work identically to the more conventional design. Experience indicates, however, that large amounts of rf-level compression work best in very quiet systems. The compression needed at the rf level without TGC places the system noise close to the smaller signal levels, making the SNR often too small for effective separation.

Although we have devoted a significant portion of this chapter to studying the rf amplifier passband, alterations of the signal can also occur if the video amplifier passband is too small. Inappropriate video filtering spreads out the video signals, making them appear broader than they really are. The trade-off is between video signal shape and noise, where a narrower passband admits less noise but a wider passband permits better video signal representation. Once past such an amplifier, the signal can be somewhat restored, however, by differentiating the signal and adding this derivative back to the smoothed signal to sharpen the leading edges of the envelope. This process is called edge enhancement, and has been used often to bolster a sagging signal stream. A desire for higher-fidelity signals has decreased the use of edge enhancement. Although edge enhancement is not often employed in the newer designs, the technique is hidden in older machines and new productions of older designs.

The video amplifier emits video signals that represent the stream of echoes received on each pulse-listen cycle. The signals are still some distance from the signals that make up the displayed, two-dimensional image, but are quite useful to depict signal amplitude and range. Although the eye can be fooled sometimes on a gray-scale display, it cannot be fooled on relative signal amplitudes on an A-mode display, which clearly shows signal range, individual amplitudes, and any signs of signal alterations in the signal stream to that point (Figure 2-4). The relationship between signal levels and TGC is quite evident and is often displayed along with the TGC curve, which relates back to the tissue-ultrasound interaction. An A-mode display and a standard signal source can show whether the TGC is working properly or not. Nonlinear TGC responses are seen easily on an A-mode display, as well as any unusual signals characteristic of the tissue. Still, these signals are not the image, which is the desired result.

If A-mode signals are altered slightly and collected together, a two-dimensional image results. Where to place the signals on the display is determined from the positional information relayed from the next segment of the machine, the scanning arm.

Scanning Arm

In addition to displaying the stream of signals that flow from the detector, the sonograph must correlate signal position on the display with the transducer position in space. The scanning arm provides this position information.

The scanning arm has a set of articulations, or joints, with position encoders located either at the joints or connected to the joints through a set of wires (Figure 2-13). The encoders follow the changes in joint angles as the scan is made. The encoders carry voltages that are used to calculate the transducer position in the scanning plane.

The encoding can be analog or digital, depending upon the design of the machine. Analog encoders are large, precision potentiometers. Digital encoders represent an attempt to more completely digitize the B-scanner [5]. Experience shows, however, that digital encoders have not markedly improved overall arm-position accuracy. The reasons for this lack of improvement are not entirely clear, except that analog technology may currently be too advanced and too stable to improve arm-position accuracy simply by applying digital techniques. Accuracy is enhanced, nevertheless, when the encoders are located in the arm, as shown in Figure 2-13, rather than connected to the arm through wires.

Additional encoders in the arm base mark the position of the scan plane itself. Thus, we can reference examination scan planes to a patient's external anatomy. These positions appear on the display screen in centimeters, left or right of midline, or above or below the iliac crest or some other abdominal landmark. And for oblique scan-plane angles, the angulations appear as degrees on the display.

The scan arm performs two primary functions: first, confining the scan to a single plane; second, providing data on where the beam is pointed within the scan plane. In addition, when the sonographer moves the scan plane to oblique positions that are not parallel with standard anatomical planes, these oblique positions are automatically indicated on the display screen, keeping the sonologist (interpreter of the images) informed on the scan-plane position for each image. (The necessity of knowing the position of the ultrasound beam within the scan plane continues when we get into real time.)

With signals positioned on the display, we can look at the display in more detail.

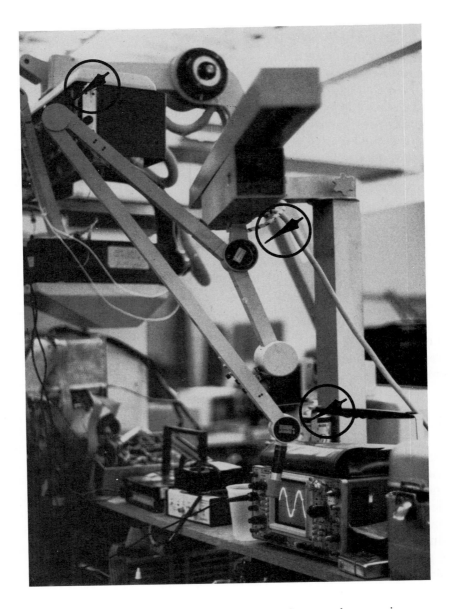

2-13 Scanning arm encoders to determine transducer position. A B-scanning arm requires position encoders that measure
the position of the transducer in the scanning plane. Here the
position information comes from potentiometers in the joints of
the scanning arm (arrows). Courtesy of Technicare Ultrasound
Division, Englewood, Colorado.

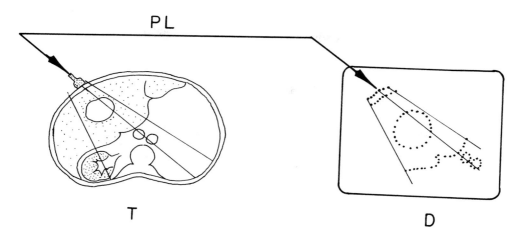

2-14 Linking transducer position to the display. Forming an image from B-mode traces requires positioning the trace on the display *D*, just as the transducer is positioned on the body *T* through a mechanical or electrical link *PL*.

Display

A limitation of all transducers is that they lack a memory. As a result, we can move transducers about to make the data for a two-dimensional image, but the transducers remember none of it. To make the image, the sonograph must assemble the signals in storage and bring them to a common display, as shown in Figure 2-14. The memory for signal storage is most often contained in the display portion of the machine.

Besides storing information to make an image, the display is also a transducer, changing electrical energy (signals) into light (gray-scale dots) that we can see and use for analysis. Formation of the B-mode display is shown in Figure 2-15. The display transducer still used for this is the cathode ray tube. Other display transducers are now available, such as light-emitting diodes and liquid crystals, but the CRT continues to dominate the displays for ultrasound.

The CRT is made from an evacuated glass cylinder with a source of electrons at one end and a nearly flat, phosphor-coated face at the other end, as shown in Figure 2-16. Between the two ends is an array of elements designed both to form the electron beam into a small, nearly inertia-free writing stylus and to move the beam in response to electrical instructions. Beam movement in a straight line is called a trace. The beam position along the trace is indicated by a bright spot on the CRT screen, provided the beam is moving slowly enough. With fast beam motion, the spot smooths into the characteristic bright line of a trace. Because the amount of light emitted from either the dot or the trace is proportional to the

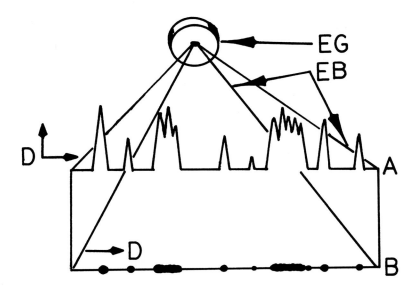

2-15.   Forming a B-mode trace. An A-mode trace, A, shows echo-signal amplitude versus time or distance. A B-mode trace, B, turns the electron beam, E3, on and off in proportion to the signal strength. Again, the display shows echo-signal position and amplitude in gray scale. EG is the electron gun.

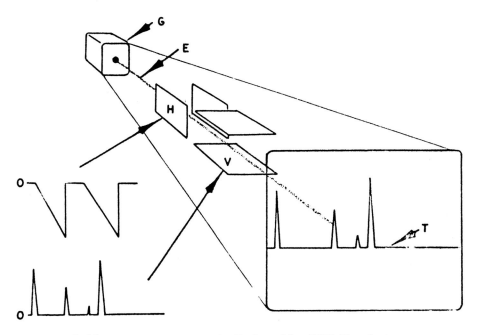

2-16.   Forming the A-mode display with a CRT. The electron gun, G, emits electrons to form the beam E that is moved over the CRT face by electrodes H and V. The phosphor at the CRT face changes the electron energy into light, making the trace, T, visible.

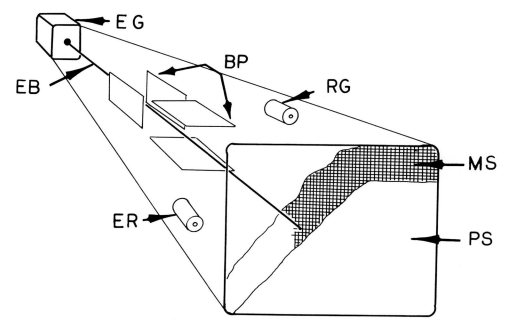

2-17 The variable persistance CRT. The electron gun *EG* forms an electron beam *EB*, moved inside the CRT by the beam-moving plates *BP*. The electron beam writes onto the memory screen *MS*, selecting which electrons can reach the phosphorous screen *PS*. The reading electron gun *RG* floods the *MS* with electrons that pass through to the *PS*, making the stored image visible. The erasure gun *ER* replaces electrons on the *MS*, erasing the stored image. Balancing writing, reading, and erasure changes image persistance.

number of electrons in the electron beam, controlling the beam current means controlling the intensity of the spot formed by the electron beam-phosphor interaction.

Because the beam is formed from electrons, it is charged and can be moved by applying electrostatic forces to the beam through beam-moving plates inside the CRT. Alternatively, because the electron beam is made of moving charges, outside magnetic fields can apply forces to the beam. This is a popular technique for CRTs in TV monitors. Whether the forces are internal-electric or external-magnetic, the accurate reproduction of the signals brought to the display will depend upon accurate beam positioning and predictable electron-phosphor interactions.

Within the sonograph and the display, we assume a constant propagation velocity. In reality, this proves to be only partially true, but the propagation velocity is adequate for the display process. The average velocity within the tissue is 1540 m/s. If we assume this constant, then, the sonograph shows distance by counting time. The clock for this process is the CRT trace, which moves against a reference of markers separated 13 μs apart to represent centimeter intervals in the tissue.

Because it is hard to build a meaningful two-dimensional image from an A-mode display, a B-mode display is used instead. A moving electron beam forms the B-mode trace, but rather than modulating movement for signal strength, as in the A-mode display, we modulate the beam on and off in response to the echo signals (Figure 2-15). If the electron beam current changes in proportion to the video signal amplitude and the phosphor can respond, the trace takes on gray-scale qualities. The image appears from the collection of all the pulse-listen cycles comprised by a scan, shown simultaneously. Clearly, the display needs a memory.

A short-term memory can result from choosing the right phosphor for the CRT. Mixing different phosphors together gives different colors to the trace and different retention times for the CRT. Long-persistence phosphors, for example, can retain an image long after the electron beam has passed, ranging from a few milliseconds to several minutes. But this is not the sort of memory that offers a chance to interrogate an image in detail over a long period of time.

A much-longer-term memory is photographic film, used early in ultrasound as both a memory and for making records of the examination. Because in the past the phosphors of most CRTs were short-persistance, the sonographer built the image on film by opening the camera shutter and scanning "blind" with no immediate visual feedback. However, the sonographer needed a high level of skill to make uniform movements of the transducer over the body surface in a compound scan. Although photographic film was an effective memory, its use in this mode was too demanding for the average sonographer to make the images repeatable. Ultrasound therefore needed another technique.

The next technological advancement placed a memory onto the CRT face. Using a layer of insulating material between the electron beam and the phosphor, the electron beam left a pattern of charges, storing the electron beam positions and echo patterns during the scan. The electron beam knocked electrons out of the insulating material, leaving a trail of positive charges across the insulating material. Then, by flooding electrons toward the screen, the positive-charge distribution was made visible, since the flooding electrons could reach the phosphor only through the positive-charge locations. The result was an effective memory, but it had only bistable qualities, that is, only two shades of gray were possible. Furthermore, the charges on the dielectric were not stable and would "leak" into the surrounding insulating material, causing a bleeding quality to the image. And using electrons to "read" the image meant the electrons could combine with the distributed positive charge and erase the image. Ultrasound thus needed a better memory.

Next to appear was an insulating layer displaced from the phosphor onto a separate screen, but still located between the electron beam and the phosphor, as in Figure 2-17. This system stabilized many of the problems associated with the storage CRT, but retained all those characteristic of a physical memory system. Still, the variable persistence CRT, as this system is called, did give some gray scale in the display, and, of significance, a more stable image. But like its predecessors, the variable persistence CRT lacked a major capability: it could not interface with the outside world on a standard format. Each of these displays—the standard CRT, the storage CRT, and variable persistence CRT—is an X-Y display, unable to interface directly with outside recording devices such as videotape recorders, multiformat cameras, and additional monitors. These problems found their solution, in part, in a recombined form of CRT technology that provided

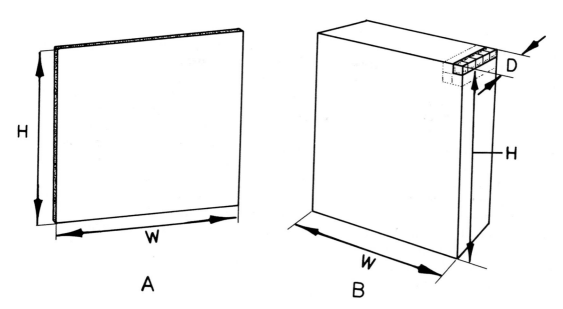

2-18   Comparison of analog and digital memories. The analog memory *A* has a physical height, *H,* and width, *W,* with signal amplitude stored as charges on the memory plane. The digital memory *B* not only has height, *H,* and width, *W,* but also a thickness, *D,* representing the size of the digital word used to store signal amplitude.

a standard output to the outside world. The device is called an *analog scan converter* (ASC). Briefly mentioned here, it is discussed in more detail in Chapter 4.

The ASC combined the physical memory with an ability to read the stored information off the memory in a standard format. Analog scan conversion, however, still carried the curse of all physical memory systems: instability due to varying voltages, temperature, and component aging. Nevertheless, the ASC produced a gray-scale image from the signals and offered a standard TV output. When it worked, the system was outstanding, providing some of the best imaging ever. But it seldom worked well or for long. The B-scanner was thus forced into the next level of technology, the digital scan converter. Ultrasound again found a better way.

Aerospace technology clearly showed the advantages of digital storage and digital image processing, even though the technique was more expensive and was not well known in the ultrasonic imaging industry. Acceptance came quickly, however, and in a short time, digital scan converters ruled the B-scanner imaging community. A strong motivation for accepting the digital scan converter was the availability of digital random access memories (RAM) at a quality and cost that permitted building large digital memories for ultrasound.

The *digital scan converter* uses the RAM for data acquisition and storage at one rate and data fetching and display at another rate. The result is scan conversion, but with a stability not previously available. Central to the process is the conversion of the analog signal coming out of the detector into a set of binary numbers that can be stored. Storage occurs according to rules that permit later image reconstruction from the digital data. But along with stability came a new set of problems, concerns, and capabilities—aspects that are explored in Chapter 5.

It should be mentioned here, however, that going digital uses a much smaller number of gray levels to depict the range of signals than were formerly used in the continuous range of gray intensities that are fundamental to the analog scan converter. The manner in which the analog video signals are assigned the available numbers is a process called preprocessing. Although a great deal of controversy surrounds preprocessing, the central concern is not the presence of preprocessing, but the issue of linearity. All digital systems must have preprocessing. Disagreement occurs, however, when considering whether or not the transfer from an analog signal to a digital number is linear or not. The need for nonlinear preprocessing depends upon the number of values available in the scan converter, that is, the number of bits that make up the computer "word" and the dynamic range of the signals being divided into digital segments. Further complicating the process is the question of which range of signals should receive finer or coarser division. This issue is treated further in Chapter 5.

In the signal stream, our immediate concern is the *analog-to-digital converter* (ADC), whose function is to convert the analog signals that arrive at one input port into a set of binary numbers out of another port. Preprocessing can be introduced at this level. Alternatively, the preprocessing can be introduced by shaping the analog signal range being brought to the ADC, leaving the ADC linear. This is an analog preprocessor, and like all analog circuits, it has both limited stability and range.

Out of the ADC is a set of binary numbers that change in value according to the signal amplitudes presented to the ADC during a single pulse-listen cycle. Also, positioning the numbers into the RAM depends upon where the transducer is pointed in space. The scan-arm encoder information is used to assign data position. Thus, a "ray" of information maps over the memory as if we were dealing with a rectangular flat memory like the analog scan converter memory plane (Figure 2-18).

Once stored in memory, the signals can be retrieved without destroying the memory contents. They are fetched out as if an electron beam raster-scan were being carried out over the stored image. The result is a series of digital numbers representing image components, streaming out at a standard TV rate, completing the scan conversion. The data, however, are still digital and lack the control signals needed to make a TV monitor respond properly. Consequently, control signals are often added digitally, and then are run to the next function in the signal stream, the *digital-to-analog converter,* or DAC.

The purpose of the DAC is to convert the stream of digital signals coming from the RAM into a set of analog signals that meet the signal range requirements of the TV system. But once more, we are faced with a small dilemma. How are the intensity ranges of the TV, or gray-scale levels, to be allocated to the digital signals? Thus, the signals from the memory need to be processed again, and because the processing occurs after the memory, it is called postprocessing. As before, the finite set of digital numbers must be matched to an analog, continuous set of gray levels. The results are not continuous, however, but become a finite set of gray intensity levels. As in preprocessing, all digital machines must have postprocessing. The controversy seems not to be the existence of postprocessing, but the sort of processing used. In addition, postprocessing that uses variable assignment curves or manual controls does not work well when too few gray levels are available. For example, 16 gray levels are too few to effectively use variable postprocessing. Once the DAC makes the conversion, the signals are ready to be placed on the TV screen.

Because the output from the scan converter is a standard TV signal, the output can interface with additional monitors, videotape recorders, or other storage devices. The image finally brought out will depend upon the assignment of signal to number (preprocessing) and the assignment of number to gray level (postprocessing). Often these assignments are under operator control. Some ways of rationally handling these controls are discussed in succeeding chapters.

Conclusion

We have traced the signal from its first excitation by the transmitter, through reception, transduction, amplification, detection, digitalization, storage, reconstruction, reconversion to analog, and finally to the display. Along the way, the signal has been altered in energy, shape, and character, changing finally into light.

Such a signal stream can be built to describe any available sonograph. In attempting to understand the events leading to the image on the screen, questions that an operator asks can be guided by the limits imposed by a specific machine's design. Machine instruction books—both the operator's manual and the electronic design and repair manual—can help to fill in knowledge gaps. The salesperson from whom the machine was purchased, as well as the marketing department of the corporate home office, can provide additional answers (many corporations now have educational programs, and the instructors within these programs are a good information source). By exploring all routes of inquiry, the sonographer is that much more likely to take advantage of the machine's potential, rather than having it be an inexplicable black box that stands between sonographer and patient.

The organization and operation of a sonograph can hardly be compressed into one chapter. To provide further enlightenment on the information load just presented, succeeding chapters will more fully address particular aspects of the machine. With the general concepts in hand, the specifics of a sonograph, of whatever make, should now be easier to grasp.

References

1. Wells, P.N.T., and K.T. Evans. October 1968. An immersion Scanner for two-dimensional ultrasonic examination of the human breast. Ultrasonics 220–228.
2. Havlice, J.F., and J.C. Taenzer. April 1979. Medical ultrasound imaging: An overview of principles and instrumentation. Proc IEEE 67:620–641.
3. Melton, H.E., Jr., and F.L. Thurston. 1978. Annular array design and logarithmic processing for ultrasonic imaging. Ultrasound Med Biol 4:1–12.
4. Wells, P.N.T. 1969. Physical principles of ultrasonic diagnosis. London and New York: Academic Press.
5. Waxman, A. The use of microprocessors in gray scale ultrasound. Santa Clara, CA: Searle Ultrasound (2270 Martin Ave., Santa Clara, CA 95050).
6. Powis, R.L. 1978. Ultrasound physics . . . for the fun of it. Denver: Technicare Corp.
7. McDicken, W.N. 1976. Diagnostic ultrasonics: Principles and use of instruments. New York: John Wiley & Sons.

Chapter 3

Making and Receiving Ultrasound: Transducers and How They Work

The Transducer as an Interface

The transducer is a central component in the production and reception of ultrasound. By enabling us to produce and "hear" ultrasound, the transducer acts as an interface between the body being scanned and the machine electronics that provide an image. Like any transducer, the transducer in a sonograph quietly changes one form of energy to another. On the body side are all the events connected with ultrasound as a mechanical wave: propagation, refraction, reflection, scattering, and attenuation. On the machine side are the electronics, which regulate the events needed to convert the ultrasound information into an image: amplification, detection, shaping, storage, and display. The task in designing the ultrasound machine is to make the display represent the events within the tissue as accurately as possible. The transducer and its characteristics are the first step in this process.

The division of events at the transducer interface involves more than changing one form of energy into another. On the tissue side, sonographers have no real control over the events. On the electronics side, however, it is possible to exert a great deal of control. Through knowledge of the electronic events and their influence on the display, the mechanical events that form transduction are also analyzable, allowing the sonograph to be used to better advantage in depicting the events within the tissue.

This separation of the mechanical and electronic events means that the controls that influence the final image have little or no effect on events within the tissue. For example, a common misconception is that changing time-gain compensation (TGC) controls will somehow change the focal point position or some other aspect of the transducer beam. Such a change could only happen if the transducer is a phased array (linear or annular), with the appropriate front panel controls, of course, and TGC would not be the control to change. For machines with single-element transducers, this is not possible. We must change transducers in order to move the transducer focal point.

As stated in Chapter 2, the term *probe* has been used often in the past in place of *transducer;* however, in our view, *probe* is an inaccurate and out-dated label. Another name often applied to the transducer is "ceramic crystal," because of the material used to make the transducer. The words *transducer* and *crystal* are used interchangeably in this book to describe the source and sensor of ultrasonic, mechanical waves.

Piezoelectricity

Ultrasonic transduction occurs as a result of piezoelectricity, which literally means "pressure electric." A pressure field applied to one of these transducing materials causes an electric field to be generated within the crystalline material. If the pressure is rhythmic, the electric field will change in a corresponding rhythmic manner, as well. Quartz and tourmaline exhibit this property naturally, as do a wide range of synthetic materials. It is from these synthetic materials that transducers are made for diagnostic ultrasound.

The property of piezoelectricity also carries a sort of reciprocity, in which the application of an electric field produces a change in the physical shape of a crystalline material. By virtue of this capability, a transducer can be excited into vibration by hitting it with a sharp electrical pulse. On the other hand, if the electrical excitation is rhythmic, the change in shape will also be rhythmic. Both of these excitation techniques are used to make the transducer produce ultrasound.

Transducer Materials

Most of the synthetic materials that have piezoelectric properties are called ferroelectrics. Ferroelectrics are materials that carry a small net electrical charge at the molecular level [1], much like the ferromagnetics made of molecules that carry a small net magnetic dipole. Aligning the molecules together forms a large net magnetic field for the ferromagnetic material and a large net electrical field for the ferroelectric material. From this net charge orientation, the ferroelectric acquires the property of piezoelectricity [1].

By mutual alignment, small groups of molecules can gather and act together. These small regions of alignment are called domains (Figure 3-1). If all the domains are randomly positioned in a ferroelectric, it will have no piezoelectric properties. To bring all the electrical fields into alignment, the ferroelectric is heated until the domains are free to move in response to an outside force. A large outside electrical field forces all the domains in the heated material into the same direction. With

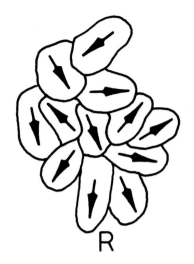

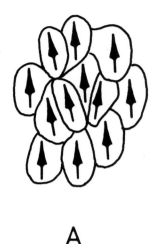

3-1   Aligning ferroelectric domains. Ferroelectrics have small regions with net electric dipoles called domains. To make a ferroelectric transducer, the random domains *R* are aligned, *A*. If the transducer is later heated above the Curie temperature, the domains become random again, and the material loses its transducer properties.

the electrical field still applied, the material is allowed to cool, leaving a permanent electrical field in the ferroelectric [1]. The result is a piezoelectric material, able to transform one form of energy into another.

The material produced is also sensitive to temperature. If the new transducing material is heated again above a certain temperature, this time without the external field, the domains become mobile once more and assume a random pointing pattern. This transition temperature is called the *Curie temperature,* and represents a transition between nonmobile and mobile ferrorelectric domains [1]. Hospital autoclaves can easily reach the Curie temperature for most of the transducing materials now available, and an autoclaved transducer is usually dead when it is taken out. This destruction occurs by thermally disrupting the crystal domain organization.

Transducers have to operate in two directions, that is, changing mechanical to electrical energy and vice versa. But not all transducer materials respond to an applied electrical field with the same reliability as when they respond to an applied mechanical pressure. Standard quartz, for example, can receive mechanical energy very well, but responds poorly to rapidly changing electrical fields [2]. Most of the materials currently used for transducers have a firm balance between the two transduction processes. Examples of these materials are lead zirconate titanate (PZT), and barium titanate [2].

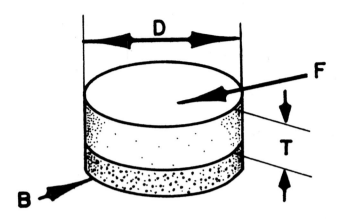

3-2 Components of a damped transducer. A damped transducer has a diameter, *D,* and a thickness, *T.* A backing material *B* is placed on the transducer to shorten the vibrational period. Vibrating in the thickness mode, the transducer emits energy from its front and back surfaces. Ultrasound travels to the tissue from the face *F* and at the same time, into the backing material *B.*

Transducer Vibration

Making ultrasound is simply a matter of setting the transducer into vibration. Like most solid materials, a transducer will vibrate at a natural frequency that is determined by the physical dimensions of the transducer. Most transducers are a thin wafer of material, with the vibration occurring along the wafer thickness (Figure 3-2). The natural resonant frequency of the transducer, therefore, is determined by the wafer thickness. The lowest natural resonant frequency possible for the transducer is when the wafer is equal to half a wavelength thick.

As noted earlier in the discussion of mechanical waves, the wavelength of ultrasound in any material is a function of frequency and the velocity of propagation. Most transducer materials have a high propagation velocity, so most thicknesses are not too small for reliable manufacture. For example, the velocity of propagation in PZT-5 is 3,780 m/s. A 5.0-MHz transducer would then have a thickness of 0.38 mm, with a wavelength of 0.76 mm in the PZT.

If the diameter of the transducer is much larger than the thickness, a thickness mode of vibration is easy to establish. When these two dimensions approximate each other more closely, however, the ability to exclude other modes of vibration lessens. The mixed frequencies and modes of vibration then begin to dominate transducer vibration, as the dimensions of the transducer in other directions can support ultrasonic vibrations (Figure 3-3) [3]. In phased arrays, these additional modes of vibration appear to affect the intensity of the transducer beam during the beam-steering process [3].

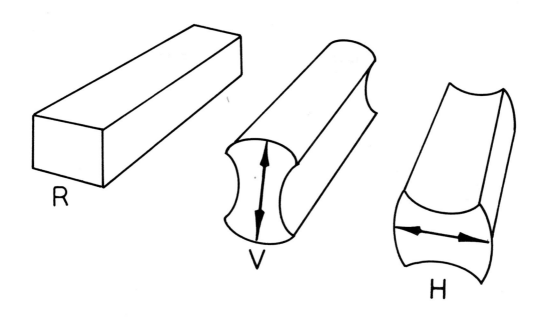

3-3   Vibration modes in rectangular transducers. Transducers cut into small rectangles *R* can have unusual vibrational modes. Thickness vibrations *V* and horizontal vibrations *H* are possible in the same transducer, producing complex ultrasound emissions that can affect phased and linear arrays.

Transducer Excitation

The electrical forces used to excite a transducer into vibration can originate from various shaped pulses, ranging from very sharp electrical spikes to sine waves at the transducer resonant frequency. Because the transducer acts like an aggregate of capacitors, inductors, and resistors, it responds differently to varying voltages and current-phase relationships. Furthermore, it will respond to the impedance it sees during the excitation and ringing processes. To better match the transducer to the transmitter in the sonograph, special inductors, capacitors, or resistors often are placed in the transducer current path. However, as stated in Chapter 2, no two manufacturers makes the same transmitter, and it is difficult and often unwise to trade transducers designed for one sonograph for another.

Along with the current-voltage relationship, the shape of the pulse also plays a role in transducer events. Some transducers respond well to a soft spike with a slow rise and fall in voltage. Others require fast rise times. This response is a function of several parameters discussed later in this chapter. The primary need at this point is to know that these sensitivities exist.

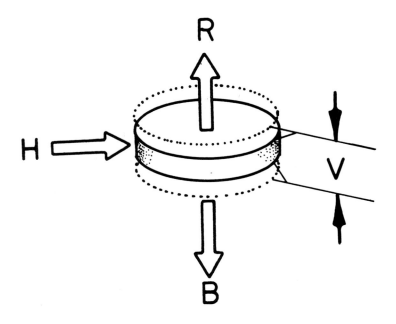

3-4 Energy loss in normal vibration. A transducer cut as a wafer will vibrate in a thickness mode *V*. Energy losses from a transducer include radiation from the front face *R* and the back *B*, as well as that resulting from internal heating *H*.

Damping in Transducers

Once the transducer is set into vibration, the amplitude of the vibration could remain the same with no loss of energy. But energy is lost from the transducer both in the form of internal heat and the ultrasound energy that is radiated away (Figure 3-4). Thus, the start and finish of a vibrational process form a vibrational envelope. In the imaging system, this envelope is used to represent the returning echo within the system electronics. If we seek a high-resolution imaging system, that envelope needs to be as short as is practical. One way to shorten the envelope is to remove energy from the vibrational process as rapidly as possible. This technique of quickly subtracting energy is called damping, and the material used to absorb the energy is called a damping material.

To remove energy efficiently from a transducer requires a close coupling between the damping material and the transducer. The damping material is usually placed on the back of the transducer, away from the direction we want ultrasound to leave the transducer (Figure 3-4). The material is typically an epoxy substrate with metal powder inside to produce a highly energy-absorbant substance. Like the shocks on a car that take the oscillating mechanical energy of the car's springs and

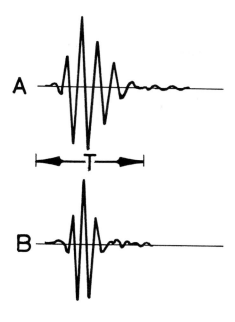

3-5 Decreasing pulse length with increasing frequency. The damping process in transducers produces nearly the same number of vibrations, regardless of frequency. Comparing the vibrations of a 3-MHz transducer *A* with a 5-MHz transducer *B* shows a shorter pulse length with higher frequencies. *T* is 2 μs.

converts it to heat, the damping material takes the mechanical energy of the transducer and converts it to heat. In a properly damped transducer, the vibration can start and stop in four to six cycles—or even shorter, if the transducer is excited with a carefully controlled sine wave. Regardless of the method, the end result is the same: very short envelope of ultrasonic vibration, as shown in Figure 3-5.

The time needed to start and stop the transducer vibration determines how long the ringing envelope will be, and therefore, the resolution of the echo-ranging system along the beam axis. This resolution is called *axial resolution*.

Because damped vibrations are almost frequency independent, nearly the same number of cycles will go into a transducer vibration, regardless of frequency. And because each cycle is faster for a higher frequency, moving to a higher frequency shortens the total length of the vibrational envelope. From this relationship is derived one of the basic tenets of ultrasound: Increasing transducer frequency improves axial resolution. This relationship does not hold true, however, if the damping on the compared transducers is not the same. A well-damped 2.25-MHz transducer, for example, could have much better axial resolution than a poorly damped 3.5-MHz transducer. Clearly, transducer damping and transducer frequency strongly influence the axial resolution of an echo-ranging ultrasound system.

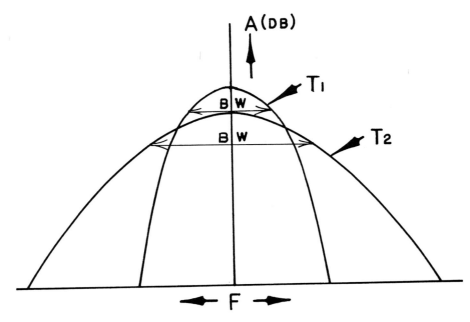

3-6 The frequency response of a damped transducer. Graphing the frequency component amplitude A as a function of frequency F shows the transducer frequency response. Band width BW represents a decrease in amplitude of 6 dB. Increasing the amount of damping usually decreases the amplitude response, T_1 to T_2, but increases the band width BW.

Transmitted Frequency Content

Clearly, increasing the damping process of the transducer shortens the vibrational envelope, but it also changes the frequency content of the transmitted ultrasonic wave train, as shown in Figure 3-6. Chapter 1 stated that the shape of a mechanical wave train determines its frequency content. The steeper the starting and stopping slopes on a wave envelope, for example, the larger the number of frequencies outside the fundamental frequency that are present in the wave train. And with an increasing number of frequencies, the amount of energy distributed in the frequencies also increases. As a result, the steep starting and stopping slopes of a well-damped vibration will produce a much wider band of frequencies than expected. In effect, by damping the transducer vibration to shorten the pulse duration, we have increased the Fourier components of the wave train. The parameter used to describe this increase in frequency components is the *transducer passband*.

One method of measuring the degree of damping in a transducer is by a quality of the transducer called Q. Q is the ratio of the amount of energy contained in a vibrational cycle to the amount of energy lost in that cycle. Generally, higher Qs yield narrower frequency passbands, and lower Qs yield wider frequency passbands. For example, a system vibrating with little energy loss can have a Q of 500 or more. In contrast, diagnostic ultrasound transducers commonly have Qs of 2 to 6 [2]. The result is a broad range of frequencies present in the transmitted ultrasonic wave train.

The passband of a transducer can be explicitly stated as the range of frequencies that are present above a certain energy level; alternatively, the passband can be implied by stating the Q of a transducer. Obviously, stating the passband is a more informative way of understanding what frequencies are present. The frequency limits of the passband are often expressed as the 3-dB points, that is, where the frequency spectrum energy drops to 3 dB below maximum. A more useful expression is the 6-dB points, where the energy of the frequencies present decreases to 6 dB below the maximum level. This larger value is better to use because of the typically high gains and dynamic ranges used in sonographs. In addition, the passband limits can be expressed as a percentage of the center operating frequency of the transducer. For example, a 5.0-MHz transducer with a 50% passband means that the range of frequencies measured from the transducer range from 3.75 MHz to 6.25 MHz and have amplitudes greater than 50% (6 dB down) of the highest amplitude present. Clearly, then, the transducer frequency marked on the side of the housing is not what is present in the transmitted energy. All these frequencies away from the fundamental frequency will have an influence on image quality in different portions of the image.

Transmitted Field Geometry

The unfocused transducer and its field are the starting points for looking at transducer beams and beam characteristics. Fortunately, the unfocused transducer with a diameter much larger than its operating wavelength is well behaved. As a result, we can model this particular transducer on a computer. The results, measured experimentally, correlate well with theoretical predictions.

A look at the field generated by driving a transducer with a continuous sine wave close to its natural resonant frequency provides some primary indications of events within the field. To begin with, the field close to the transducer has a width close to that of the transducer itself (Figure 3-7). As we move farther from the transducer, the width of the field changes little. Proceeding farther still, we pass a boundary where another process takes over, and the field begins to diverge steadily. The portion of the beam close to the transducer with a nearly constant width is called the *near field*. The steadily broadening field beyond the near field is called the *far field*. The location of the transition boundary between these two field segments is a function of the transducer frequency and the diameter of the transducer face. Generally, as the diameter of the transducer increases with a constant frequency, the far field is moved farther from the transducer. On the other hand, holding the transducer diameter constant and lowering the transducer frequency pulls the far field closer to the transducer face. Some mathematical relationships using these parameters are developed later in the chapter. As it happens, these two segments

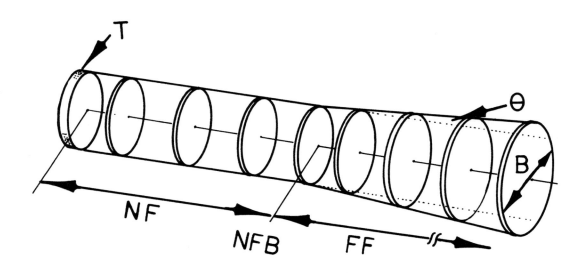

3-7 Model of an unfocused transducer field. The transducer *T* produces a zone close to the transducer with a beam width *B* nearly equal to that of the transducer, which is the near field *NF*. At the end of the near-field boundary *NFB*, the wave fronts become planar and expand with increasing distance at a steady rate Θ, forming the far field *FF*.

of the ultrasound field represent two different mechanical wave processes that have a major influence on the utility of diagnostic ultrasound.

The near field is also called the *Fresnel zone*, after the 19th-century physicist and mathematician Augustin Fresnel, who investigated light diffraction with the light source close to a diffracting aperature [4]. The field close to the transducer acts as if the transducer were an aperture and the real source of ultrasound a point located behind, but close to, the aperture. Thus, the wave fronts leaving the point source are not planar, but curved, and the rays passing through the aperture are not parallel (Figure 3-8). In fact, the wave fronts are spherical, and interact with the aperture in a complex manner. The events within the near field are quite complicated and do not permit easy modeling [4]. Nevertheless, the near field plays a central role in the solution to some resolution problems in imaging.

In contrast to the Fresnel zone, the region beyond the first divergence of the beam is called the *Fraunhofer zone*. This region was named after Joseph von Fraunhofer, a 19th-century physicist and mathematician who described diffraction processes in which the rays through the diffraction aperture are parallel [4]. One way to make rays parallel is to move the source of the waves some distance behind the aperture, or, in other words, to move the observation point for the beam far enough from the aperture so that the waves become planar. Thus, the central characteristic of the Fraunhofer zone is a plane wave front for the advancing ultrasound. And the geometry of the ultrasound beam in this region is predicted

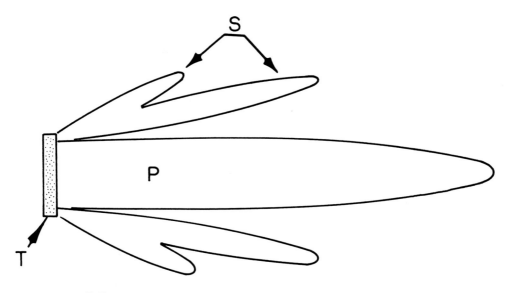

3-8 Transducer side-lobe formation. Because the transducer
T acts like a diffracting aperture, the beam forms into a primary
lobe *P* and lower-energy side lobes *S* that radiate energy away
from the primary lobe axis.

by the Fraunhofer equations for diffraction. Fortunately, the behavior of the beam in this region is sufficiently good to permit calculations that can reasonably represent measured events.

As noted in Chapter 1, diffraction processes are a result of looking at only a portion of the total wave front advancing from a wave source. Consequently, the exact nature of the diffraction will depend upon the size of the aperture relative to the wavelength of the mechanical wave. The resulting diffraction pattern varies both across and along the beam. If the pressure exerted by the ultrasound beam were graphed as a function of distance, the near field would appear quite complex, with a series of high positive and low negative pressure regions (Figure 3-9). Close to the transducer, these variations are rapid, but as the pressure waves advance farther from the transducer, the pressures oscillate less and less, until the *last axial maximum pressure* appears. Beyond this maximum, the pressure field falls off regularly, as if the wave fronts were all planar. This last axial maximum, then, represents the transitional region between the near field and the far field. We will refer to this range from the transducer face as the *near-field boundary* (NFB). Proximal to the transducer from the boundary is the near field; distal to the boundary is the far field. From the model of the transducer field pressure, the last axial maximum is calculated to be:

$$NFB = (D^2 - \lambda^2)/4\lambda, \tag{3.1}$$

where *D* is the diameter of the transducer (the effective aperture), and λ is the wavelength. But the wavelength for the higher frequencies now used in diagnostic

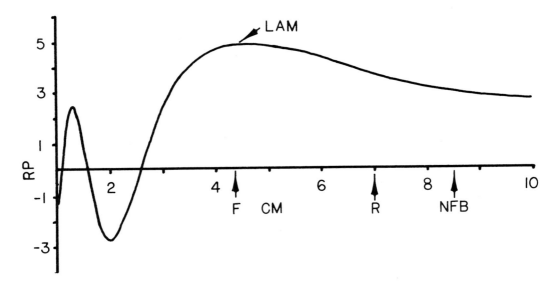

3-9   Relative pressure amplitude with distance from a focused transducer. Steady-state pressure field for a focused transducer. At the focal point *F*, the focused wave fronts become planar, forming the last axial maximum *LAM* in the pressure field. Note that the focus is less than both the calculated near-field boundary *NFB* and the radius of curvature on the lens *R*. *RP* is the relative pressure; *CM* is the distance from the transducer in centimeters.

ultrasound is very small; thus, the squared wavelength term does not significantly change the NFB calculation and can be ignored. The final equation looks like:

$$NFB = D^2/4\lambda. \tag{3.2}$$

This is the form of the equation best used to determine the near-field boundary location for any transducer with a given diameter and central operating frequency.

Let's look at some calculations from the near-field boundary equation, starting with a 13-mm, 3-MHz unfocused transducer. It has a near-field boundary at $(13^2)/4(0.5) = 84.5$ mm. At the same time, a 13-mm, 5-MHz unfocused transducer has a near-field boundary at $(13^2)/4(0.3) = 140$ mm. These calculations mean that the ultrasound field of the 3-MHz transudcer is going planar at about 8.5 cm, and the same is happening for the 5-MHz transducer at about 14 cm. (This boundary and where it is located will assume greater importance later when we try to focus the ultrasound beam.)

If the transducer is treated as a flat piston oscillating at the resonant frequency of the transducer, we can calculate the pressure waveform as a function of distance. These calculations show oscillations in the near field, as well as the location of the last axial maximum. Examples of two of these calculations are shown in Figure 3-10.

The first question that arises from examining the form of the pressure field is: Why do we not witness the null points in the field that are present in the calculation

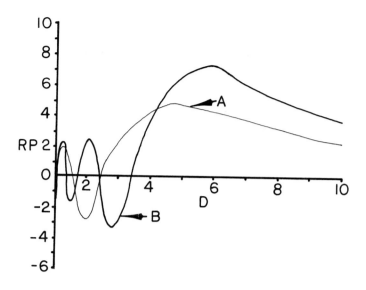

3-10   Effects of frequency on pressure field. Two pressure fields from transducers with the same radius of curvature on the lens and diameter. *A* is a 3-MHz transducer and *B* is a 5-MHz transducer, both with 1.3-cm diameters, and a 7-cm radius of curvature on each lens. Increasing the frequency moves the focal point farther from the transducer and increases the relative pressure at the focal point. *RP* is the relative pressure; *D* is distance in centimeters.

when we use an unfocused transducer on a B-scanner? The answer comes from two areas. First, the transducer is being pulsed, and the interaction of field components is temporally limited. As a result, the field of the pulsed transducer is close to, but not exactly like, the field from a continuously driven transducer. Second, pulsing the transducer provides a wide range of frequencies in the pressure field, filling in the nulls formed at each frequency. The result is a more uniform field than predicted by the model, but one not entirely constant over the range of the transducer near field. Once into the far field, the wave fronts adhere very well to predictions.

A test for our model is to measure the intensity of the unfocused transducer field using a beam profile machine. The results show a rather constant beam width and intensity all the way to the calculated near-field boundary (Figure 3-11). At the boundary, a slight increase in intensity is present, which is why the boundary is often called the natural focal point for the transducer. Beyond the NFB, the intensity of the beam falls off in a regular fashion, representing, as we now know, the geometric advancement of plane wave fronts.

Although unfocused transducers are used for special purposes, they usually produce some obvious problems in making estimates of lateral size, determining the number interfaces (echo sources) that are really present, or just making range measurements on objects with curves within the beam diameter. The task is clearly

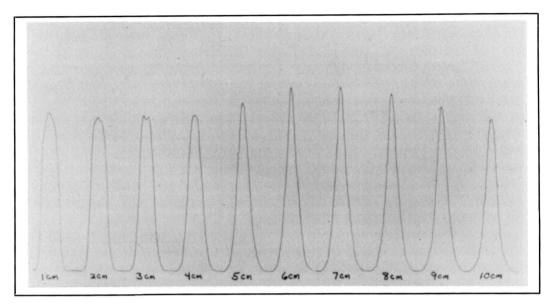

3-11   Beam profile from an unfocused, 2.25 MHz transducer. This transducer has a 13 mm diameter, which places the natural focal point and near field boundary at 6.2 cm. The profile shows an increase in beam intensity at the near field boundary.

one of narrowing the ultrasound beam width to permit better estimates of size, shape, and range of the echo sources. Narrowing the beam utilizes methods of concentrating the beam that are common to all waves and are included under the general heading of *focusing*.

Transducer Focusing

Fortunately, ultrasound, even with a wave formation different from transverse waves, carries the same properties as any mechanical wave. As a result, methods developed for directing electromagnetic radiation in both the radio and light spectrum to a focus will also focus ultrasound.

The first focusing technique is to use a lens. The lens simply applies an uneven bend to the ultrasound rays, forcing them to converge toward a point. The wave fronts are bent by the lens to form a concave wave front that advances geometrically toward a common point. Because this same technique is used to focus light, the optical lens is a good model for the ultrasound events. In fact, the first surface lens equation that predicts the focusing of light also predicts the focusing of ultrasound [2]. The lens is formed from a material with a velocity of propagation different from the transmitting medium. If the velocity in the transmitting medium is lower than in the transducer, which is usually the case, the converging lens will appear

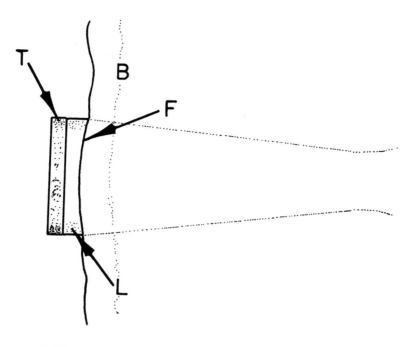

3-12 Forming the transducer lens. Because the velocity of propagation in an acoustic lens is higher than the tissue, the lens is concave. The interface between the lens *L* and the body *B* forms a first-surface lens *F*. *T* is the transducer.

as a concave surface at the lens-medium interface (Figure 3-12). The curvature has, in fact, formed a first surface lens, converging the ultrasound beam to a focal point.

A lens is not the only means of forming a curved wave front from the transducer face. The transducer can itself be curved, forcing the curved wave front from its physical shape (Figure 3-13). As before, the curvature causes the wave front to advance toward a focal point. Focusing is also possible by transmitting from an unfocused transducer into a curved mirror that can focus the beam. These three methods—lens, transducer curvature, and mirror—represent mechanical methods of focusing in which the ultrasound interacts with some sort of curved surface. Nonmechanical technique is also available, in which a curved wave front is formed from the superposition of several smaller wave fronts. This focusing technique, used in phased and linear arrays, is discussed later in the chapter.

We can now divide the focusing processes into two divisions. The first category includes those techniques that do something external to the transducer, such as a lens or mirror. These involve *externally focused transducers*. The second category includes those techniques that do something internal to the transducer, such as curving the transducer or synthesizing a curved front from many wave fronts. These involve *internally focused transducers*. The type of focusing of a transducer, either internal or external, is often indicated on the transducer housing.

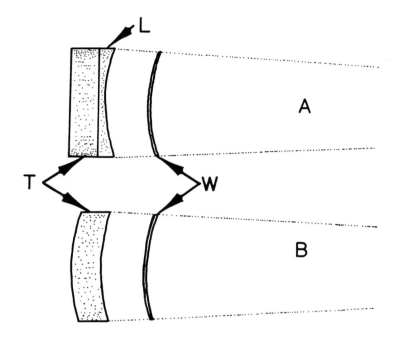

3-13 Two methods of focusing. The goal in focusing is to curve the wave front *W* from the transducer *T*. Methods include a lens *L,* as in Part A, or bending the transducer, as in Part B.

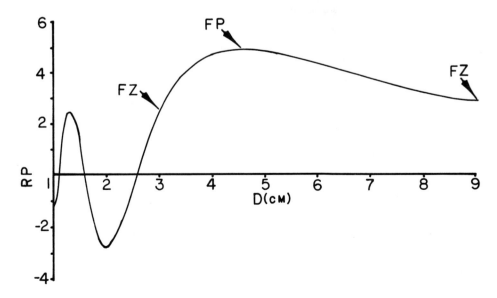

3-14 Focal zone in a pressure field. The focal zone *FZ* extends over a region defined by a decrease in the pressure field to one-half the maximum value *FP*. *RP* is the relative pressure; *D* is the distance from the transducer in centimeters.

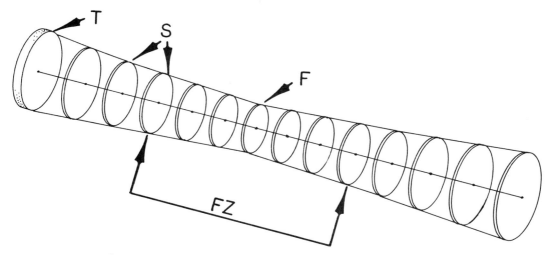

3-15   Model of focused transducer beam. Focusing forms a three-dimensional beam (visible through the sections *S*), which converges to a focal point *F*, forming a region of narrowness extending along the beam axis. This region is called the focal zone, *FZ*. *T* is the transducer.

As in the case of an unfocused transducer, the beam from a focused transducer can be modeled and calculated. In this focused transducer model, the transducer is curved (internally focused), with an aperture equal to the projected transducer diameter. Elements in the model include the diameter of the transducer, its operating frequency, and the radius of curvature for the transducer. Just as in the earlier unfocused transducer, the pressure field is calculated as a function of range from the transducer. The model is simple and makes no distinction between focusing from a lens on the transducer face or a curved surface. It is the advancing curved wave front that is the primary event.

In the pressure profile shown in Figure 3-14, the pressure undergoes a series of rapid oscillations about the ambient pressure, then reaches a maximum, which falls off steadily. A glance back at the profile from the unfocused transducer (Figure 3-10) shows a similar pattern for field behavior at the near-field boundary. It appears that focusing in this case moves the transition between the Fresnel zone and the Fraunhofer zone closer to the transducer. At the same time, the focusing concentrates the ultrasonic energy into a smaller area, increasing the pressure amplitude at the focal point.

The physical process of focusing never really forms a tight focal point, but instead, a region of narrowness equivalent to the region of least confusion used in light focused by a lens [4]. The regions of highest pressure and geometric narrowness coincide, forming the focal spot for the beam. A plane perpendicular to the beam axis at the narrowest portion of the beam forms the *focal plane* (Figure 3-15). On both sides of the focal plane is a region of narrowness called the *focal zone*. Because the focal zone holds the narrowest portion of the ultrasound beam, we can expect the best lateral resolution for structures within that zone. The boundaries of the focal zone will also be known as the *depth of focus,* corresponding to the depth of focus used in physical optics.

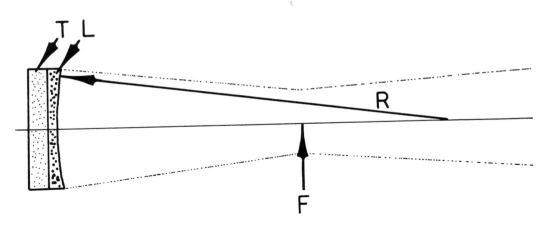

3-16   Relation of focal point and lens curvature. Focusing a transducer *T* with a lens *L* usually brings the focal point *F* closer to the transducer than the radius of curvature *R* on the lens. This shortened focal range is due to the diffraction processes of the transducer.

The change in the pressure profile that appears with focusing suggests that the transition between Fresnel and Fraunhofer regions is moved closer to the transducer. This appears to be equivalent to changing Fresnel diffraction to Fraunhofer diffraction in physical optics by adding a lens to the diffraction aperture [4]. In terms of the lens, the maximum distance a lens could focus nonplanar rays would be its own focal length. But the waves in the Fresnel zone are not planar, so applying a lens to an unfocused transducer means that focusing will occur at a range shorter than the focal length of the lens. And the focusing can be applied only in the near field of the transducer.

Stated another way, focusing makes the curved wave fronts of the Fresnel zone planar, and the wave fronts in the Fraunhofer zone cannot be made more planar than they already are. Clearly, focusing is confined to the near field. Thus, previous calculations of the NFB establish the outer limit of transducer focusing. And focusing farther out means moving the NFB farther out by using larger transducers.

Looking at the model again from still another point of view, we find that the expected point of focus, which should be the radius of curvature on the transducer or lens, and the actual point of focus do not coincide (Figure 3-16). In fact, diffraction processes are operating here, too, bringing the real focal point closer to the transducer than anticipated. We can acquire some understanding of this process by looking at the Fraunhofer diffraction problem in Chapter 1. A lens will focus light at its focal point if the light rays entering the lens aperture are parallel. But we know from the Fresnel diffraction problem that the rays are not parallel. The diffraction processes at the transducer place the virtual wave source behind the lens or transducer curvature, with a net effect of pulling the transducer focal point closer to the transducer than expected. Not long ago, this fact was not widely known, and the radius of curvature of the lens was used to cite the focal point of

TABLE 3-1
Some typical focused transducer parameters.

Frequency	Diameter	Focal Point	NFB	HMBW
2.25 MHz	19 mm	75 mm	133 mm	3.3 mm
3.0	13	45	83	2.2
3.5	13	60	96	2.5
3.5	19	90	205	2.5
5.0	13	60	137	1.7
5.0	6	20	29	1.3

NFB is the near field-far field boundary
HMBW is the half maximum beam width at the focal point

the transducer. When beam profiles came into use, the truth was revealed, and transducers long thought to be focused at 7 cm to 8 cm were in fact focused at about 6 cm. There is little chance of being fooled again. Our improved understanding of transducers, together with some simple calculations, can be used to verify any suspicions.

With our current grasp of the limitations on focusing, a logical question might be: Just how small can I make the focal spot? The answer lies in the combined effect of focusing and diffraction. Because curving a transducer or putting a lens out front is a mechanical replication of the Fraunhofer diffraction problem, the equations used to predict the spot size in the optical case can be applied to this mechanical wave. The radius of the effective spot can be calculated from the equation:

$$R = 1.22 \, \lambda \, L/D, \tag{3.3}$$

where R is the radius of the spot, λ is the wavelength, L is the focal point range from the lens or transducer, and D is the diameter of the aperture (transducer). This equation often appears in the ultrasound literature as the *half maximum beam width*, or HMBW. Because it describes the radius of the spot, it will also describe the effective beam width in which the beam intensity is 50% or more of the maximum intensity.

Equation 3.3 begins to offer some insight into the factors controlling transducer beam narrowing. For example, as the focal range, L, increases, the degree of focusing decreases because R varies directly with L. But by increasing the transducer diameter, D, the spot size, R, can be reduced at any given range. We already know that the NFB is directly proportional to the square of the transducer diameter, and effective focusing must stay within this boundary. Thus calculations of HMBW can provide some expectations on effective transducer focusing. Some typical values for HMBW and other parameters are shown in Table 3-1.

In a classical sense, the depths of focus for a transducer and a lens are similar but not exactly alike. Because of diffraction processes in the near field, a simple application of geometry cannot accurately predict the transducer depth of focus; a more general approximation is used instead. In terms of beam geometry, the depth-of-focus limits are when a standard reflector produces an echo reduced in amplitude by 50% from the maximum value at the focal point. This will nearly coincide with doubling the effective beam cross section as we look at the beam width on both sides of the focal plane. The equation for the approximation looks like:

$$DOF = 7 \lambda (L/D)^2, \tag{3.4}$$

where DOF is the depth of focus, λ is the wavelength, L is the focal length, and D is the diameter of the transducer.

In this equation, the trade-off is obvious between the degree of focus, that is, the narrowness of the focal spot, and the depth of focus. As the beam width is narrowed, the ability to keep the beam narrow over some distance on either side of the focal point is reduced. Much like the camera problem of aperture size and depth of focus, the transducer is unable to handle all problems by a single combination of parameters. Consequently, a large range of transducer parameters, focal points, depths of focus, and frequencies are available for the B-scanner and some real-time systems.

A parameter frequently used to talk about transducers is the so-called f-number. This is a ratio between the focal point range of a transducer and its diameter. Both of the previous equations for focusing and depth of focus can be reexpressed in terms of the f-number, or $f_{\#}$. They appear as:

$$HMBW = 1.22 \lambda f_{\#} \tag{3-5}$$

and

$$DOF = 7 \lambda (f_{\#})^2. \tag{3-6}$$

Because we are dealing with transducer wave diffraction, most of the equations for spot size predict a spot that contains about 85% of the total energy. What happened to the remaining 15%? The remaining energy went into radiation patterns that were not along the beam axis. This off-axis radiation is known as *side lobes,* and represents a loss of central energy due to diffraction. Side lobes also represent an opportunity for imaging artifacts. A three dimensional diagram of side lobes in normal beam formation is shown in Figure 3-17.

We know from the organization of the sonograph (Chapter 2), that the machine has no way of accounting for off-axis radiation patterns. It simply includes the off-axis echoes into the display trace along with on-axis echoes. If the side lobes are too large, the beam can appear to be far wider than expected, as revealed either in a beam profile or in calculations of the expected lateral resolution. Visual effects include filled-in cystic structures and strong specular reflectors where none should be. The problems with side lobes become major when we begin to deal with phased arrays.

Having achieved some understanding of transducer focusing and the means of describing the process, we next take up methods of improving transducer function.

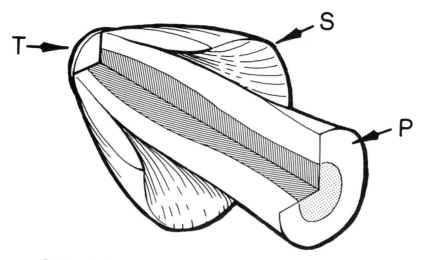

3-17.   A three-dimensional view of the primary beam and side lobes. The diffraction processes of the transducer, T, forms a primary beam, P, and side lobes, S, that extend outward at an angle. In addition, most of the energy (shading) is in the primary beam center.

Improving Transducer Efficiency

In spite of all its seeming activity, the transducer is really a large passive device, responding to electrical stimulations and pressures applied by the returning ultrasonic waves. Its ability to do this is a function of transducer diameter. The transducer can be thought of as an acoustic sail, collecting ultrasound like a sail collects wind. The larger the sail, the greater the amount of energy collected. We can improve returning energy concentrations by focusing the transducer; in addition, as described in the previous section, focusing is also a function of transducer diameter. Thus, a first step in improving the transducer's efficiency is to increase its size. At the same time, if the transducer has to be used in intimate contact with the patient, some practical limitations exist on the final dimensions of the crystal. On the other hand, if the transducer is placed in a water bath some distance from the patient, the transducer can be much larger, improving sensitivity, focal spot size, and depth of field.

The information collected by the transducer is not over an infinitely thin line in space, however. It is a volume in space with boundaries determined by the geometry of the ultrasound beam. From the superposition principle, we know that the pressure seen by the transducer, and therefore the electrical output from the transducer, will be a function of the amplitude and phase of all the mechanical waves reaching the transducer surface at the same time. If the sum of the amplitudes is zero at any time, the result will be a zero voltage out of the transducer, despite all the ultrasonic energy that may be passing through the transducer. Because of this phase-dependent superposition of waves at the transducer face, the transducer is called a *phase-sensitive device.*

The summing process at the transducer face depends upon the amplitude, phase, and frequency of the returning ultrasonic energy. And each of these parameters depends upon the nature of the interfaces within the ultrasound beam. Thus, each tissue has a characteristic speckle that is a function of the organ's micro- and macro-architecture. By measuring some elements on the display with a small millimeter ruler, it can be shown that the displayed tissue texture components are less than three wavelengths long (the time taken to effectively start and stop transducer vibration), and less than a beam's width wide. Image dot production in both the axial and lateral directions depends, obviously, upon the transducer phase sensitivity.

Another method of improving transducer efficiency is by improving energy coupling into and out of the transducer. Reflection at an interface occurs because of a change in acoustic impedance across the interface. If the change is large, the amount of energy reflected is also large, and little energy passes through the interface. This is precisely the situation in trying to get ultrasonic energy out of a transducer and into the body. The impedance change over the interface is so large that most of the energy hitting the interface is reflected back. A method of reducing this reflection problem is to divide the overall impedance change into a series of smaller steps. We can do this by placing a material with an intermediate acoustic impedance value between the transducer and the body (Figure 3-18). Furthermore, by making the material a quarter wave thick, we can gain another benefit from a constructive interference pattern within the quarter-wave layer [5]. The result is a better transfer of energy out of the transducer for the same amount of electrical energy into the transducer [5]. At the same time, the quarter-wave layer improves the coupling of ultrasonic energy back into the transducer. Understanding how these techniques work requires knowledge of some concepts developed in Chapter 1.

Consider a transducer (Figure 3-18) that is a half wave thick, coupled to a material on one side that is a quarter wave thick. It has the same velocity of propagation as the body, but has an acoustic impedance between that of the tissues and the transducer. We previously used the reflectivity equation to indicate not only the amount of reflection but the phase of the reflection. A positive numerator indicated no phase shift; a negative numerator indicated a 180° shift. With these conditions, let us now examine the movement of ultrasound leaving from and returning to the transducer.

Consider first a traveling wave with the positive portion in the transducer and the remainder of the wave extending through the quarter-wave layer into the tissue. At the quarter-wave layer-tissue interface, the change in impedance is positive, meaning that at the interface, the reflection will be in phase with the incident wave. The traveling reflected wave is shown as line B in Figure 3-18, traveling back toward the transducer quarter-wave layer interface. At the transducer quarter-wave layer interface, the change in acoustic impedance is upward, which means the reflectivity equation becomes negative. The reflection is inverted and starts traveling back toward the tissue, but now it is in phase with the traveling wave from the second half of the cycle that was formerly within the transducer. The

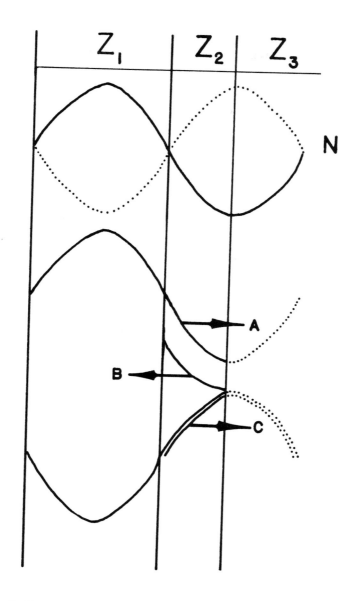

3-18 Quarter-wave layer on transmission. N is the normal vibrational mode, alternating between the solid and dotted line. The transducer is a half-wave thick, Z_1, with a quarter-wave material, Z_2, coupled into the body, Z_3. Decreasing impedance values are Z_1, Z_2, and Z_3. Traveling wave A is proceeding from left to right. At the Z_2-Z_3 boundary, a portion of the incident wave is reflected back toward the transducer B without a phase shift. At the Z_1-Z_2 boundary, a reflection occurs with a 180° phase shift, but in phase with the traveling wave moving toward the tissue C. The waves, both incident and reflected, add together to increase transmitted energy.

traveling waves add together, producing a wave that is the sum of the two individual waves. The result is an increase in the forward traveling energy, as well as a higher amount of energy coupled into the tissues. In this manner, we have increased the effective transmitting efficiency of the transducer.

On the receiving portion of the cycle, the quarter-wave layer will have a similar effect, increasing the amount of energy entering the transducer by constructive interference. We can follow events in the same fashion by looking at Figure 3-19. Line A shows the traveling wave returning to the transducer. The wave has traveled through the quarter-wave layer and just reached the transducer. At the transducer quarter-wave layer interface, a portion of the incident energy is reflected, but because the wave sees a transition from a low to a high impedance, the reflected wave is phase shifted 180°. That traveling wave is shown on line B. At the quarter-wave layer-tissue interface, reflection again occurs, but this time the reflection is positive, and no wave inversion occurs. The primary traveling wave has now advanced one-half of a wave, and the reflection and traveling wave are now moving in the same direction with the same phase. As before, superposition occurs, increasing the amount of energy reaching the transducer. Thus, we have improved the transducer sensitivity without changing any of the material characteristics of the transducer, and have altered only the ability to couple energy into and out of the transducer.

Increasing the sensitivity of the transducer by using a quarter-wave layer also enforces a frequency preference defined by the thickness of the coupling layer. This spatial filtering changes the shape of the transducer frequency response, as shown in Figure 3-20. The relative amplitudes of the frequencies away from the center operating frequency are reduced. And as we will find out later, the presence of lower frequencies will affect the ability of the sonograph to penetrate into tissue. The changed passband that accompanies a quarter-wave layer will change the ability of the transducer to penetrate and to be focused. Some of these changes can be made closer to the standard transducer by adding still another quarter-wave layer, with a thickness (therefore, frequency) different from the first layer. The result is a partial recovery of the lower frequencies that play a central role in tissue penetration. The layer thicknesses to be chosen are not immediately obvious but require some primary calculations through computer simulation [5]. Double quarter-wave technology is still new, but should provide some interesting returns when the technology is better controlled and understood.

So far, we have considered the ultrasound beam not so much in tissue, but in a homogeneous fluid. This setting is a useful way to understand the simple formation of the beam and the manner in which beam geometry changes with distance from the transducer. Things become more complicated when a nonhomogeneous tissue carries the ultrasound. Some of these added complications can be dealt with if the beam is well behaved in its formation and physical characteristics. When the beam formation is not according to expectations, however, the results can cause confusion and artifacts that have little or no connection with what is happening in the tissue.

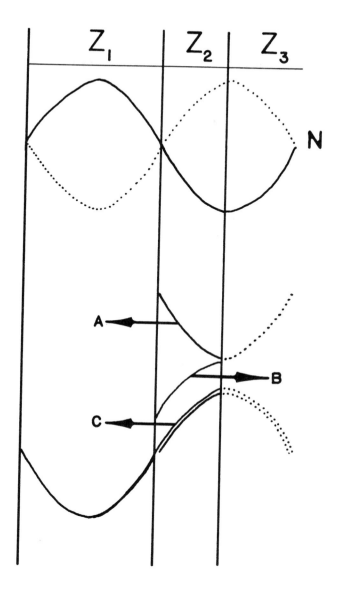

3-19 Quarter-wave layer on reception. The same conditions exist as in Figure 3-17. Now, however, the returning energy *A* passes through the Z_2-Z_3 boundary, moving toward the transducer. At the Z_1-Z_2 boundary, a reflection occurs with 180° phase shift, which moves toward the Z_2-Z_3 boundary *B*. At the Z_2-Z_3 boundary, a reflection without a phase shift occurs, timed to add to the remainder of the incident wave, and causing an increase in received echo, *C*.

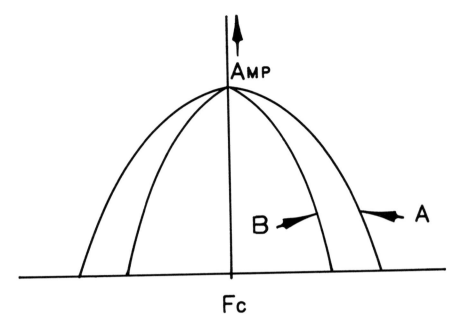

3-20 Transducer frequency response with quarter-wave layer. Adding a quarter-wave layer to a transducer with a frequency response, as shown with curve *A*, will narrow the frequency response, as shown with curve *B*. *Amp* is amplitude; *Fc* is the transducer center operating frequency.

Synthesizing Transducer Wave Fronts

Focusing in the phased array is quite different from mechanical manipulation of the transducer or beam. The array is composed of a set of individually unfocused transducers that are aligned into alternate forms, such as a linear array, a rectangular array, or an annular array. A curved wave front is synthesized by adding together the individual wave fronts from unfocused array elements. As in the single-element transducer, the curved wave front advances to a focal point. The summing mechanisms are guided by the normal superposition of waves and the arrival of the individual wave fronts at the summing region in space. The arrival times are controlled by the excitation sequence of the individual elements relative to one another. Generally, this is called a phasing technique, although *phasing* is not an accurate descriptor here. *Phasing* correctly used refers to changes in wave relationships that are less than or equal to one cycle (the phasing in phased array timing exceeds this one-cycle limit). However, to try to change the name would be a hopeless endeavor; thus, it is best simply to remember the special meaning of phased arrays.

To understand some of the focusing techniques used with these transducers, we refer to a small model consisting of five elements, as shown in Figure 3-21. Each element is unfocused, and about one-quarter of a wavelength wide. A NFB calculation for each element shows that it would be about one-quarter of a wavelength

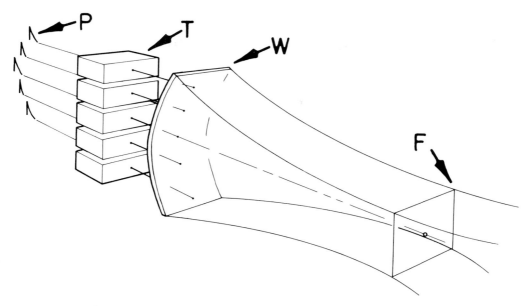

3-21   The beam from a linear phased array. A linear phased array (T) forms a curved wave front (W) to focus (F) the ultrasound with a shape determined by the timing among transmitter pulses (P). The phasing focuses only along the array.

from the transducer face. The beam synthesis, then, uses the Fraunhofer zone from each transducer to form the final beam. This is a good choice because the wave fronts are linear and well behaved, and the synthesis comes about in a more predictable manner.

According to Figure 3-21, elements 1 and 5 can be pulsed together, then 2 and 4, and finally 3. When summed together, the wave fronts form a common wave front that mimics the timing differences among the transmitting pulses. In this case, the two limbs of the wave front are linear because of the linear relationship among the transmitting pulses. The wave advances from the synthesized wave front in a normal manner, converging to a focal point and forming a focal zone at the same time. By changing the timing between the limbs, the focal point can be changed. (This can be controlled from the front panel on many sonographs.) When the focal point position is changed automatically in a pattern, the technique is called *dynamic focusing.*

Focusing and beam steering can also be carried out by timing events on the receive side of the pulse-listen cycle. In this instance, we are interested in making the unfocused linear array act as if it were curved and focused at a point. The "curving" process is achieved by timing the summing of the signals from each element as if the elements were physically curved in an array. Only signals from the synthesized focal point will have the correct timing at the transducers to sum together maximally. Because we are using a timing process again, the focal point can be moved by changing the timing. In addition, by changing the delay among the elements, the beam can be steered. Thus, a phased array can be focused on transmit or receive or both by changing the summing of waves on a time base.

If the individual elements of a linear phased array are increased in size, the result is another transducer arrangement called a linear array, with a different set of properties. In the linear array, the number of elements included in the focusing processes is smaller, but each element is physically larger. The object of this arrangement is to form a linear scan along the array, while using no moving parts in the scan. The technique incorporates functions from both the single-element transducer and the phased array that merit closer examination here.

Generally, the linear array does not form a sector scan along the array axis, although a combined linear and sector scan derived from a linear array to form a compound scan of the tissue has been demonstrated recently [6]. The linear scan provided a single pass over the tissue that could demonstrate tissue-ultrasound interactions such as enhancement and shadowing. The compound scan increased the field of view of the system and improved the delineation of boundaries over the linear scan. The combination of both techniques in the same instrument is a result of combining phased-array and linear-array techniques.

The linear scan requires forming a set of beams from array elements, then switching a single pulse-listen cycle along the array elements, one at a time. Each beam is formed separately and used in a linear sequence to form the linear scan. To add focusing to the beams, the timing techniques used in phased arrays are applied to the linear-array beam. Coincidentally, enough scan lines must be formed to provide good spatial image resolution. This requires techniques that form more scan lines than the number of elements in the linear array. Each of these techniques is discussed in turn below.

Take, first, a set of linear elements, each unfocused, but each larger than the phased array (a schematic array is shown in Figure 3-22.) We can form the first line of sight from the linear array by exciting elements 1 and 5 together, then 2 and 4, then 3. As in the phased array, the individual wave fronts add together to form a wave front that is focused toward some point in space in front of the transducers. Once a single pulse-listen cycle occurs, the control grouping of transducers is switched down the array one transducer. Now transducers 2 and 6 fire together, then 3 and 5, then 4 to form another scan line. The first scan line centers on element 3, the second on element 4. This form of control can be switched down the array to form a linear scan, with each beam centered on an array element. If the array has 64 elements, the top two and bottom two are usually not used to center a scan line, leaving 60 formed scan lines. We will need 60 more to complete the required scan-line density.

Regrouping the transducer elements forms a second set of scan lines, but which are displaced from those formed earlier. In the first sequence, we grouped the elements into odd-numbered sets that centered the scan line on each of the 60 interior elements. Using an even number of elements centers the scan-line axis between array elements. For example, if elements 1 and 4 are fired together, then 2 and 3, the scan line will be centered between elements 2 and 3 (Figure 3-22). As before, this control grouping can be transferred down the array, forming another set of scan lines. But these scan lines are centered between transducer elements, and therefore are displaced from the first scanning set using odd-numbered groups.

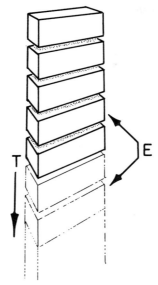

3-22   Linear array organization. A linear array consists of a set of individual elements *E* collected into a line. Linear arrays range from 20 to 120 elements, with typical values around 60 elements. *T* is the transducer.

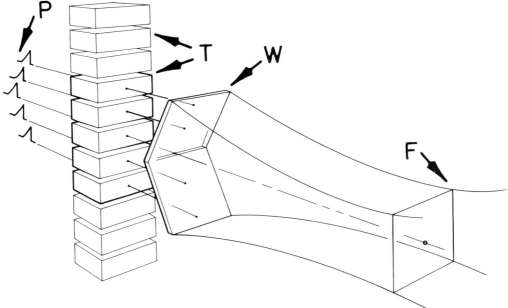

3-23   Focusing in a linear array. A linear array can use many of the same techniques as a phased array to focus the beam. Here five elements combine to form an axicon focus that can be switched down the array to linearly sweep a focused beam. Like the linear phased array, focusing is possible only along the array length. Focusing transversely to the array length requires other special efforts. P, transmitter pulses; T, transducer elements; W, focused wavefront; F, focal point.

If again the top two and bottom two elements are not used for scan-line centers, another 60 scan lines can be formed, but, as before, they are displaced from the previous grouping. Thus, by alternating odd- and even-numbered groups of transducer elements, the linear array can produce nearly twice as many scan lines as transducer array elements.

From another viewpoint, we can see that linear-array focusing is not symmetrical around the formed beam axis (Figure 3-23). Transverse to the array, the beam is not focused, with the result that the array has good lateral resolution in one axis but poor lateral resolution in the other. One obvious solution to this decrease in performance is to place a cylindrical lens on the array to focus the beam transversely to the array axis, and, at the same time, use electronic focusing along the array axis. An alternate solution is to use more than one linear array, creating a large rectangle of elements. By using multiple elements in two directions, the array can be focused along and transversely to the array's long axis. To decrease some of the electronic control, the transducer array could also be bent along the short rectangle axis, physically focusing the array beams in one direction and electronically focusing in the other. Often several of these techniques are combined to form a beam as symmetrical as possible.

Linear-phased arrays have a similar problem. Like the larger linear array, mechanical designs circumvent this limitation either by applying external focusing to the transducer array transversely to the electronic focusing or by using a rectangular array. Still another transducer arrangement can eliminate this problem simply by forming the transducer elements into concentric rings [7]. The device is called an *annular array*. By controlling excitation timing like the linear array, but now among ring elements, we can form a focal point, ranged electronically as before. The symmetry of the focusing, however, is greatly improved in the annular array.

Despite these rather exotic modes of beam formation, these transducer arrays are all guided by the same events that occur in any single-element transducer: The NFB is still a function of frequency and effective transducer diameter as either a single element or in groups; the transducing elements, either singly or in groups, are still passive receiving devices, and therefore, are phase sensitive; the formation of the beam still requires a curved wave front that can advance to a focal point; and the degree and depth of focusing will still depend on the transducer frequency, aperture size, and focal point range. Knowing these realities permits the user to perform simple and direct evaluations of new transducer technologies.

Evaluating Transducer Performance

With some of these facts in hand, we can ask: How might we use them to evaluate transducers? The answer is straightforward.

One of the more informative sources of information for evaluating a transducer

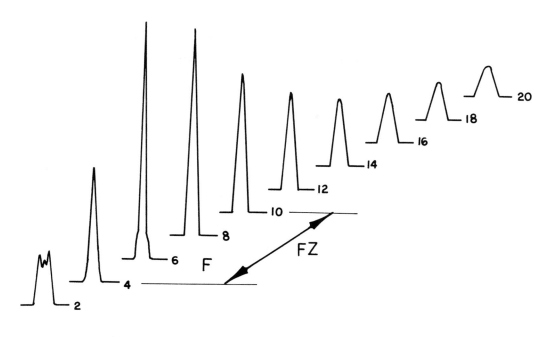

3-24 Multitarget beam profile for focused transducer. By placing identical wire targets at fixed distances from a transducer, a beam profile will show relative signal strength from different portions of the ultrasound field. Indicated are: focal point position F; focal zone range FZ; rate of gain into focus; rate of intensity loss out of focus; and effective beam width at various ranges.

is the beam profile. This graph (profile) in Figure 3-24 shows the transducer beam mapped as a function of echo amplitude from a standard reflector at regularly spaced distances. Several manufacturers supply such beam profiles as a standard part of machine information. The profile is often made by presenting a set of equally spaced wire targets to a transducer that is coupled to a calibrated transmitter and receiver. The result is a profile such as that shown in Figure 3.24. The field can also be mapped by moving a small spherical target, such as a ball bearing, in the field and mapping the transducer response as a function of the ball-bearing position. An alternate profile display is a set of isointensity lines that show the axial and lateral dimensions of constant intensity (Figure 3-25). As in the first profile form, many of the normal and abnormal beam characteristics are visible.

A typical beam profile supplies information on such things as 1) the focal point location, 2) the focal zone range, 3) the rate of intensity increase into the focal point, 4) the rate of intensity decrease out of the focal point, 5) the centering of the beam along the geometric axis of the transducer, and 6) the effective change in beam width as a function of range. These data are integrated into the discussions on image formation and resolution later in this book.

The output from the transducer is ultrasound, but how much ultrasound? The answer comes from a measurement of the transducer output. The efficiency of the transduction process is central to this measurement, which means the transmitter

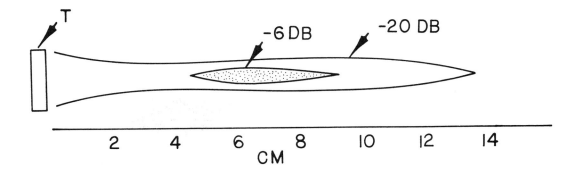

3-25 Contour beam profile. This method of showing beam width and character displays isointensity curves for the beam as function of distance. *T* is the transducer; *CM* is the range along the transducer axis in centimeters.

that is normally used to excite the transducer must be used during this measurement. In addition, the transducer beam geometry will influence any measured intensities. In analyzing the transducer power measurements, the total energy output and the beam geometry must be included.

The primary power measurement is the total power output from the transducer. This measurement is usually made using either a calibrated hydrophone for a calibrated force balance. The hydrophone measures the pressure applied by the ultrasonic energy at a small point in the field, and the force balance measures the collected force from the whole field. Because of the problems in making very small hydrophones, the force balance technique seems currently the best for calibrated, reliable measurements. Because the force balance has a slow response, however, the power measurement is a temporal average over many pulse-listen cycles. The unit for this measurement is usually the watt or if this is too large, the milliwatt.

Having measured the total power of a transducer and with some knowledge of the beam geometry (Figure 3-26), we can average the power over the effective cross section of the beam to form the *spatial average time average* (SATA) expression of beam intensity. These power and intensity relationships are discussed in detail in Chapter 10.

We learned earlier in this chapter that transducers are formed from ferroelectrics that have small domains with a common net electrical dipole. A similar situation occurs for ferromagnetics, but the domain has a small magnetic field. The magnetic power of a ferromagnetic can be reduced by randomizing the domains so that they do not point in a common direction. We can do this by heating the magnet or by striking the magnet repeatedly with a hammer to physically jar the domains into disorganization. The domains of ultrasound transducers can also be randomized. Aging occurs in ultrasound transducers not because of heating (excluding an episode in an autoclave), but because of repeated excitation, which can be viewed as an electrical hammer.

As the domains become random, their ability to physically pack together decreases, and the transducer can become slightly thicker, lowering the center operating

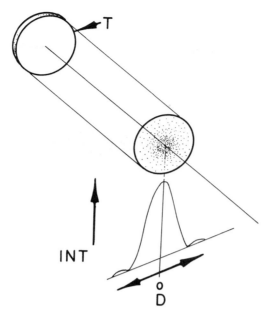

3-26 Lateral beam intensity pattern. Because the transducer acts like a diffracting aperture, the beam intensity is greatest in the center of the beam, decreasing to the outside. *T* is the transducer; *INT* is the beam intensity; *D* is the lateral distance away from the beam axis.

frequency at the same time. Because the domains are increasingly random, the piezoelectric properties also fade, resulting in reduced penetration. The user observes and increased dot size (lower frequency) and a decreased penetration (decreased transduction). It appears that transducers do not violate the second law of thermodynamics, but increase in randomness along with the rest of the universe.

Transducers are unique devices for the most part. Thus, transducer aging is individual, some transducers seeming to go on forever, others vanishing after only a short period of use. Transducers now being manufactured seem to be longer lived because they are better made and better matched to the sonographs. A few of the "old timers" are still in operation and are treated often as laboratory standards of reference. While improvements in transducer technology are apparent when we compare the old to the new, the older, still-working transducers remain standbys to many.

Some of the older transducers show a different characteristic when connected to new sonographs. The older sonographs were low-gain devices, which meant they were not very sensitive to the radio frequency environment of the hospital. The transducers were often unshielded as a result. Modern sonographs, however, are high-gain machines and are sensitive to the rf environment of the modern hospital. To prevent the outside rf from entering the sonograph receiver, the transducer and signal-carrying cable must be electrically shielded. Often this shielding is a conductive paint on the inside of the transducer housing and coaxial cables to move the signal about the machine. A transducer should always be examined for proper rf shielding to prevent the superposition of outside noise on the image.

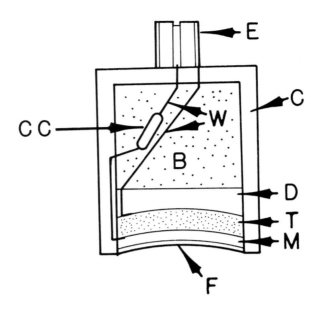

3-27   Putting all the components of the transducer together for the finished product. *T* is the transducer, *D* is the damping material, *M* is a quarter-wave matching layer, *F* is the transducer housing face, *B* is the backing material to support the transducer in the housing, *C* is the housing for the whole assembly, *W* is the transducer wires, *CC* is an electrical compensating component, and *E* is the electrical connector to the outside.

Conclusion

We can now look at the components of a transducer in cross section (Figure 3-27). Sandwiched between the backing material and the quarter-wave layer is the transducer itself. It is covered with conducting materials to allow an exciting electrical field to reach the transducer and to pick up, as well, the small electrical voltages produced by the returning echoes. The large electrical excitation and the small electrical voltages are conducted to and from the transducer by electrical wires, which span the distance between the outside connector and the transducer faces. Further surrounding the transducer is the rf shielding, which is also connected to the machine's grounding system. The damping material on the back of the transducer decreases the vibrational envelope during transmission and reception. The quarter-wave layer on the face of the transducer improves the transfer of energy into and out of the transducer. A plastic cap or other facings are used to shield the patient from the voltages that excite the transducer. Within the housing are additional electrical components that shape the transmitting pulse to match the characteristics of the transducer. And the transducer is usually focused, internally and sometimes externally, to improve lateral resolution. Thus, from front to back, the transducer has no unused components; all contribute to the transducer function of making and receiving ultrasound.

The central role of the transducer has not changed significantly since the beginning of ultrasound. We still depend heavily on its reliable production and detection of ultrasound. A bad transducer will guarantee a bad image, and no amount of manipulation of the machine electronics will improve the situation. Technologically, transducers have also changed little in the last five years. In the last year, however, transducers have gained recognition as a key to success in imaging. As a result, a great deal of money and effort is being devoted to improving this critical link in the imaging technique.

As noted earlier, a recent improvement in transducer function has been the addition of one or more quarter-wave layers. On the materials side, new and different materials offer stable and inexpensive high-frequency transducers above 7.5 MHz. Material improvements in the lower frequencies also forecast better production techniques, perhaps lowering the transducer cost while increasing the quality. Great strides have already been made in image display. Perhaps now the other end of the signal stream will experience a similar improvement.

But whatever shape these improvements take, we will be in a much better position to appreciate their applications and clinical significance, given our current knowledge and understanding of transducers.

References

1. Kittel, C. 1976. Introduction of solid state physics. 3rd ed. New York: John Wiley & Sons.
2. Wells, P.N.T. 1969. Physical principles of ultrasonic diagnosis. London and New York: Academic Press.
3. Smith, S.W., et al. May 1979. Angular response of piezoelectric elements in phased array ultrasound scanners. IEEE Trans, Sonics and Ultrasonics 26:185–190.
4. Halliday, D., and R. Resnik. 1960. Physics for students of science and engineering. 2nd ed. New York: John Wiley & Sons.
5. Effects on diagnostic imaging: Multiple matching layer theory and application. Aero Tech 1(5).
6. Carpenter, D.A., M.J. Dadd, and G. Kossoff. 1980. A multimode real time scanner. Ultrasound Med Biol 6:279–284.
7. Melton, H.E., Jr., and F.L. Thurston. 1978. Annular array design and logarithmic processing for ultrasonic imaging. Ultrasound Med Biol 4:1–12.

Chapter 4

Charges and Images: The Analog Scan Converter

We learned in Chapter 2 that the scan converter provides a memory for the system, producing a complete image from the temporal integration of individual pulse-listen cycles. The information is acquired at the transducer scanning rate, and is stored and read out at a standard television rate. Storing the signals provides an opportunity not only to see the completed image but to manipulate the data into a preferred display form. Such image manipulation occurs after image storage and is therefore, termed postprocessing. During the early applications of gray-scale ultrasound, the best device for storing and displaying acquired signals was the analog scan converter.

However, a glance through a current buyer's guide for diagnostic ultrasound shows almost no analog sonographs left on the market. Why study a system no longer in use? For several reasons. First, a number of ultrasound departments still have analog systems. For some, it is a purposeful decision, while others simply have not yet purchased new equipment. Second, many departments have used equipment with analog scan converters (ASCs), purchased as second-hand machines because of a limited budget. Third, the organization and signal handling of the analog scan converter gives insight to cathode ray tube (CRT) displays in general. And fourth, the analog scan converter sets the stage for the operating requirements of the digital scan converter.

Understanding the analog scan converter requires information, first, on the organization and function of a standard cathode ray tube, the starting point for this chapter's discussion.

Organization of the Cathode Ray Tube

Despite the numerous types of CRTs that surround us in the form of oscilloscopes, displays, and televisions—each with different exteriors and controls—the fundamental organization of the CRT has undergone only minor changes since the original experiments with cathode rays [1]. The operating technology used within

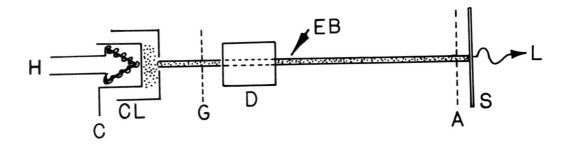

4-1 Basic elements of a cathode ray tube. Heater *H* heats the cathode *C* to produce a space charge of electrons. A beam columnator *CL* forms the electrons into a small beam *EB*. Control grid *G* controls the amount of current in the beam. *D* represents the deflection plates that move the electron beam in space. *A* represents the anode, charged to a high positive voltage to attract the electrons. *S* is the phosphor-coated screen that converts the electron kinetic energy into light *L*.

the CRT has changed, however, and these alterations are responsible for the wide variety of displays now available. Displays can have varying colors on the tube face; moreover, the face can be flat or curved, square or round, hold an impression of an image for a long or short time, and even be split into sections, each portion with a different persistence time. Yet, all such CRTs share a common set of events.

The first functional event within a CRT is the freeing of electrons. Electrons do not stay liberated very long in the presence of electron-accepting molecules; thus, the electrons must be set free in a molecule-free space or vaccuum. The cathode ray tube contains a vaccuum for the free passage of electrons.

Within the CRT is an electric heater called a filament (Figure 4-1). Surrounding this heater is a metal oxide electrode. When the filament heats this metal, electrons are freed from the metal and form into a cloud around the metal. These electrons are liberated in every sense of the word and can be moved about by applying an outside force. Because they are charged, they respond naturally to an applied electric field. Once freed from their metallic world, the electrons need to be moved in preferred directions.

The free electrons carry a negative charge, and if a positive charge is set some distance from the electrons, the electrons will be drawn toward it. The vaccuum tube can now change shape, increasing length to become long and narrow, with a metallic screen at the end opposite the filament (Figure 4-1). A positive charge on the screen will pull the free electrons toward the screen. To make the screen positive relative to the filament, we connect a battery, with the metal oxide coating attached to the negative terminal and the screen attached to the positive terminal (Figure 4-2). The positively charged screen is called an *anode* and the negatively charged metal oxide electrode, a *cathode*. In this configuration, the battery can supply new electrons for those lost from the metal cathode. The electrons streaming off the cathode toward the screen form a "ray" of electrons, hence the traditional name, *cathode ray tube*.

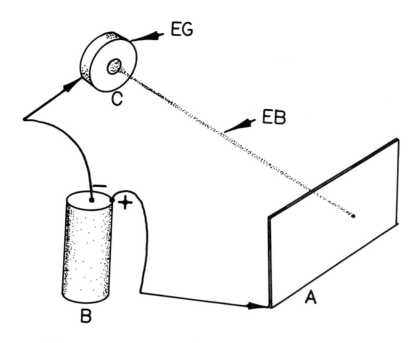

4-2   Current loop for cathode ray tube. The cathode ray tube for a close current path, extending from the electron gun *EG* and cathode *C* to the anode *A*. Charging the anode positive and cathode negative with a battery *B* permits current to flow through the circuit. *EB* is the electron beam.

In general, the farther away the screen is from the cathode, the smaller is the force applied to the electrons and the greater is the voltage required to move the electrons down the tube at a constant rate. Thus, to use a lower voltage battery, the screen would have to be moved closer to the electrons coming off the cathode. This would allow the electrons to move using lower voltages on the tube. The screen that accelerates the electrons is called an *accelerating anode,* and several of these can be stationed along the electron path to provide a uniform motion to the electrons.

Until now, the moving electrons have been fairly undisciplined, moving in a great streaming cloud toward the anode. To use the CRT for a display, the beam needs a smaller diameter. A large portion of the internal CRT technology is thus dedicated to focusing the electrons into a tight beam. One method of forcing the electrons tightly together is to apply a uniform circular force, for example, by sending the beam through a metal opening that is charged negatively. In this manner, the outlying electrons are forced toward the center of the beam. An alternative method is to apply a uniform magnetic field from the outside. Orienting the field properly forms a kind of magnetic lens that bends the outlying electrons toward the center of the beam. A third method is also possible in which the cloud of electrons simply passes through a metal cap with a hole that limits the number of electrons in the cloud that can reach the other side. This is like using a pin hole in a piece of paper to limit the amount of light beyond the paper. The result with light is a diffraction pattern. Electrons, too, behave as if they were waves, producing a diffraction pattern in the emerging electrons [2]. Thus, part of the internal technology of the CRT will be to correct for this diffraction produced by the electrons passing through the aperture. In most CRTs, all three of these methods are applied to form a tight, well-focused beam of electrons.

With a focused beam of electrons, the next task is to move that beam around in space with one end of the beam "tethered" to the cathode. Once more, we use the charge properties of the beam to move it about by applying outside electrical forces to the beam. The electrical forces reach the electron beam through plates positioned parallel to the path of the electron beam (Figure 4-1). Negative charges repel the beam; positive charges attract the beam. By positioning four plates properly in the CRT, the beam can be moved around according to outside electrical instructions (signals). Because the electrons that compose the beam are moving, they will also respond to an outside magnetic field. The magnetic field can be produced by a set of coils called a deflection yoke, positioned around the CRT to apply directional forces to the electron beam. The final product is a nearly inertia-free writing stylus made of a focused electron beam.

The movement of the beam can assume nearly any form or direction within the confines of the CRT display face. A common method of directing motion is to establish a pattern of movement along a straight line called a trace (Figure 4-3). The electron beam moves steadily along the trace, then rapidly snaps back to the starting position. During the repositioning, the electron beam is nearly turned off. The result is a steady velocity along the trace that can be used to display time-dependent information. In addition, the trace can be positioned anywhere and at any angle within the geometry of the CRT face.

Given a writing stylus, we next need something on which to write. The "paper" for this writing is a thin layer of phosphor coated on the face of the CRT opposite the cathode. The striking electrons cause the phosphor to give off light, converting the kinetic energy of the accelerated electrons into electromagnetic energy (light). If the light falls into our visible spectrum, we can see it outside the tube. Thus, light on the face of the CRT shows the position of the electron beam within the CRT and any motion of the beam over time. This organization forms an *oscilloscope* that lets us visualize an electrical signal by following the motion of an electron beam in response to a signal (Figure 4-4).

The phosphor on the face of the CRT comes in a variety of mixes to obtain a desired color of light, a desired amount of light emitted by the phosphor in response to the electrons, and a desired length of time that the phosphor will continue to emit light after the beam has passed. These three parameters are color, luminosity, and persistence, respectively.

A number of technical considerations about the overall performance of the CRT should be mentioned here. Many of its performance capabilities depend as much on the electronic support for the device as on the physical technology within the glass envelope. Along with an ability to move the electron beam, the time taken to effectively turn the electron beam on and off should be considered. The amount

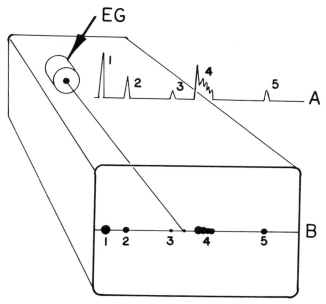

4-3 Ways of modulating the electron beam. Signals can appear on the CRT screen as either an X-Y display *A* or as an intensity display *B*. *A* is commonly called an A-mode display. *B* is commonly called a B-mode display. *EG* is the electron gun.

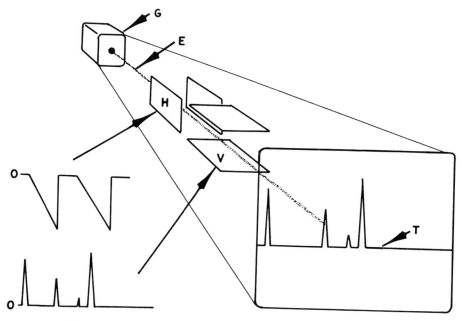

4-4 Control signals to form an A-mode trace. Forming an A-mode trace requires moving the electron beam *E*, with signals applied to the beam-moving plates *H* and *V*. The result is the A-mode trace *T*. *G* is the electron gun.

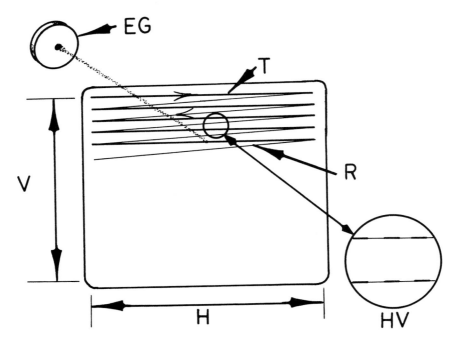

4-5 Cathode ray tube TV raster scan. To create an image on a cathode ray tube, the electron beam is moved over the CRT face with a raster scan. The scan begins at the upper left with a trace *T*, from left to right, then a retrace *R* to reposition the beam to the left, one line down. Within the trace, the beam intensity is changed *(HV)* to create the final TV image. *EG* is the electron gun; *V* is the vertical dimension; *H* is the horizontal dimension.

of current in the electron beam needed to obtain a certain luminance, as well as the persistence time, are also valuable considerations. And, of course, the electron beam spot size on the face of the CRT will affect the display of events.

Each of the above parameters relates to familiar aspects of physical optics and electrostatics. Yet, the ability to turn on and off the electron beam is described by the seemingly unrelated terms "display line density." To understand the connection, consider an electron beam moving across the screen in a regular fashion, forming what is called a *raster scan* (Figure 4-5). This scan pattern begins in the upper left corner of the screen, moves across steadily, then snaps back to the left, but has been moved down slightly. The result is a pattern of beam movement over the tube face that forms a set of horizontal lines. The display line density is related to how fast the electron beam can be turned on and off to produce a set of vertical lines in the raster scan, and is seen as individual lines. For example, a 400-line display refers to the ability to put 400 changes in beam intensity across the face of the display in a manner that enables them to be seen as individual vertical lines. A 1,300-line display can put 1,300 of these intensity changes on the display, all of them seen as individual vertical lines.

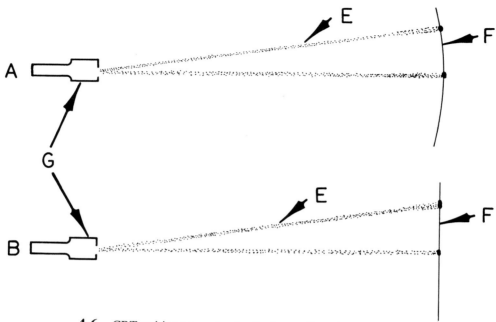

4-6 CRT writing geometry for the beam. In order to maintain image quality over the whole face of the display, many CRTs have a curved face *F*, as shown in Part A. The lateral smearing of a flat-faced CRT (uncorrected) is shown in Part B. *G* is the electron gun; *E* is the electron beam.

The movement of the beam within the CRT is anchored at the cathode, which means that it circumscribes an arc rather than a straight line (Figure 4-6). As the angle between the face of the CRT and the beam becomes something less than 90°, the beam projection onto the face widens much like a beam of light broadens when a flashlight is projected at an angle onto a flat surface. In order to keep the spot projection as small as possible, CRTs often have spherical faces rather than flat faces. But photographing a curved-face CRT causes a distorted image on film, so a flat-faced CRT is preferred. Clearly, another technique is required to keep the dot size as small as possible on flat-faced tubes that are to be photographed. One solution is to place another magnetic field around the CRT, close to the face of the tube that bends the electron beam. The field is placed around the CRT just as the beam is about to strike the phosphor, thus forcing the beam to hit at 90°. These additions are called *collimators* and make the source of the electron beam appear to be infinitely far from the CRT face. The result is a flat-faced tube with a dot size that does not significantly change over the face from the center to the edges.

These techniques are hardly ever perfect. Therefore, the amount of distortion still present is expressed as a percentage between the center and edges of the display. Two percentages are used. The first describes the ability to form the electron beam display spot, and the second describes the ability to move the electron beam in a linear fashion. These, then, are the parameters essential to the function of any CRT. They apply also to the function of the analog scan converter, as well as to the television monitors used with sonographs.

Analog Scan Converter Organization

An examination of the basic structure of an analog scan converter shows that the formation of an electron beam follows the same procedure as in a standard CRT. The electrons are freed from the cathode by heat, they are accelerated to the "front" of the tube by a high positive voltage, and form the electron beam by a combination of electrostatic and magnetic forces. Beam movement, as in the CRT, originates from electrostatic forces projecting from beam-forming plates or from magnetic forces exerted by a beam-moving yoke. The same scientific knowledge and ability that formed and moved the electron beam was applied to the development of the analog scan converter.

The only real difference between the standard CRT and the analog scan converter is the target at the far end of the tube. Instead of a phosphor layer, the analog scan converter uses a special target that is designed to store the signal information presented to the tube as a set of electrical charges. Once stored, the electrical charges are "read" and the information brought to the outside on a standard signal format. We will be concerned with the storage, that is, the writing and reading phases of the scan converter cycle. The storage plane for the tube is described first.

The target is an insulating, dielectric material that can capture and hold local charges. A dielectric material contains electrons that are held fast within its molecules, unable—except by a high external voltage—to be moved out of the firm, molecular grasp. The target is divided into a set of small islands of dielectric material, with conducting metal in between the islands [3]. A typical composite target is rectangular, with about 10,000 small islands on each side of the rectangle, producing about 10^8 islands for the whole target [4]. With these dimensions, even the most narrowly focused beam will spread over several of islands. All of the metal surrounding the islands is connected together to form the signal output electrode (Figure 4-7). The total formation is much like a fine-meshed metal screen, with the dielectric material occupying the holes. These dielectric materials are often lithium based, and the scan converter tube is called a *lithicon tube* as a result.

The task is to put charges on and off these islands. To help control the electrons in the space close to the dielectric target, an element called a collecting mesh sits close to the target. This screen is designed to catch the electrons that will be knocked off the target in order to prevent them from collecting as a space charge in front of the target and interfering with the electrons traveling from the cathode (Figure 4-8).

With the physical organization of the scan converter thus outlined, we can examine the events of the writing and reading cycle.

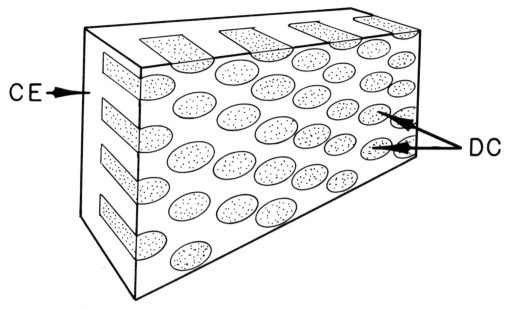

4-7 Elements of an analog scan converter memory. The memory plane of an analog scan converter consists of a large common conducting element *CE*, with small islands of dielectric materials *DC*, distributed over the plane. The dielectric elements do not touch or otherwise connect to one another.

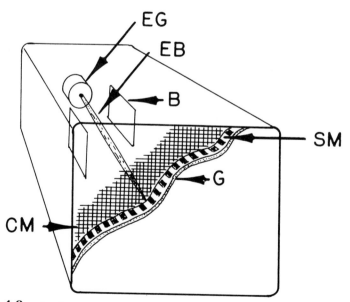

4-8 Analog scan converter tube. The analog scan converter tube is a CRT with a modified target. Over the face of the tube is the scan converter memory *SM*, with a collecting mesh *CM*, to remove any space charge from in front of the memory plane. *EG* is the electron gun; *EB* is the electron beam; *B* represents the beam-moving plates.

Scan Converter Function

If we look at the electrons coming to the lithicon target, two aspects of the beam must be considered. The first aspect is the number of electrons that are arriving at a given time, which is called the electron beam current. The second aspect is the kinetic energy of the electrons as they arrive at the target. A situation can exist whereby the current in the beam is very high, but the kinetic energy of the electrons is very low. Conversely, the current can be low, but the kinetic energy high. The kinetic energy controls the type of interaction that occurs between the dielectric material and the electrons, whereas the beam current determines how much of that interaction occurs. In other words, the electron beam kinetic energy dictates the quality of the interaction, and the beam current the quantity of the interaction.

A useful analogy to events between the dielectric and the electron beam is a circular plate with marbles stuck to the surface with a soft, sticky glue. If we lightly "shoot" free marbles into the collection of already stuck marbles, the moving marbles will interact with the stationary marbles by bouncing around and will finally get stuck along with those already present. On the other hand, we can shoot in free marbles with a great deal of energy. If these fast-moving marbles strike an already-stuck marble, the stationary marble may be freed from the surface. At the right energy between these two extremes, just as many marbles can be knocked off the surface as added by shooting. Two groups of free marbles are present. Those shot in are *primary* marbles, and those knocked out are *secondary* marbles. Let us now look at the electron-material interaction.

The electrons in the dielectric are held in place by a sticky molecular glue. Electrons from the outside gather kinetic energy in proportion to the accelerating voltage inside the tube. If the arriving electron kinetic energy is low, then they will be stuck onto the surface of the dielectric, caught like the previous low-energy marbles. The ratio of the number of electrons arriving at the surface to the number of electrons leaving the surface is a large positive number, indicating that the primary electrons outnumber the secondary. The result is an accumulation of electrons and the formation of a negative charge on the dielectric. This process is called *negative writing* (Figure 4-9).

Because negative writing is energy dependent, we can hold the energy of the electron beam in a very narrow range, and by modulating the beam current, change the amount of charge accumulated in proportion to the beam current. Thus, as the current increases, more and more charge is stored on the dielectric. As earlier, the energy determines the character of the interaction, and the current determines the amount of interaction.

By further increasing the energy, some of the arriving electrons are given enough energy to knock out electrons held by the material molecules. An energy-balance point can be reached at which the number of electrons arriving at the surface equals the number leaving the surface; at this point, also, the storage plane acquires no net charge. This is called the *zero writing point*.

By raising the electron energy still further, the secondary electron population is increased to beyond the number of arriving electrons (Figure 4-10). The result is

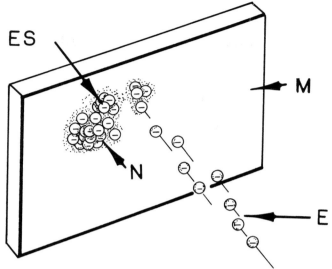

4-9   Negative writing for an analog scan converter. Negative writing onto the memory plane *M* results in the incident electrons *E* sticking to the memory plane to form negative charge distributions, *N* that store the echo signal *ES* as a charge.

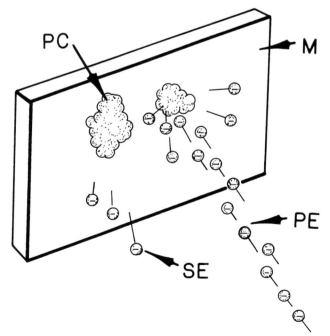

4-10   Positive writing for an analog scan converter. In positive writing on the memory plane *M,* the incident primary electrons *PE* knock off secondary electrons *SE,* leaving a positive charge, *PC* on the memory plane.

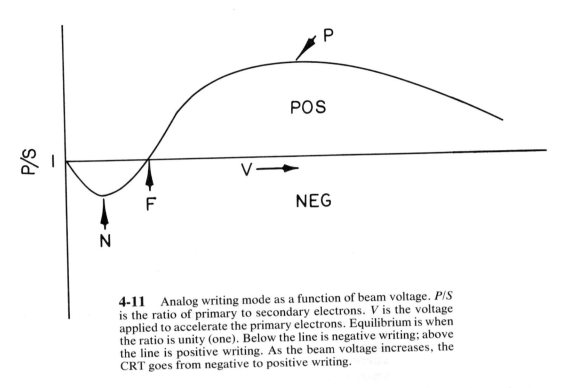

4-11 Analog writing mode as a function of beam voltage. *P/S* is the ratio of primary to secondary electrons. *V* is the voltage applied to accelerate the primary electrons. Equilibrium is when the ratio is unity (one). Below the line is negative writing; above the line is positive writing. As the beam voltage increases, the CRT goes from negative to positive writing.

a net positive charge on the dielectric plane when dielectric electrons are lost as secondary electrons. The quantity of charge on the dielectric follows the beam current as before, with the resulting amount of charge proportional to the beam current. This ratio between the secondary electrons and the incident electrons increases up to a point as the energy is increased, and then begins to decrease again. Because of the positive charge left on the lithicon plane, this process is called *positive writing*. Additional increases in beam energy will bring about another zero point between incident and secondary electrons, but none of the diagnostic ultrasound converters operates in that energy range. These different writing points are shown in Figure 4-11.

The scan converter cycle involves placing a charge on the storage plane with a distribution and density proportional to the signals that came into the scan converter; reading the stored charge distribution; and then erasing the memory in preparation for the next image. Writing the image involves use of a negative writing mode, and erasing uses a combination of a positive writing mode with a subsequent negative writing mode to set the dielectric charge back to zero. Between writing and erasure is reading.

In displaying a gray-scale image, the signal amplitudes from the video stages in the sonograph are used to modulate the intensity of the electron beam. Thus, strong signals will put a denser electron charge on the lithicon tube than will weaker signals. Movement of the electron beam over the storage plane is guided by the ultrasound beam-position information, which sets the starting point for the formation of the image trace and the angle of motion over the memory plane. From that starting point, the beam moves along the trace at a rate related to the assumed speed of ultrasound in tissue. The result is a charge distribution over the lithicon plane that mimics the body in cross section, with the larger echo signals portrayed as a greater charge. If electrons were visible, we could look in on the plane and see a charge distribution that exactly matched the time and amplitude information received by the ultrasound machine during the scan. But because we cannot see electrons, the information must be "read" off the storage area by the machine. The same beam used to make the charge distribution is used to read the charge distribution.

In the reading mode, the electron beam moves over the charge distribution in a raster scan. The beam moves from left to right, starting at the left top of the storage plane and moving down a line at the start of each beam scan. This motion is exactly the same motion used to form the image on a television monitor. The number of scan lines made in reading the whole memory plane is also equal to the number of scan lines used to make a TV image. And the number of whole-plane scans made each second equals the number of images formed in a TV every second. In other words, the electron beam moves over the image plane in a fashion that imitates a standard TV-format raster scan.

As the electron beam moves over the image plane and charge distribution, the electron beam interacts with the stored charge. The writing was negative, leaving a negative-charge distribution; therefore, the stored charge tends to repel the oncoming electron beam. The electron beam energy is set low in order to let the charge on the plane repel the electron beam. If the stored charge is dense, the electrons in the beam can be completely deflected back to the collecting mesh. When this happens, no current can reach the output electrode. On the other hand, if no charge is present, the electron beam can easily reach the metal surrounding the dielectric islands, and the highest output current appears at the output electrode. With charges between these two extremes, the amount of current reaching the output electrode and the collecting screen changes value in proportion to the amount of stored charge. Thus, by following the output electrode current—in other words, by considering the beam current as a function of the stored charge—the charge distribution is interrogated (or read) by the electron beam and transferred to the outside. The transfer to the outside world is at a standard television rate.

Because both the stored charge and the electron beam are negative, the interaction between the electron beam and charge is minimized to prevent destruction of the image during readout. This process, termed *nondestructive reading* [3], permits repeated scans over the charge for reading (60 frames per second) without having the electron beam alter the stored charge. One method of enhancing this process is to feed back a portion of the output signal onto the cathode, taking care to decrease the possibility of further interaction. A delicate balance is sought to keep the reading process from altering the image being read.

The signals used to position and sweep the beam in the scan converter tube are also used to sweep and position the electron beam in a more conventional CRT, which is the TV monitor (Figure 4-12). The signals taken from the scan converter via the output electrode are used to modify the electron beam current on the TV

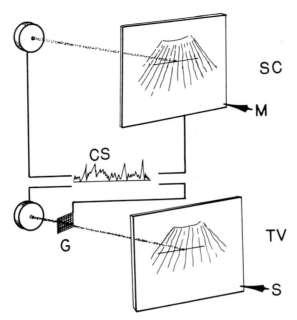

4-12 Transferring an analog scan converter image to a display. The stored image on the memory plane *M* in the scan converter *SC* affects the reading electron beam, forming the signal *CS,* which controls the electron beam through a grid *G* in the TV. Thus, the pattern of stored charge is transferred to the TV screen *S* through a common signal.

monitor; thus the charge distribution is read out, having been converted to a set of video signals that any TV monitor can accept. Now the scan conversion is complete, with the scanning rate of the image formation converted into a set of video signals that can be used by any external monitor, camera, or other video device.

But setting charges onto a lithicon plane takes time. The storage is not instantaneous, but requires several pulse-listen cycles in order for the stored charge to acquire a value that is in equilibrium with the writing electron beam. This process is called *equilibrium writing* [3] and is essential to the representation of equal signals with equal charges, and thus, equal gray scale. It will take about 100 ms to achieve equilibrium in many systems, which represents about 10 pulse-listen cycles in the sonograph. In addition, the erasure process requires first knocking all the stored electrons off the storage plane, then a writing process that brings the net charge on the dielectric back to zero. The timing for this process is typically one TV frame for the first erasure, one TV frame for zeroing, and a complete erasure with the converter ready for the next image input in as long as four TV frames. It was, in fact, the long times such as the above that are required for many of the primary scan converter functions that prevented analog scan converter use in real time.

Because the number of storage elements involved in forming the image on the dielectric plane is large, an effective image-amplifying technique can be used after the image is stored. This is called a *read-zoom* function. By confining the sweep area of the reading electron beam to a specific region on the memory plane, the TV monitor can look at only a portion of the stored image. The converter can "zoom" in on image segments without changing the stored charge distribution. Even with this zoom function, the number of elements composing any given image is so high that the image can be amplified up to nine times the original size with no major loss in image resolution. This permits a technique where several images can be stored on different areas of the memory plane at the same time. In some systems, as many as nine images can be placed on the memory plane and transferred to a camera in one step. Although the picture-element density is not a problem for the analog scan converter, it is a central issue in the digital scan converter.

An overview of the reading-writing cycle is as follows: First, the electron beam is set into a low-energy form, and a negative writing format is used to place a negative-charge distribution on the memory plane as the echo signals come into the scan converter. The amount of charge stored on the plane is proportional to the echo-signal amplitude. Once stored, the image is read by the same beam, but in a still-lower energy level. The current that reaches the output electrode is controlled by the amount of charge placed on the dielectric islands, with the stored charge generally repelling the electron beam. This forms the nondestructive reading process. To remove the image, the energy of the electron beam is raised to a positive writing level, which is then scanned over the stored charge, removing the electrons until a net positive charge is formed. Then a negative writing cycle brings the stored charge back to a net value of zero.

Input and Output Signals for the Scan Converter

Signals brought to the scan converter usually come directly from the detector in the sonograph [4]. In early scan converters, these signals were shaped and modified into a voltage range of 0.0 V to 0.7 V, but were stepped into a finite number of signal levels. The process was almost digital in terms of the separation of the signal levels into established steps. The result was 10 to 15 gray levels on the analog display. Considering the prevailing belief that the eye could see only 10 shades of gray, this was considered enough gray levels for effective use of the sonograph.

The signals into and out of the scan converter were designed to be compatible with most of the established monitors, although, without a memory, the input signals could not be effectively displayed. Nevertheless, these standard signal levels were understood by service personnel, making setup and service relatively easy.

If the signals into the scan converter are set into a finite number of gray levels, the output from the scan converter will follow the character of the input. Ten steps in will yield 10 grays out. And if we could see into the interior of the scan converter

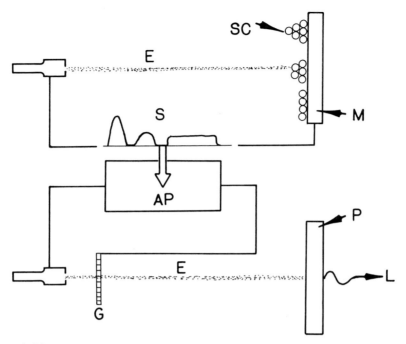

4-13   Converting stored charge to gray scale. The reading electron beam *E* passes over the stored charge *SC* on the memory plane *M*. Scanning the reading beam produces the signal *S*, which controls the amount of beam current *E* reaching the phosphor of the TV screen *P*.

to the lithicon target, the various signal levels would appear as layers of charge representing any given echo-signal level.

Still, the output from the scan converter can be modified, provided the signals are divided into a large enough number of steps. This provision will modify the video signal out of the scan converter to change both the range of signals that will write on the display from black to white, as well as where these signals happen to be located in the overall range of available signals. The process is called postprocessing and lets the user modify the visual qualities of the display to better separate and enhance signal differences.

The first technique is to "window" signals within the total range of output signals, and within the window to set the minimum signal to the lowest intensity of the display and the largest signal to the highest intensity of the display (Figure 4-13). Window sizes range all the way from the widest dynamic range of output signals to bistable. Although no quantities can be derived from the technique, the immediate payoff is an ability to change the visual contrast among signals. At the display level, the contrast and brightness of the display seem to be changed. But appearances can be deceiving. In fact, the monitor contrast and brightness are not being changed at all. It is the assignment of video signal levels to the stored charges that is being altered.

The position of the amplitude window can also be changed with a front panel control. Thus, the range of stored signals to be displayed can be set by the window width, and the second control sets the window position over the range of signals from the scan converter (Figure 4-13). These features appear again in the digital scan converter, but with a stability that will permit quantitative techniques.

The Thorny Side of the ASC

Stability inside the scan converter is built on controlling the quality of the electron beam. For example, a writing electron beam needs to be thin, with a tight average kinetic energy, that is, very few electrons can have an energy far away from the specified energy needed to stick the electrons onto the storage plane. On the other hand, the erasure beam must be highly energetic and broader than the writing electron beam in order to be able to erase the memory contents quickly. Again, the reading beam must be small and not very energetic. Beam focusing for erasing, reading, or writing is different for each function and must be automatically set for each. But often the control can become electronically confused or drift out of adjustment. When this happens, the image can be correctly made but incorrectly read or erased. One of the earliest recognized difficulties with the analog scan converter was the drift in the focusing and energy levels for each of the scan converter functions. Because these functions depend so much on the physical characteristics of the scan converter tube, the differences among scan converters can be large. Not until the digital scan converter were these differences reduced substantially.

The dielectric material at the memory plane is made of extremely small pieces that have a poor ability to transfer heat away from the memory element. As a result, a scanning electron beam that stops for a long time at one location can burn out the memory at that spot. Further, writing only onto a small portion of the memory can degenerate the dielectric, leaving a permanent spot in the image field. Thus, with the analog scan converter the electron beam needs to be in constant motion or turned off.

The writing electron beam that stores electrons on the dielectric can also cause local heating of the material. The kinetic energy of the incident electrons must be released in some manner, and that means transforming the kinetic energy into heat. Thus, local writing will cause local heating. At the same time, the electrons can absorb heat as kinetic energy, reducing the ''stickiness'' of the scan converter memory. Consequently, a slower scanning rate will cause local heating and change the charge content and thereby the gray-scale representation at that location. In addition, the overall temperature of the memory plane will change as heat trans-ferred into the scan converter from other parts of the machine is added to the heat generated by the scanning process. The result is a temperature change over time that will again alter the stability of the charges. Thus, the display gray scale will change over time as the temperature of the memory plane changes. Once more we are dealing with a mechanical system that cannot handle energy very efficiently, producing heat as a by-product.

Delivering the electrons to the scan converter memory requires that the electrons fall within discrete energy ranges for the electrons to interact correctly with the memory material. In turn, the electron energy is controlled by the accelerating voltage applied to the internal electrodes. The stability of these accelerating voltages will change the effective memory plane-beam interaction. Also, the electrons do not all respond to an acceleration voltage in quite the same way, and a wide range of electron energies is often present in the electron beam. The ability to carry out equilibrium writing and nondestructive readout depends upon the energies present and the narrowness of the range of energies within the beam. As a consequence, writing will not always come up to equilibrium and the reading process will not always be nondestructive.

The writing and reading cycle entails putting charges on the memory and then removing them—on again and off again. The cycle is never completely efficient, leading to a net accumulation of electrons on the dielectric. In effect, the electrons wear out the dielectric, and the dielectric ends up with mobile electrons. Soon the insulator begins to act like a conductor. And if the charge distribution is left on the memory for a long time—for example, over night—the electrons can migrate deeply into the memory material, leaving a permanent ghost image on the memory plane. The only alternative when this occurs is to buy a new scan converter tube, which is an expensive purchase. This problem happens as the result of a physical memory system defect that can never really be eliminated without a major redesign of the analog scan converter.

We noted earlier that the time required to write to equilibrium is about 10 ms or about 10 pulse-listen cycles for most B-scanners. This slows down the rate at which data can be reliably acquired for storage. But another problem quickly emerges that is fundamental to the analog scan converter. The writing and reading processes use the same electron beam; thus, writing and reading cannot happen simultaneously. Nevertheless, we need to see the image in formation to determine if the scan is proper. This requires quickly switching between reading and writing to permit image evaluation during the scan. The switching process produces a bright flicker and retrace lines in the image that cannot be removed until the writing mode is turned off. Once more we are dealing with an inherent limitation to a physical memory system.

Erasure in the analog scan converter has a similar time requirement as the writing time. The beam must be focused to a new width and energy level and scanned quickly over the memory plane to remove the stored electrons. The energy is high enough for the memory plane to be left positively charged. Then the second erasure step is used to bring the charge on the memory plane back to zero. This whole cycle takes over four TV frames to complete, and the erasure is not regional. A portion of the memory, such as a single ray, cannot be selectively erased and written back into quickly. As mentioned earlier, these cycle times, plus a lack of selective erasure, have prevented analog scan converter use in real-time imaging.

Conclusion

The analog scan converter has provided the needed storage and display of images for a significant portion of the time gray-scale ultrasound has been in use. The result has been some of the most aesthetically pleasing images yet to be produced because of the combined dynamic range of gray-scale levels in the ASC and the small elements that compose the image. The analog scan converter carries images that can be transferred to multiformat cameras, other monitors, videotape recorders, and even hand-held cameras. And it has provided a standard of image quality still applied to other scan converters and image-storage forms.

Despite its advantages, however, the analog scan converter was unable to compete with the digital scan converter. Within two years of the introduction of the digital scan converter, the market had almost completely changed to digital. The reasons become clear in Chapter 5.

References

1. Halliday, D., and R. Resnik. 1962. Physics for students of science and engineering. 2nd ed. New York: John Wiley & Sons.
2. Loeb, L.B. 1938. Atomic structure. New York: John Wiley & Sons.
3. Scan conversion memory, Model 639H. 1976. Carlsbad, CA: Hughes Aircraft Co., Industrial Products Division.
4. McDicken, W.N. 1976. Diagnostic ultrasonics: Principles and use of instruments. New York: John Wiley & Sons.

Chapter 5

Bits, Words, and Images: The Digital Scan Converter

Chapter 2 described the role of the scan converter in the static B-scanner organization. The scan converter performs a variety of activities, including storing image information gathered during the scanning process and retrieving that information in a format for communication to the outside. The scan converter must also have a gray-scale capability that converts the signal amplitude coming into the converter into a dot intensity on the display. And, if possible, the relationship between the signal level and the dot intensity should be variable and operator controlled.

Until a few years ago, the above functions were filled by the analog scan converter (ASC), described in Chapter 4. The analog scan converter stored the image as a set of charges distributed on a dielectric matrix. The charge was placed into and read out by an electron beam that made image formation dependent upon qualities unique to each scan converter.

When the digital scan converter (DSC) became commercially available, the analog scan converter lost its position in the marketplace in a flash of "going digital." Although at that time few users really understood the implications of the digital equipment, experience with other digital products had established the belief that *digital* meant *better* because it was stable and repeatable. A few companies sold both scan converters for a while, but finally went solely to digital scan converters as orders for the ASC vanished.

Although the digital scan converter performs the same role as the analog scan converter, events within the digital system are quite different. The digital scan converter takes the incoming analog signal from the detector and converts it into a set of binary numbers that are used to represent signal levels. The location of these numbers in the scan converter memory decides which echoes the numbers will represent. The rate at which the numbers are slotted into memory is determined by the physical scanning rate of the transducer. Once in memory, the numbers are read out nondestructively from the random access memory, or RAM, in a television format, completing the scan conversion. The digital signals are then modified and converted back to analog signals, which are then sent to the standard TV monitor. Along this pathway, shown in Figure 5-1, are some rather complicated technolo-

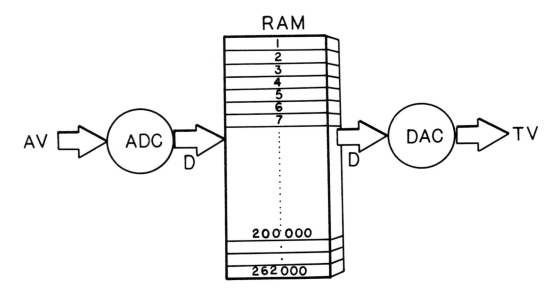

5-1   Digital organization of digital scan converter. The digital scan converter represents a digital signal processor for the analog video signal *AV*. *ADC* is the analog-to-digital converter; *D* is a digital, binary number; *RAM* is the random access memory; 1, 2, . . . 262,000 represents addresses within the *RAM; DAC* is the digital-to-analog converter; and *TV* is the composite TV signal for display.

gies. Understanding them not only makes the digital scan converter a more useful tool, but dispels much of the mystery surrounding "going digital."

With this general overview as a guiding tool, we can now deal more thoroughly with the steps of conversion.

Analog-to-Digital Converter

We learned earlier that the envelope of the transmitted ultrasound signal is used to represent the echoes received by the sonograph. Detecting this amplitude is often a matter of rectifying and filtering the radio frequency (rf) generated by the returning echo. Because of the phase-sensitive qualities of the transducer, the individual signals that result from the journey through the tissue are complex. These video signals occur after the application of time-gain compensation; thus, they have a dynamic range of 30 dB to 45 dB, depending upon the design of the particular machine. Because these signals are changing amplitude sharply, the range of frequencies within the video signals is large. A 5-MHz band width is not uncommon, and this band width places an effective limitation on the character of the signal conversion from analog to digital.

The signals are stored in a memory as numbers; consequently, the first activity required of the scan converter is to convert the analog signals into a set of binary numbers. The conversion happens in a special circuit called the analog-to-digital converter (ADC), which samples the incoming analog signal at a fast rate, ranging from 10 MHz to 20 MHz, and converts each component of the signal amplitude into a binary number representing the signal amplitude at that time. These digital numbers are then stored in the memory to represent the amplitude variations of the signals over time.

The numerical values available for the digital numbers are a function of what is called the *word length,* which refers to the number of elements, or bits, that are used to make up the numbers stored in the memory. For example, a ADC with a four-bit word has an output that uses four binary digits to describe all its values. Each bit can have two values, hence the term binary, giving a value minimum that is all zeros and a maximum that is all 1s. The smallest value is, of course, zero and the maximum value is four digits of 1s, or decimal 15. That range offers 16 values that can be used to represent signal amplitudes ($2^4 = 16$). Because the output is digital, no intermediate values, like 12.5 or 4.8, are possible. Only whole numbers between zero and 15 are permitted. The addition of one more digit doubles the number of values available, for example $2^5 = 32$, and one more digit doubles the value again to 64. A more detailed description of binary mathematics is found in Chapter 6. For most of the current systems, the output from the analog-to-digital converter is a set of 4, 5, or 6 digit binary numbers.

Referring again to the analog scan converter, the signal amplitudes in the early analog systems were placed into a finite set of values before being stored in the scan converter. Later, the video signals were set into a range of voltages compatible with the input to the scan converter, providing an almost continuous set of gray levels. This continuous gray scale is in marked contrast to the events within the digital scan converter.

The signals entering the digital scan converter are divided into a finite set of values. If, for example, we have a 40-dB video dynamic range, corresponding to a 100-to-1 range in relative signal amplitudes, the signal range must be divided into however many digital numbers are available at the analog-to-digital converter. Later, the numbers will become gray-level intensities, and the result is a finite number of grays available to the digital system.

Because of the wide range of signals that must be represented by a finite set of numbers, the division of analog signals uses rules that lead to an adequate image at the display. The input analog signals are set to each of the digital numbers by taking a group of signal values and assigning them all to the same digital number. This signal processing can be carried out at the analog-to-digital converter by a series of look-up tables or other techniques, guided by a set of digital instructions on a programmable read only memory (PROM) [1]. This signal processing occurs before the information is stored in memory, and is called preprocessing for that reason. Although all digital systems have preprocessing, preprocessing is not the same in all digital systems. Alternative signal handling philosophies revolve around

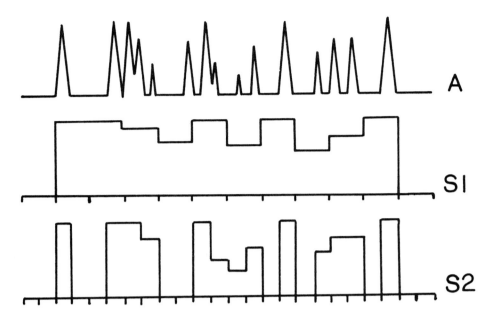

5-2   Digital sample rate and signal fidelity. *A* is a set of analog signals, sampled at two different rates, *S1* being one-half the sample rate of *S2*. An accurate reproduction of *A* with digital sampling would require a much-higher sample rate, but *S2* is clearly better than *S1* in representing *A*.

the number of bits in the analog-to-digital converter. These philosophies and their applications are examined later in Chapters 14 and 15.

The sampling rate of the analog-to-digital converter is determined by the number of memory locations used to store the information from a given pulse-listen cycle and the field of view of the sonograph. For example, if the field of view is 20 cm, all of the echo information will arrive into the analog-to-digital converter in $20 \times 13 \times 10^{-6}$ s. Let us assume the transducer is pointed straight down and 512 memory locations are used to store the pulse-listen cycle (Figure 5-2). The resulting 260-μs period will be divided into 512 parts, with each sample made in 260/512 = 0.51 μs. Inverting this number gives 1.96 MHz as the sample frequency. Decreasing the field of view to 5 cm increases this sample frequency to nearly 8 MHz. Special views and writing across the memory can increase the sampling rate to nearly 20 MHz [1, 2]. It follows that a fast ADC is the first requirement for a digital scan converter.

Once we have the signal sequence of a given pulse-listen cycle, the sequence must be stored in the memory in a fashion that will permit later reconstruction into an image. That means information must be stored into memory according to the transducer position in space when it acquired that signal sequence. Clearly, part of the information input to the scan converter involves where the transducer is pointed in space.

In turn, transducer position is identified by a set of arm encoders that can be analog or digital. The decision of where to place the data into memory is handled by a circuit in the digital scan converter that takes the encoder information and converts it into digital addressing data. These data are then used to direct the image information to the proper memory locations. Thus, the incoming data are addressed for storage according to where the transducer is pointed in the scanning plane. Knowing the rules of storage assures that the operator will later be able to logically retrieve it to produce an image.

Storing Information in the Memory

At the heart of the scan conversion process is a memory system that permits acquisition of information in one format and retrieval of that information from memory in another format. Further, the memory must be accessible randomly as the transducer moves through the scanning plane during various scanning procedures. The memory device of choice is a random access memory, or RAM.

The working-level subunit of the memory is the large-scale integrated circuit chip. On each chip, up to 16,000 bits of information can be stored. (The chips are called 16K RAMs for that reason.) In turn, the chips are mounted on circuit boards, with each memory location on each board specified by an addressing number. Comparing this memory system with that of the analog scan converter system yields little similarity between the two, although the memories assume the same role within the sonograph. If we could see the charge distribution stored on the analog scan converter memory, we would see the image. But if we tried to look into a digital scan converter for the same information, we would see nothing but a confusing set of "on" and "off" states distributed among a large number of chips. Such a difference is the result of physical information storage and the manner in which we treat that information after storage.

One way to treat the microorganization of the RAM is to think of the memory locations as if they were in a plane. The dimensions of this plane are defined by the number of memory locations available to store information (Figure 5-3). For example, a square memory plane can have 512×512 addressable locations, giving 512^2, or 262,144, memory locations. At each location is a word that can be 4, 5, or 6 bits deep. From these considerations, we can think of a three-dimensional matrix, $512 \times 512 \times 4$ or more bits deep. The writing and reading sequence can be visualized, then, like the analog scan converter, with the image distributed over the matrix and filled-bits representing signal amplitudes.

Fundamental to this idea is a separation of memory locations from the pixels on the display screen. Although memory locations and pixels will often have a one-to-one relationship, they are indeed different. Confusing the two can cause problems in trying to extend the utility of postprocessing. The memory location is a component part of the memory, at which a portion of the image information is stored as a digital number. A pixel, on the other hand, is the irreducible basic element of the digital *image,* a small area on the display screen that has a constant gray intensity. The intensity of the gray level at any pixel is defined by the number

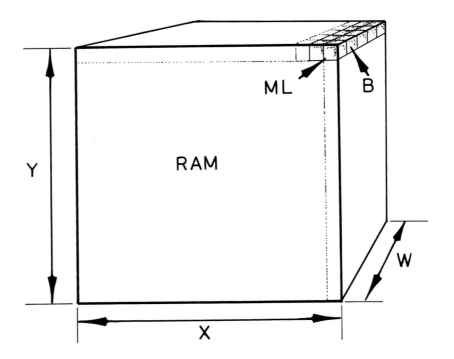

5-3 Mathematical organization of the scan converter RAM. The physical organization of RAM is closer to Figure 5-1 than here, but data is entered and read as if it were organized as shown in this figure. *Y* is row addresses; *X* is column addresses; *W* is the digital word length; *B* is a digital bit; and *ML* is a memory location.

stored in a corresponding memory location. The image, stored as numbers in the memory, is produced by mapping, on a one-to-one basis, the contents of the memory locations onto the display screen with varying gray levels (Figure 5-4).

Now we can think of the memory plane in the digital RAM in the same terms as the memory plane in the analog scan converter. We can fit the image information into this plane with higher numbers representing larger signals, just as higher charge densities represented larger signals in the analog scan converter.

The information entering the digital scan converter is received at a very high rate, with each equivalent 1 mm of tissue acquired every 1.3 µs. This rate is faster than most RAMs can accept large amounts of information, so the incoming signal is placed first into a high-speed buffer that can accept the high data rate [1]. The stored information is then transferred to the RAM for storage at a reduced rate.

The format for storing the information is as if the cross section were laid out over the memory plane. With the buffer available to store the incoming information for a few microseconds, the addressing can be carried out to decide where in memory to insert the information. All the interrelated timing for placing data into the memory is now complete.

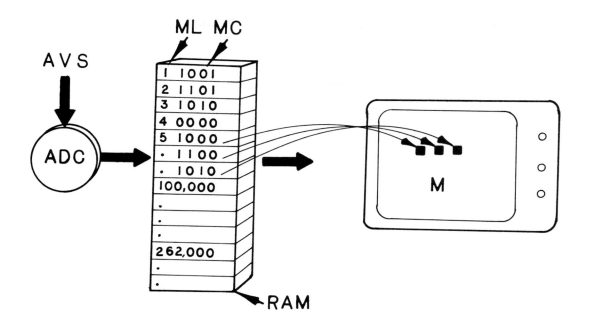

5-4   Mapping RAM memory locations on the display. The digital scan converter maps memory locations within RAM onto a fixed display location. *AVS* is the analog video signal; *ADC* is the analog-to-digital converter; *ML* is a memory address or location; *MC* is the memory contents; and *M* is the display monitor.

   The process of retrieving information from the memory must be synchronized with that of storing incoming information [2]. Synchronization is required because the RAM cannot handle reading and writing at the same time. Each step must thus happen individually, but quickly. The result is a cycle of writing, modifying, and reading information within the RAM. The time required to read the image out of memory is guided by the TV rate. For example, the U.S. TV format is 525 lines of raster scan, of which 480 lines are actually displayed. The time taken to scan one TV display line is 63.5 μs, which includes a reading and writing segment. To keep the timing correctly coordinated, a buffer is used again to store outgoing information [2]. Thus, the information read out of the RAM is brought to a buffer, and from the buffer onto the display. Now the rapid operations within the RAM can be timed to happen within the TV line formation.
   The timing of events within the scan converter thus involves regulating the TV format on one side and the transducer scanning rate on the other. The timing for the input to the digital scan converter must also be controlled by the DSC. The result is that all the major information timing management, including the pulse repetition frequency in the sonograph, is set by the digital scan converter, which becomes the major synchronizer within the sonograph.

Fetching Information Out of the RAM

The first real advantage in switching to a digital memory system is its ability to retrieve stored information nondestructively. Unlike the analog scan converter, the reading process in the digital memory does not impose a physical balancing act between the reading and writing processes. And keeping the information in the memory for a long time period does not affect the memory adversely. The information stored in the RAM can be refreshed at a regular rate by the RAM control circuits, or, if the memory is nonvolatile, the information can stay in memory without any additional power. The memory can be erased hours, days, or even weeks later with no damage to the memory. Thus, the RAM presents a truly nondestructive situation—not only in terms of the stored data but also the storing memory.

But the processes of reading, writing, and modifying cannot happen simultaneously. Rather, they happen in a sequence, one event at a time. Fortunately, the RAM is fast for each of these events, and nothing is lost by this sequence requirement. The image appears on the screen in real time as the transducer is scanned over the body. None of the image is lost, and the image does not flicker during the acquisition and reading processes. The absence of flicker is a primary difference between analog and digital scan converter operation.

Regardless of the internal timing cycle, the information coming out of the scan converter must be synchronized with the activities of a standard TV monitor. The data are selected from the memory, address by address, at a standard TV rate as if we were moving an electron beam over the memory plane. Because the retrieval is at a TV rate, the stream of data coming from the reading process requires only a minimal amount of modification to be ready for the TV monitor.

To retrieve data from the RAM memory address by address, we have to know where the information was stored in the image plane in the first place. Knowing the memory locations and treating the memory as if it were a plane means using a mathematical mapping technique to produce something that does not really exist, that is, the memory plane. A look inside a digital scan converter clearly shows the physical realities of the memory. Inside are four or five circuit boards, with the image placed at locations distributed among the boards. To construct the image, bits of information collected one at a time are brought to the display, with each location in the scan converter memory represented as a small area on the screen. The gray level seen on the screen, however, may not have the same relative weighting as that stored in memory. Each gray level is assigned to a stored number, controlled by postprocessing. This assignment of gray level to stored number is often nonlinear and selectable by the operator using front-panel postprocessing controls.

Once the information is read out of the memory, it is still not yet ready for the display TV monitor. First, it is still digital, which is not compatible with most

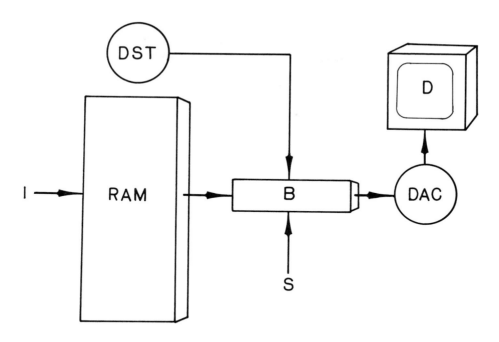

5-5　Signal flow and control to the display. The ultimate timing control for the sonograph comes from the digital scan converter. *DST* is the scan converter timer. The digital echo-signals *I* enter the memory, *RAM,* and are read out into a signal buffer *B,* under *DST* control. Additional control signals *S* are added to control the monitor *D*. The composite digital signal is converted to analog through the digital-to-analog converter *DAC*.

display TV monitors. Second, the signals that control the electron beam position inside the TV are not contained in the raw digital information read out of the memory. The first order of business after the signals are read out of memory is the addition of control signals that position the electron beam and turn the beam off during the retracing of the electron beam in the cathode ray tube (CRT) (Figure 5-5).

In order to make sense of the digital scan converter organization, we need to remember the process carried out by the analog scan converter. The electron beam in the analog scan converter is synchronized with the electron beam in the display CRT. As the scan converter electron beam scans the stored charge distribution, the display TV electron beam scans the phosphor. The information stored in the charge distribution can be mapped onto the display screen as a set of dots of varying intensity. The digital scan converter does the same sort of thing, except that the interrogation of the stored information does not use an electron beam. Nevertheless, the CRT electron beam and the data-fetching process are synchronized in the digital scan converter, linking the two together as closely as is the link between electron beams and TV display in the analog scan converter.

The Digital-to-Analog Converter

Once the control signals have been added to the data streaming out of the memory, the machine is almost ready for the display. The TV monitor will accept only analog signals. The task now is to convert the digital video signals back into analog signals.

The conversion of digital signals to analog signals happens in a circuit called a digital-to-analog converter (DAC). The conversion, however, is under the influence of the postprocessing circuit (Figure 5-1). In addition, the postprocessing can be modified in some systems with front panel controls, offering major manipulations of the image by the sonographer.

Postprocessing occurs in every digital system because the digital numbers coming out of the memory must be assigned to a corresponding gray level on the TV display. These gray levels are bounded by the intensity range of the TV monitor. The assignment of numbers to gray levels can be used to separate small signals in the low signal-level range, to compress middle range signals, or to compress or separate visually the larger signals. The assignment can be easily modified to match the intensity variations characteristic of the TV display, or just to show a very narrow range of signal levels. And all this can be carried out without rescanning the patient. As in the case of preprocessing, the question is not whether pre- or postprocessing is present, because they are present in all digital machines. The real question is what shape the processing curves take.

Nature and Organization of the Display

Chapter 4 pointed out that the TV monitor moves an electron beam in a motion pattern called a raster scan. When the electron beam is at the end of the scan, it must be quickly moved back to the left-hand side of the screen. During this retrace period, the current in the beam must be turned off to prevent the sweeping beam from putting diagonal lines through the image. The command used to turn off the beam during this retrace period is called the *blanking voltage*. Thus, a composite video contains not only the intensity instructions for the electron beam but also the retrace and blanking instructions as well. This is the complex signal mix brought to the TV monitor.

At the TV, the image is made into a series of composite images called fields. Each field uses one-half the available display lines. For example, the U.S. TV format is 525 lines, with 480 lines actually displayed. One-half of the displayed lines, or 240 lines, are shown as one field, then the second field is shown with the remaining 240 lines interlaced with the first field. Each of the fields is individually shown at a 60-Hz rate and is interlaced, producing an overall image renewal at 30 Hz [3]. In contrast, the European standard format is 625 lines, with 580 displayed at 50 Hz and with a similar set of rules governing the production of image fields.

Beyond the number of lines used to make the display, the monitor needs to have a gray-scale response. Monitors used for such things as computer graphics have a very high image contrast that is proper for the display of computer-generated letters or numbers, but unsuited for the display of gray-scale information. Good gray-scale monitors that have a well-understood response to the intensity instructions are expensive. At the same time, they offer the best chance to see gray-scale changes that can be hidden by less able monitors.

Along with the gray-scale capability, the monitor must produce a clean image with no video ringing that leaves "ghosts" trailing behind very large signals. Furthermore, the spatial distortion should not exceed 3% over the face of the display. And the display should have at least a 500-line resolution. This means that intensity variations in the electron beam during the sweep over the face of the tube should be able to produce 500 resolvable vertical lines. Combining these capabilities with good overall stability will improve the transfer of visual information from the TV screen to the visual system of the sonographer and sonologist.

With these contributing factors from the display in mind, we can look more closely at some of the scan converter events in order to better grasp scan converter function.

Memory Size and Preprocessing

The range of signals resulting from variations in tissue interface reflectivity is 50 dB to 60 dB, which is compressed or suppressed to 30 dB to 45 dB. At the analog-to-digital converter, the continuous analog signal range is divided into a set of binary numbers that must span the range of analog signals. If a 40-dB dynamic range is divided linearly into 16 numbers, for example, each digital number value would have to represent a range of 40 dB/16 = 2.5 dB. As a result, the analog signal level would have to change by at least one-third (33%) to move from one digital number to the next. Unfortunately, the signals change much more gradually than that in a biological signal mix. The result is a blocky- and coarse-appearing digital image. To smooth out the image, signal separations must be in the order of 1 dB/step in the medium to low signal levels. And that sort of signal separation forces the digital signal spacing to be closer than that in the larger signals. The result is a nonlinear assignment of numbers to the incoming signal levels, in other words, nonlinear preprocessing (Figure 5-6).

In most machines with 16 gray levels, a nonlinear preprocessing technique is used to restore the image quality lost to too few grays. The region of compression and expansion can be set by a front panel control to separate close signals in the range of interest. For example, a preprocessing curve that has a high slope in the low signal levels and a lower slope in the medium and high signal range will better separate the low signal levels. Another curve can be used to compress the middle signals and expand the top and bottom end of the signal spectrum (Figure 5-7). And where the signals reside relative to the preprocessing curve will depend on

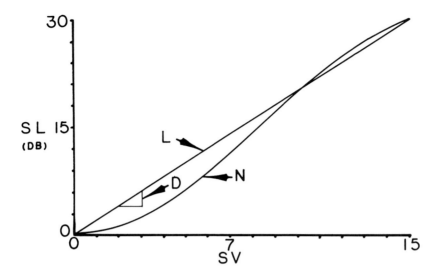

5-6 Linear and non-linear preprocessing. Preprocessing is an assignment of the numerical values available to the scan converter to the analog video signal. *SL* is the analog signal level expressed in dB. *SV* is the RAM-stored digital value, in this case for a four-bit system. *L* is the linear relationship; *N* is a nonlinear relationship. *D* is the amount of analog signal levels assigned to a single digital value in the RAM.

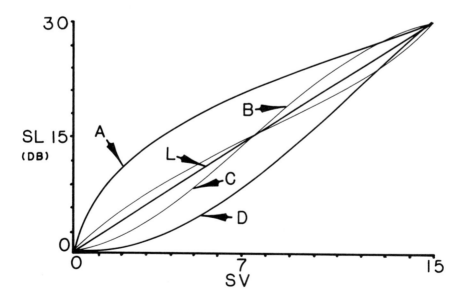

5-7 Typical specialized preprocessing curves. the preprocessing assignments can greatly influence the image quality and ability to extract clinical information. *SL* is the analog signal level in dB; *SV* is the stored digital value for a 16 gray-level system; *L* is a linear assignment; *A* is a curve that enhances high-signal separation, spreading most of the digital numbers over the higher signal levels; *D* enhances low signal levels; *B* deemphasizes the medium signal levels, visually compressing high and low signals together; *C* enhances the middle range of signal levels.

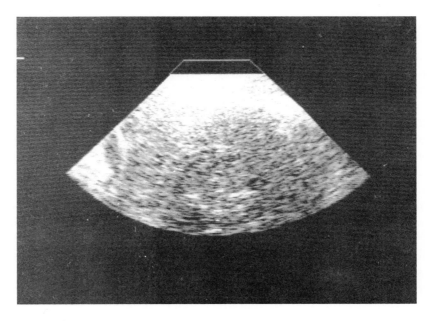

5-8 Subjective contouring in a limited gray scale image. Operating with fewer than 32 gray scale intensities in an image can cause subjective gray scale contouring where normal unlike echo-signal amplitudes appear as the same gray scale intensity. As a result, the echo-signals form contours of like intensity within the image and can give the impression of masses.

how the TGC and system response is set up. As a result, the same preprocessing curve will not work for all patients, unless the setup of the sonograph is carefully considered. (The strategy for selecting appropriate preprocessing curves is the central theme of Chapter 15.)

In addition to the problem of adequate signal separation, 16 gray levels produces another visual effect called subjective gray-scale contouring. This phenomenon results from trying to display a complex signal mix with too few grays. More specifically, the contouring appears in the image as regions of constant gray intensity that would normally be different but that now appear the same because not enough digital values are available to describe the range of signals completely [4]. The signal dots run together on the screen, giving the impression of layers, or steps, within the image (Figure 5-8). The image looks as though it had been painted by the numbers. Further, the contours can run together at times, forming what looks like structures within the image, but which are really artifacts. On a smaller scale, the contouring can produce very large-appearing dots in the image, a problem often described as "blobby dots" by many users. More often, the contouring causes the image to look incomplete, but in a manner difficult to describe. The contouring also causes abrupt changes in the gray levels at boundaries and structures, increasing the spatial frequencies in the image. The image is often then described as "digital" and judged as poor by the experienced observer, who at the same time may not be able to explain why.

If most of the image information is in the lower signal levels, the preprocessing curve can be used to provide appropriate signal separation there, and at the same time, accept poorer separation in other parts of the signal range. This is how the various preprocessing curves work; they properly separate signals in one range at the expense of the remaining signals.

Increasing the number of digital values to 32 or 64 improves the ability to divide the incoming signal range into even smaller parts. For example, 40 dB/32 steps = 1.25 dB/step, which is close to the desired signal separation over the whole signal range. Going to 64 values divides it even further to 0.625 dB/step, eliminating any chance for observable gray-scale contouring. In these systems with larger digital numbers, preprocessing is much less complicated. The full dynamic range of the biological signals is divided into 32 or 64 steps in a log-linear manner, in which the signals are divided linearly (evenly) according to decibel levels (a logarithmic function). This sort of preprocessing is possible only in systems with 5 or more bits in the storing RAM word.

Because preprocessing changes the image signal-to-number assignment in a nonlinear way for systems with 16 or fewer grays, the stability of this circuit becomes pivotal to the overall machine image quality. If the preprocessor is temperature dependent, images will look different as the machine warms because the assignment of numbers to signal levels changes. Discrete component failures in the preprocessor can also adversely affect image quality. Often one of the first signs of system failure is gray-scale contouring in a machine that normally did not.

Managing Output Signals with Postprocessing

As noted earlier, the process of assigning gray levels to the stored numbers is called postprocessing. The assignment can be complex, but is easily handled by the machine because the assignment is in the digital domain. Programmable read only memories (PROMs) can be used to store instructions about the assignments. Different assignments can be used to rapidly evaluate the image for acoustic enhancement and shadowing or other qualities without rescanning the patient (Figure 5-9). The assignments can be even more flexible than just a few curves selected by a front panel switch. Postprocessing can be quite variable and controlled by the user.

The assignment of a digital number to the display gray level can be exact because it is digital. Thus, variable postprocessing can provide discrete information about the signals stored in memory. Comparisons are possible between adjacent signal levels or other signals in the image. And if the separation of the signals is known, that is, the preprocessing is known (or linear), numerical comparisons are possible.

Making numerical determinations means the postprocessing must be able to separate individual signal levels stored in memory. This is possible by forming a digital "window," which can admit any range of signals, from a single value to the

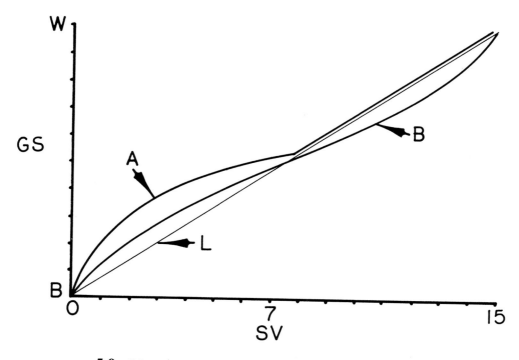

5-9   Linear and non-linear postprocessing. Post processing is an assignment of the stored value *SV* to a gray-scale intensity on the display. This is a 16 gray-level example. *L* is a linear assignment; *A* is a nonlinear assignment, which elevates the brightness of the lower signals but keeps the upper signals normal; *B* is a compressing assignment that places most of the gray-scale changes in the large and small signal levels. *GS* is the gray-scale intensity range.

whole range of stored values (Figure 5-10). Furthermore, the window needs to be movable over the entire range of signals available. Like the analog postprocessing from the analog scan converter, the signals within the window must be linearly cast over the intensity range of the monitor from black to white. The result is that barely discernible signals under normal gray-scale conditions can be visually separated in intensity, producing an unusual contrast enhancement.

But beyond the ability to enhance neighboring signal levels, variable postprocessing can be used to make numerical evaluations that can contribute to clinical comparisons. Because signals from like interfaces are a function of the material in front of the interfaces, the influence of the intervening material can be estimated by comparing the signals from two like but separated interfaces. Behind a shadowing mass, signals will be smaller than those from a like reflector with normal tissue in front. Conversely, reflectors behind a less-than-normal attenuating mass will have larger reflections than similar reflectors with normal tissue in front. Comparing like reflectors both around and behind a mass provides clues on the amount of attenuation caused by the mass. This sort of analytical power comes only from a variable postprocessing system. (Chapter 14 is devoted to variable and selectable postprocessing.)

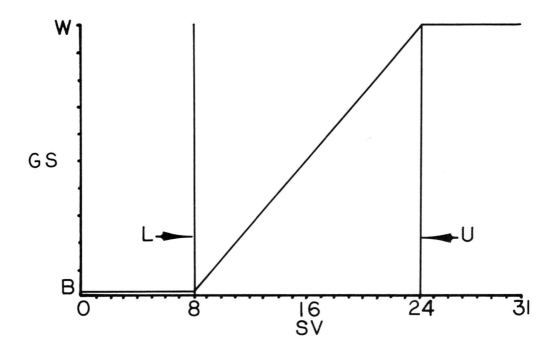

5-10   Variable postprocessing window. With a variable post-processing window, any range of stored values SV can be spread over the full intensity range GS of the display. L is the lower edge of the window; U is the upper edge of the window. Here the middle 16 values in the RAM are spread over the full display gray-scale range.

The ability to use variable postprocessing effectively depends upon the amount of information stored in memory. In turn, the amount of information stored is a function of the word size. A four-bit system does not have enough signal amplitude information to effectively use any sort of analytical postprocessing. Variable post-processing is most effective on systems with 32, 64, or more gray levels, and these systems most often have variable postprocessing.

Zoom Functions in the DSC

We often want to expand a portion of the image to better evaluate a lesion or structure. In an A-mode trace, the portion of the trace under interest can be expanded by delaying the start of the display trace until echoes from the start of the desired region just appear, and then moving the trace faster than usual over the screen to the end of the region. In between, the depth can be indicated by centimeter marks that are 13 μs apart. We have thus "zoomed" in on the region of interest by amplifying one segment of the trace and limiting the display to only that region.

The same sort of delay can be applied to B-mode signals entering a scan converter memory. By delaying the start of entry of the signals into the memory and moving the writing process faster, the region of interest can be amplified *into* the memory. Nothing changes in reading the information out of the memory. We have "zoomed" in on one portion of the tissue and displayed that portion over the whole storage area (Figure 5-11). This process is called *write zoom,* named for the amplification that is applied *before* physically writing into the memory.

The technique can be applied to analog or digital scan converters, but carries some limitations in the analog system. The analog scan converter writes into memory with an electron beam, and the fast electron beam motion required in write zoom limits the ability of the electron beam to write to equilibrium. As a result, write zoom is not normally used in analog scan converters. This same writing limitation does not occur, however, in the digital scan converter. The writing limitation in the digital system is the analog-to-digital sampling frequency, and is not a problem for the digital scan converter.

An alternate form of image amplification is that of limiting the reading scan to only a small portion of the stored image. In the analog scan converter, the reading electron beam scans over the whole memory matrix (Figure 5-11). Amplifying a small area of the memory means scanning the reading beam over just this small portion. The electron beam scans in the TV monitor, however, are spread over the whole display. As mentioned in Chapter 4, the process is called *read zoom* because we are amplifying the signal for display during the reading process. In the digital scan converter, read zoom is accomplished by limiting the addresses brought to the display TV. We are effectively restricting our display to only a few memory locations and displaying these locations as large pixels on the screen.

In the analog scan converter, the image elements used to store and represent the image are very small. Thus, the electron beam spot size and image dot size are the real limitations to image resolution. Furthermore, by using the whole memory plane, the electron beam can write to equilibrium; thus, the gray-scale information is still distinct and reading the data off the memory plane will be close to nondestructive. But in the digital scan converter, another mechanism begins to take over that limits the utility of read zoom. The digital memory elements are substantially fewer than the analog memory, and expanding a portion of the memory for reading increases the size of the display pixels. The result is a blocky, often unreadable image if the amplification is much over two times. Clearly, part of the smoothness of the digital image we are used to seeing comes from the very small pixels used on the display. In a read zoom, the pixels become large and visible, producing a digital-looking image.

In each type of scan converter, a preferred technique of amplifying, or zooming, emerges from the basic nature of the storage techniques. The analog scan converter uses the read zoom better than does the digital scan converter. Conversely, the digital scan converter uses the write zoom better than does the analog scan converter. Still, some digital scan converters will have a read-zoom capability, but it is usually limited to an amplification of two times or less. Above that value, the pixels become too large for effective imaging.

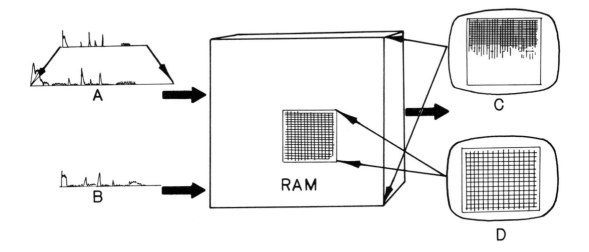

5-11 Methods of digital zoom signal processing. The zoom function is a means of expanding the size of the image. In example A, the analog signal is first expanded, then placed in the RAM. This is called a write zoom. The full contents of the RAM appear on the display, as shown in C. In example B, the analog signal is handled normally into the RAM, but only a portion of the RAM appears on the display, as shown in D. This is called a read zoom. The resulting image effects are included.

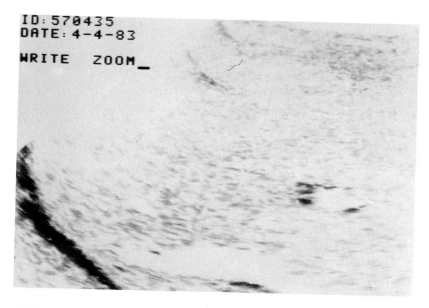

5-11   Example A

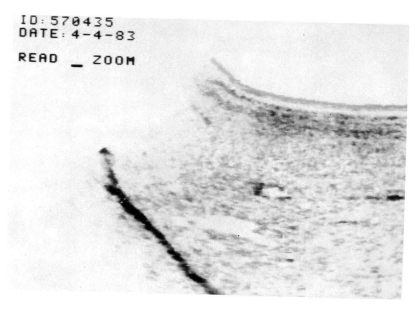

5-11   Example B

Special Writing Algorithms in DSCs

In computed tomography, the amount of information gathered into the memory is much larger than that which is portrayed on the display. The additional data are used to perform special averaging and signal-enhancing techniques within the digital memory, and only the finished results are presented to the display. A similar setup is possible for the sonograph [5]. In this technique, a large amount of information is gathered, with contributing information for a given display pixel coming from several different scans. Having gathered the data, several forms of filtering and signal-difference enhancement programs are possible, all carried out without losing the original data.

These techniques require a sizable memory in order to perform the operations. An analogous operation occurs in the smaller scan converter of the static B-scanner [1]. In this technique, the values held in any memory location are based on the largest value presented to that location. Within the scan converter writing process is a program that compares the current values in the scan converter memory location with the incoming value for that location. If the incoming value is larger than what is already in storage, the new, larger value is inserted. If the incoming value is less than what is stored, the stored value remains. Because the B-scanner overscans in most applications, more than sufficient data are available to filter the incoming information for a maximum value. This type of writing algorithm has been given a variety of names such as *peak writing* or *compound mode writing*. The end result is the same, regardless of the name, and the largest value for every memory location is what remains for display.

But the read-modify-write cycle of the scan converter can be modified to include other means of recording information. For example, the memory can accept the last value obtained from a pulse-listen cycle. In this writing method, the ray is place in memory, and the memory location accepts whatever is being received, regardless of the values previously stored. This technique is variously referred to as *survey mode* or *last value mode* of operation. Again, regardless of name, the process is the same.

Other techniques can be applied that involve spatial filtering or average-value calculations. Most of these methods require additional memory or buffering to permit operations on the data before they are stored in memory. And all this flexibility comes from using a RAM and working in the digital domain.

The survey mode represented one of the earliest modifications to the normal writing processes within the digital scan converter. Aside from presenting the last value at any location, the survey mode opens the door to a faster use of the B-scanner. Values are replaced on each pulse-listen cycle, permitting rapid movement and image updating wherever the transducer is scanning the body. Thus, the survey mode, as the name implies, can be used to rapidly survey the body, rivaling some real-time systems in survey speed. Most of the digital B-scanners have slow modes in scanning arm movement, which lets the scan plane move over the body under power from the scan arm while the sonographer moves the transducer in a series of small rapid sectors. A skilled sonographer can survey the entire abdomen in a few minutes with this technique.

The survey mode, however, is more than just a fast way to scan. It also provides a good opportunity to see how real-time signal information is acquired, and how small movements of the transducer affect the data finally stored in the memory. For example, one of the first observations made by a sonographer is that in the survey mode, the signal levels seem to be about 6 dB lower than in the compound mode. To restore the image quality, the system response (system gain or transducer power) is usually increased about 6 dB. Every digital system with a survey mode demonstrates this sort of effect. The reasons for the decrease in system response are discussed in more detail in Chapter 7.

Digital Scan Conversion and Real Time

In the B-scanner, the survey mode of operation gathers information from the tissue on a single pulse-listen cycle. The same situation applies for real-time systems when they gather information. A real-time system carries out a single pulse-listen cycle, stores that information, and moves the beam to another location to repeat the process. Despite only a single cycle to gather information, the digital scan converter is not compromised at all. In fact, it is the speed of the digital scan converter that enables it to work so well with real-time systems.

Although real-time systems gather information "on the fly," they do not represent a random scanning process within the scan plane. Positioning the scan in the memory plane in real time is predictable. And because we are using a digital system, we do not have the physical limitations of an analog system, such as the writing time required to reach equilibrium. It is a technology blend that uses the best of both real-time and digital technology—the moving transducer of the real-time scanner and the writing speed and dependability of the digital scan converter. Adding a scan converter to a real-time system means the image can be frozen for detailed examination and photography; moreover, the output of the scan converter connects to all sorts of standard recording devices, including a videotape recorder. This last transfer to a video recording system allows the image to be stored and later examined from an imaging as well as a dynamic point of view.

Real-time systems can be divided into two basic fields: rectangular fields and sector fields. The rectangular field is produced by a linear scan. Loading this information into a scan converter is accomplished by letting each scan line occupy a fixed memory column. The image information can then be read out by rows to produce the scan conversion and a TV video output. With the rectangular field, data management is relatively uncomplicated.

Loading image information from a sector scan into a memory can be managed in two ways. The first simply treats the sector information in the same manner as would a standard B-scanner. The position of the information in the memory is constant, as is the position of the information ray within the scan plane. The sector information is then cued by the position of the ultrasound beam in the scanning plane, and the ray is written across the memory like a standard B-scan. The sampling rate will change with the amount of angulation across the memory, which means the ADC must know where the ray will be placed in memory. Segments of the memory outside the sector are not used to form the image, but can be used for write zoom in a sector field, annotation, and additional displays such as time-gain compensation curves or gray bar patterns. The process of reading information out of this configuration is unchanged, as fetching performs a raster scan over the memory scan plane at a TV rate.

The second method of loading information from a sector scan is to place the incoming rays of information into columns as if the scan were linear. This technique eliminates writing across the memory and having to deal with the Moiré patterns that result from missing pixels when writing across a memory plane [1]. On the other hand, the information must be read out of memory in a nonstandard way in order to reproduce the sector field on the display. Image synthesis can occur by reading the information out of memory by rows and changing the size of the pixels on the display, with small pixels at the top of the image and larger pixels at the bottom. Even then, the formation of the image may not be adequate to handle a sector angle greater than 60°. Because the more anterior part of the sector is badly overscanned, redundant information in this region can be removed, improving the ability to form large sector angles. The information taken away is redundant, so no clinical capabilities are lost in doing this. The return for this sort of management is a more efficient use of the memory than in the first technique. Both techniques are successful, however, and produce images that are stable and clinically useful.

Bringing Image Information to the Outside

The first transfer of information from the sonograph to the outside world is through the display CRT. The digital data stored in the DSC appear as a gray-scale image depicting a cross section of the body. This image is frozen in memory but refreshed on the display TV at a standard TV rate. The image can be examined and photographed directly for a permanent record.

Because the video information brought to the display is on a standard TV format, it can also be coupled to other compatible video devices. Most digital systems bring the image information to the outside through several connections that can receive a variety of recording devices. These connections are often parallel, connected to the same output amplifier on the inside, which can be quite sensitive to how many devices are connected to the output ports. Most manufacturers of these ports specify acceptable impedances and overall load capacities that will not seriously degrade the output voltages.

One of the more interesting aspects of a digital scan converter is the ability to obtain memory information directly without the intervention of DAC circuits. Because the stored information must be retrieved at a rate and voltage level that can be handled by the receiving device, a buffer is often needed to make the proper connection between the memory contents and the outside world. The data-receiving device might be a microprocessor, a microcomputer, a minicomputer, or a sizable time-shared computer common to larger hospitals and medical centers. The connection to the DSC memory is commonly called an input/output (I/O) port.

More and more laboratories are buying small personal computers, and these I/O ports may play a larger role in ultrasound evolution than currently suspected. Computer languages and machine sophistication that used to be limited to large, expensive computers are now available to the smaller computers, bringing significant computing power into the ultrasound laboratory. Outboard calculations, data manipulations for image enhancement, or specific filtering techniques are all possible with the computer coupled to the DSC memory.

The digital I/O port can be handled in another way, however. The memory contents can be read out and transferred to a floppy disc that can store many images in a digital format. These discs later can be played back into the scan converter memory and examined again with the system postprocessing. The problem with this technique is getting enough images onto a disc in a short-enough time to make the disc cost-effective. The utility of the disc, however, may not be in storing image information from the DSC but in storing information for other analytical devices that can be employed while the scanner is being used on other patients.

Despite the I/O ports that are available on many sonographs and the few computers now hooked up to scan converters, however, not a great deal is happening in special digital processing. The reason for this may be that users do not see a real need for sophisticated digital processing. Most ultrasound departments seem to feel they are getting all the information they need to carry out a diagnosis. Ultrasound experience has so far been built around a determination of size, shape, position, texture, and dynamics (if in a real-time system). Computer-assisted analysis must improve these data or add more data that are perhaps not basic to anatomical relationships. Still, the computer port remains a gateway to finding new applications of digital techniques to satisfy needs not yet recognized. It may be through a combination of sonograph and computer that quantification techniques will be most easily realized. Investigations in this area will need a DSC with an I/O port, a computer, and the organizational software to let each machine talk to the other.

Pixels and Image Quality

The displayed image is formed from the stream of digital information that comes from the scan converter and is mapped onto the display in the form of pixels. The typical TV display is divided into 512 × 512 pixels or 640 (horizontal) × 512 pixels. As noted earlier, the standard TV shows only 480 TV lines. If we now map each pixel onto the TV so that the pixels are only one line high, then only 480 pixels can be formed on the display screen. Horizontally, this is not the case, and a full 512 or even 640 pixels can be mapped over the display on each TV line. Because of the width-to-height ratio on a TV display, a square image plane of 512 × 512 locations can fill the screen vertically but not horizontally. On the other hand, 640 horizontal pixels can fill the TV, prompting a few ultrasound and digital analyzer manufacturers to go to a 640 × 512 memory plane. The advantages of the 640 × 512 architecture are an increase in the number of pixels that compose the image itself [6]. The physical size of the image also increases as more pixels are used. As always, the choice of memory size is both economic (will it cost more?) and aesthetic (how to use more of the display?).

The architecture of the memory plays a role in the perceived smoothness of the image. Any image that is produced by picture elements that have a finite size and limited intensities will be acutely sensitive to the size and character of the individual pixels. If the dots that make an image are large enough to be seen at normal viewing distance, then the image will appear too sharp and digital. The sharp edges of the pixels will dominate the image, and the more gradual trends of intensity that make up the image will be lost behind a visual flood of pixel boundaries. It seems to be a form of spatial frequency aliasing. The result is an unpleasant image to look at and analyze.

Contributing to the smoothness of an image is the number of values available to the scan converter that become gray levels. If the number of gray levels is too small, the transition among complex signals is too great, increasing the spatial frequencies within the image once again. As in the case of pixels that are too large, too few gray levels make the image look blocky and digital, and textural information is hidden behind the high spatial frequencies of the digital-appearing image. In general, then, a digital scan converter can provide its best images when the pixels are small enough not to be perceived in the image, and when the number of gray levels available to the scan converter is high enough to prevent gray-scale contouring on either a micro or macro level. (The physiology of the eye and how it applies to displaying gray-scale information is discussed in Chapter 16.)

By comparison, the analog scan converter has none of the spatial frequency problems of the digital scan converter. The elements of image storage and display are much smaller for the analog scan converter. Even when amplified, these elements are much smaller than the dots produced by the ultrasound machine itself, and the image is not compromised even with a high-amplification read zoom. In addition, the analog scan converter has available a nearly continuous gray-scale range that produces smooth, aesthetically pleasing images. In combination, these two facts enable the analog scan converter to portray subtle changes in gray scale and texture, qualities possessed only by the best digital scan converters.

Despite these characteristics, the analog scan converter was quickly supplanted by the new digital systems, by virtue of the latter's ability to offer *sustained* image quality. The stability and potential for quantification of the digital scan converter guarantee it a secure future in ultrasound.

Conclusion

We have traced signal events through the digital scan converter, from the primary conversion to a digital format to the final image dependence upon the pixels that make the image. At the analog-to-digital converter, the analog signals are converted to binary numbers. The assignment of the available numbers to the analog signal range is controlled by the system preprocessing, which divides the analog signal range into groups of values that can be equal or unequal. The binary numbers are stored in the random access memory in locations determined by where the ultrasound beam happens to be pointed in the scanning plane. Once stored, these data are read out, address by address, as if a raster scan were moving over the stored image plane. The numbers are read out of the memory in a manner that produces a stream of image information on a standard video format. Added to the image signals are control signals used to manage the display TV electron beam. The combined signals are then converted to a set of analog signals by the digital-to-analog converter circuit. At this point, the postprocessing sets the assignment of digital value to gray-scale intensities. The image is then ready for TV presentation.

Because the digital systems are fast, writing and reading times can be sequentially handled so swiftly that reading, writing, and modifying the data occur in a fraction of a second. These speeds let the digital scan converter easily combine with real-time scanning technology to extend real-time capabilities beyond simple observation.

But beyond the speed of writing and reading, the digital scan converter provides truly nondestructive reading and writing of information into a storage medium, all with a stability unachieved by analog scan converters. With the controlled conversion of analog signals to numbers and variable postprocessing, the memory contents can be analyzed numerically, not only with self-contained postprocessing, but also with computers that can be attached through an I/O port. We owe all of these innovations to the development of the digital scan converter.

References

1. Ophir, J., and N.F. Maklad. April 1979. Digital scan converters in diagnostic ultrasound imaging. Proc IEEE 67:654–664.

2. Maginness, M.G. April 1979. Methods and terminology for diagnostic ultrasound imaging systems. Proc IEEE 67:641–653.

3. Rose, J.L., and B.B. Goldberg. 1979. Basic physics in diagnostic ultrasound. New York: John Wiley & Sons.

4. Eye com handbook of image processing. 1980. Goleta, CA: Spatial Data Systems.

5. Robinson, D.E., and G. Kossoff. July 1979. Computer processing of line mode echogram data. International Congress Series 505. In Proceedings of the Second Meeting of the World Federation for Ultrasound in Medicine and Biology, ed. T. Wagai and R. Omoto. 11–16

6. Powis, R.L. August 1979. Numerical aspects of the 512×640 memory matrix. Unirad Technical White Paper No. 1. Englewood, CO: Unirad Corp.

Chapter 6

Computers and the Sonograph

In the evolution of the sonograph, few elements hold as much potential for shaping the future of ultrasound as the microcomputer. This silent partner in the image-making process looks unimpressive when first seen as a large, integrated circuit mounted among other components on a circuit board. But microcomputers have already altered significantly the organization of the sonograph, and carry an ever-increasing analytical load.

Microprocessors and microcomputers operate both inside and outside today's sonograph, controlling internal machine functions, analyzing data, or simply putting graphics on the display to label an image. Moreover, they may soon be supplying computer-based medical education to sonographers and sonologists [1].

What accounts for the microcomputer's primary influence on the design and use of the sonograph?

Things Analog and Digital

Early computers, like slide rules, were analog, relying on analog electrical or mechanical components to perform computations. What does an analog computer look like? The speedometer on a car is a good example of a mechanical, analog computer, translating the rotation of the drive shaft into miles per hour on the dial. But these are rather simple tasks, and applying analog computers to more difficult tasks is not easy. It was the digital computer that provided a major change in the nature of computing machines and, eventually of ultrasound.

We now have at our disposal digital devices of all types. What makes something digital, and what are the benefits, if any, of entering the digital world? Let us examine the analog and digital concepts in more detail.

At the outset, the analog world is a continuous world, theoretically holding an infinite number of states, or values, between any pair of defined boundaries. An easy model to illustrate this is a continuous ramp between two floors (Figure 6-1). Anyone climbing the ramp can stop anywhere between the two floors in Figure 6-1. Because the ramp is continuous, there is an infinite set of positions between the top and bottom floors.

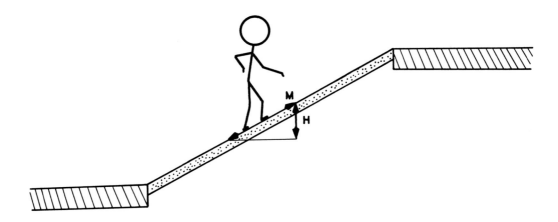

6-1   Analog system model. A ramp between two levels is a good analog model. Movement along the ramp *M* will cause a change in height *H*. Movement at a particular position on the ramp always causes a change in height, which is a good model for analog noise.

Let's leave our guest standing on the ramp for a period of time until he or she becomes a bit bored and starts shuffling around. With each shuffle, the guest moves up and down the ramp, changing height. If we think of this nervousness as noise, a primary problem in dealing with the analog world becomes evident. Noise causes an analog system to change values (or states), represented by our guest changing height on the ramp. In electronic devices, this sort of noise sensitivity can lead to large errors in operation.

The digital world, by contrast has a finite number of values. A good model for this property is a set of stairs between two floors (Figure 6-2). Now each stair represents a value, or a state, in the transition between floors. If our nervous person again stopped between floors on the stair, he or she would have to stand on one stair at a time. If, as before, our guest becomes nervous, he could shuffle back and forth on one stair or another but would not change height unless the shuffling became much larger than the stair. Thus, noise does not incur the same sort of change in this digital system as on the analog ramp. This illustrates two of the major benefits of digital systems: First, they are much less sensitive to noise than analog systems; and second, values in a digital system are discrete and well defined.

We can now develop our digital model further. Assume that the lower floor is a starting position, with the 12 feet between floors spanned by 12 steps, each step representing a value of height above the first floor. By numbering the face of each step, we could know exactly our position between the two floors simply by reading the numbers. We can therefore state a position on the stairs with representative numbers. Given this relationship between numbers and stairs, each position on the stairs can be a number between any 12 consecutive numbers. And with a fixed relationship, any number can represent a position on the stair. This system of numbers brings us to the computer.

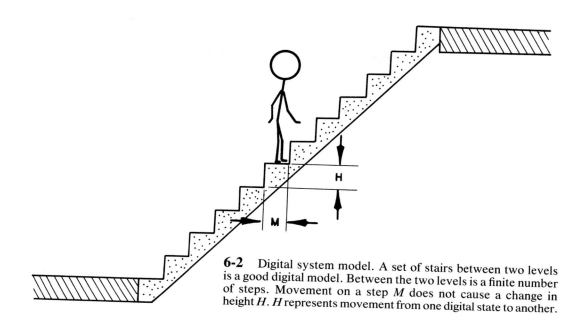

6-2 Digital system model. A set of stairs between two levels is a good digital model. Between the two levels is a finite number of steps. Movement on a step *M* does not cause a change in height *H*. *H* represents movement from one digital state to another.

Although computers run on numbers, they do not use just any number system. To simplify the internal design requirements for the computer, the system runs on a binary numbering system, using only two primary symbols, 1 and 0.

To understand the binary system, let's examine, first, the everyday base 10 or decimal system and the manner in which it codes values. The decimal system uses 10 discrete values from 0 to 9. Starting from 0 and counting to 9 covers these 10 values. At the value of 10, the primary count returns to 0, and we place a 1 to the left of the 0. This same uncomplicated system of symbolism is used in the binary numbering system.

In a binary system, the symbols for numbers are arrayed like the decimal system, but only two values are possible, 0 and 1. With only two values available, the number of elements needed to express any number will be much larger than the decimal system. For example, let us count to a value of 8, using both binary and decimal systems:

Binary	*Decimal*
0.	0.
1.	1.
10.	2.
11.	3.
100.	4.
101.	5.
110.	6.
111.	7.
1000.	8.

Clearly, each symbol in the binary system represents a multiplication of 2, just as each new symbol in the decimal system represents a multiplication of 10.

The advantage of the decimal system is writing efficiency: It takes fewer symbols to represent any number above 1. The computer, however, has a different set of needs, and the increased number of symbols needed to represent a value turns out not to be a problem because the computer is so fast. In addition, binary arithmetic in the computer makes the system logic much simpler and faster to execute.

A shorthand way of expressing large numbers is to use the "power" notation. For example, 100 becomes 10^2. Binary numbers can be expressed in a like manner using the number 2. Thus, 4 becomes 2^2, 8 is 2^3, 16 is 2^4, and 256 is 2^8. This notation is often used to describe scan converter and computer memories.

Another numbering system is often used in working with computers. This system, which is used not within the computer itself but by computer programmers, is called Octal, and, as the name implies, works on the base 8. The choice of base 8 derives from the connection between base 2 and base 8. For example, 111 in base 2 is equal to 7 in base 8. This is shown as $111_2 = 7_8$. This means that base-8 symbols can be used to represent any three symbols in binary notation. Just as in the binary and decimal system, counting and representation follow the same rules. Thus, $10_8 = 9_{10}$ and $20_8 = 16_{10}$. These relations can be easily derived by counting and using the standard rules of notation.

With an effective numbering system in hand, we can now examine the organization of the computer in general.

Organization of the Microcomputer

Any computer, including a microcomputer, is composed of three general components: 1) A central processing unit, or CPU; 2) A memory system, which includes a random access memory, or RAM; and 3) An input/output device, often called an I/O device [2]. All these components interact on a two-way basis, with information passing between them according to the operating organization of the computer. These elements and the information flow in a computer are shown in Figure 6-3.

The CPU contains all the operating logic for the computer as well as registers, arithmetic logic, timing instructions, and control circuits [2]. Instructions stored in memory are selected by the CPU and converted into a set of machine operations. The CPU controls information into and out of the memory and into and out of the whole system by controlling the I/O devices. It is the "brain" of the computer.

If the CPU is reduced in size, it becomes a micro-central processing unit, or microprocessor, containing all the same functions as the larger computer CPU. It is generally made of solid-state materials, and appears physically as a relatively large single component mounted onto a circuit board. Surrounding the microprocessor are other solid-state circuits, performing support functions for the micro-

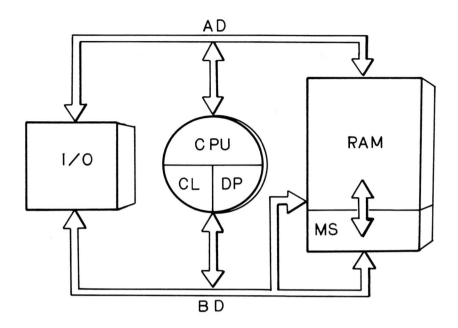

6-3 Organization of a basic digital computer. Two types of
information flow in a basic computer design: binary data *BD* and
address data *AD*. The address data keep the central processing
unit *CPU* informed on where the binary data are located. The
CPU often contains control logic processing *CL* data and arithmetic processing *DP*. Data flow into and out of the computer
through I/O devices. Data are stored within the computer system
in the random access memory *RAM* and in mass storage devices
MS such as magnetic tapes or magnetic floppy disks.

processor, including some memory circuits. If enough components are hung together,
the microprocessor board begins to look like a small computer. This has created
some confusion about the fine line between a microprocessor and a microcomputer.
Clearly, the microprocessor is a component of a microcomputer, but not the other
way around.

Essential to the functioning of a microprocessor and a microcomputer function
is a memory system, which stores digital information. To make the computer
flexible, part of this memory system needs to be accessible in a random manner.
This flexible portion of the memory is the random access memory (RAM). The
remainder of the memory system is usually less flexible, slower in accepting or
transferring data, and specialized in its use.

The fundamental memory unit is the *bit,* which can assume one of two states:
"on," representing the number 1, and "off," representing the number 0. These
bits are collected into functional groups called *words*. For most microcomputers,
these words are 8 bits long. In addition, regardless of the word size in the computer,
these 8-bit units are called *bytes*. The memory capacity of a system or any subunit
of a system is often expressed in the number of memory bytes available. For

example, a memory of 32 kilobytes has 32,000 bytes of memory, or 256,000 bits of storage. Even if some devices have 16-bit words, the memory is still expressed in units of bytes.

A memory system can contain other methods of storing information such as ROMs, PROMs, and EPROMs, specialized memories based on solid-state electronics. A ROM, for example, is a read only memory with instructions and numbers that are fixed and invariant. ROM instructions are often produced by the physical organization of the circuit and cannot be reprogrammed into another form. A PROM (programmable read only memory), on the other hand, is a read only memory that is programmable. This memory also has fixed information, but the information can be changed according to the use of the computer. Once the numbers are set into a PROM, however, they are permanent. To change the numbers, a new PROM is programmed and replaces the old one in the circuit. An EPROM, unlike the previous memory systems, can be erased and reprogrammed as needed for specialized repeated tasks. EPROM stands for erasable programmable read only memory.

Outside the physical confines of the RAM and PROMs are memory systems that accept large amounts of data for storage. Mass-data storage includes magnetic tape in the form of reel-to-reel tapes, audio cassettes, and magnetic discs that fall into two classes, *floppy discs* and *hard discs*. In their current form, floppy discs and tapes can be removed and physically stored somewhere else until the information they contain is needed by the operator. Hard discs, on the other hand, stay with the computer, and have a slightly different function. They store data that has an intermediate life, and are changed by date or need. These additional storage techniques extend the use of the computer and give it a long-term memory that a RAM alone could not provide.

Somehow the instructions used by the CPU to make the computer operate must be put into memory. Moreover, once the computer operations are complete, any new information generated by the computer must reach the outside. This transfer of information into and out of the computer is handled by the I/O devices, which are under CPU control. I/O devices can include a printer, a cathode ray tube (CRT), or a telephone line. Computers can even create music and play it through speakers.

The organization and function both of microcomputers and of larger computers appear outwardly to be the same. What, then, makes one "micro" and the other "macro?" The answer is in the nature of the CPU. The first major difference relates to size. If the processor is a small dedicated system, called a microprocessor, then the system is a microcomputer. It is not the memory size that is micro, however. Many microprocessors handle an identical or an even larger memory size than larger computers. Microprocessors, however, work more slowly. Therein lies a second important difference. The forte of the larger computer is speed. While the microcomputer is slower, however, it is also less expensive and therefore more accessible to many individuals and departments. Each machine has a role in ultrasound. The section following describes some of the computer functions that computers and microcomputers share.

Speaking "Computer"

Computers have thus far been described in terms of the functions of their *hardware*. Also essential to the computer is the set of instructions used to run the machine. These instructions are called *software*. Although the software runs the hardware, however, the software is useless without the hardware. The combination of hardware and software working together gives the computer its utility.

As noted earlier, instructions for the CPU are stored as binary numbers according to a code understood by the CPU. To the uninitiated, a list of these binary codes would be as unintelligible as were the ancient Egyptian writings without the Rosetta Stone. Thus, an "interpreter" of sorts is needed.

The human-machine interpreter takes human-generated statements and converts them into binary code for the computer. When the computer finishes its task, the interpreter converts the binary code back into words and graphics the human operator can understand. This interpretive function is put into the computer as a set of instructions that tell the machine how to deal with both types of instructions. A high-level computer language is the result [3]. Among various computer languages are COBOL, BASIC, Pascal, and FORTRAN [3]. Why so many different languages? The answer is that no single language can efficiently handle all possible applications; thus, each language is designed for special tasks such as mathematical problems, general business problems, or interactive education.

Computer languages are formal in character, with a rigid syntax. This formality prevents double meanings or confusion in the sequence of instructions programmed by the operator. The symbols within the language, however, are often standard mathematical symbols and English words.

Instructions provided by the operator can be handled in the computer in two ways. Some languages, for example, use a process in which high-level language instructions are converted into machine language on each execution of the instruction. These languages permit easy modification of the programs as they are written and executed by the computer, and are said to use an *interpreter*. Other languages take the input language instructions and assemble an efficient machine language sequence from the original instructions. When a change is made in the program, however, the whole program must be reassembled into its new form. This process is called *compiling*, and the software used to do this is called a *compiler* [3].

As the computer grows in sophistication, the associated software also increases in complexity. For example, a computer needs a number of housekeeping functions to assure that data are shuffled smoothly from device to device, or location to location. These functions require complicated instructions. To assist in this, a series of programs, called an *operating system*, is used in the computer to operate the system as a functional whole. Like computer languages, operating systems have a variety of names and purposes [4]. An operating system in fact, influences the way computers interact with their operators as strongly as do the physical characteristics of the hardware.

Software in the form of machine-level languages, operating languages, or operating systems require as much engineering ability to master as any piece of hardware. Furthermore, the development of a software design often takes as much human time and effort as a hardware design. This fact is considered later when we examine the value of computer-controlled sonographs. First, a look at what happens when a microprocessor is put inside a sonograph.

The Microprocessor Within

For a salesperson to mention that a given sonograph has a microprocessor or a microcomputer inside is an invariably effective sales pitch. Exactly what can a microprocessor do inside a sonograph, and what makes it a valuable addition to the sonograph?

One of the first things a microprocessor can do is control the routing of signals from one board to another within the sonograph [5]. This comes about because of a machine organization called a *bus system,* in which all of the input and output routes to all boards are placed parallel to each other. While the multiplicity of resulting signals could potentially cause mass confusion, the signals are routed properly to each board by making each board identifiable with an address much like the address that is used in a RAM to store and retrieve data. Thus, the circuit boards can be inserted into the sonograph in any sequence, and the signals will still find the correct routing within the sonograph. This bus system opens the door to faster and better designs for the sonograph and offers a chance to expand sonograph functions with options by simple circuit-board plug-in. It is the microprocessor that makes this design most efficient.

One of the earliest and most successful applications of the microprocessor has been that of managing the input and output from a digital scan converter [5, 6]. In this application, the scan converter RAM stores image information and the microprocessor goes to a PROM to obtain its instructions on how to handle the data [5]. Scan converter management is only a small load for the typical microprocessor, however, so the sonograph design was altered to let the microprocessor manage other parts of the sonograph as well. For example, digital encoders have been added to the scanning arm providing a B-scanner with digitally calculated, position information. Although this application requires a ''zeroing'' procedure to let the digital read-out system know where to start, the method has been integrated successfully in several B-scanner designs on the market [5].

The microprocessor furthermore assumed a more tedious yet valuable function in the sonograph, namely, generating the characters for labeling images with information like the patient's identification, scan position information, time, and date. Even the electronic calipers are under microprocessor control.

These uses of the microprocessor are examples of simple machine management. A new use is now gaining interest: numerical image analysis. To help make image analysis easier, other digital technologies are being used such as light pens, digitizing pads, or steering controls that give the computer coordinate information to make calculations such as circumferences, slopes, areas, and signal values. The operator need only outline or otherwise indicate the area of interest, and the computer does the rest. If calculations are too long, or follow a regular set of values that are complicated to calculate, the analysis can still be performed quickly by giving the microprocessor a ''look-up'' table of values to search, rather than making a calculation. The table's values are stored in a PROM, which provides rapid, easy access to the information.

''Look-up'' tables are often used with digital scan converters to manage the preprocessing and postprocessing when presenting image information. The instructions are stored on PROMs and read by the microprocessor during the scanning process to define how the data are to be presented.

Accompanying the increased processing on the inside of the sonograph, is the development of opportunities to use microcomputers outside the sonograph.

The Computer Outside

On the outside, the microcomputer often appears in the form of an analysis cart, taking on some difficult analysis normally unavailable to the sonographer and sonologist. Much of this work is new, currently presenting only a glimmer of what is to come.

A good example of one such difficult analysis is calculating the Fourier frequency components of a complex wave form on a real-time basis (Chapter 8). A dedicated microprocessor makes this rapid calculation possible. These devices have enabled new Doppler ultrasound applications, not to mention new methods of analyzing echoes from stationary sources [7].

Larger computers are also being attached to the sonograph to acquire large blocks of image information for digital manipulation [10]. These stored data are combined by the computer to obtain unusual contrast information, or they process the image to remove enhancement or shadows. We have the digital computer to thank for such new applications.

The evolution involves more than just adding a microprocessor or microcomputer to the sonograph, however. Increasingly, the sonograph itself resembles a computer.

The ''Soft'' Sonograph

An examination of the more advanced sonographs suggests that the nature of the sonograph is changing so that it now looks more like a computer with a ''data acquisition'' segment hung on the computer input. The sonograph is run on software just like a computer. The software influence extends even to the front panel controls in some sonographs, where the controls are sampled and operating values determined by a microprocessor. This sort of interaction leads to what is called a "software-driven" sonograph.

A major selling point for such sonographs is to state they are "software controlled," and are therefore easily updated. How true is this statement? To find the answer, we must look at how a soft sonograph is put together.

Most software-driven sonographs are programmed at the machine language level. A higher-level language would need a compiler or an interpreter to translate the instructions, which takes time away from the control sequence. It is thus more efficient to use machine language from the beginning. But writing machine language requires both education and experience, as well as patience. For example, the whole program is often written in parts and the parts fitted together to form the complete control package. But because programs seldom work with complete success when first written, extra time and effort must go into "debugging" them to understand where and why they are functioning improperly. The development cycle of new sonograph designs has shown that in many companies software development lags behind hardware development. Thus, a software-driven machine or any upgrade in the machine design may not arrive in the marketplace any faster than a more conventional, hardware device or design improvement.

If software does not substantially change the rate of machine evolution, then what are the benefits of a "soft" sonograph? First, using software usually means that the machine can be upgraded more easily in the field. In general, only a new set of PROMs are needed for a field upgrade and can be placed into the sonograph by the field service engineer. Second, once upgrades are decided upon, machines that are altered will look and act much like all the other upgraded machines, thus insuring a uniformity in meeting change specifications. Third, from the beginning, sonographs with the same design will have a similar appearance, reducing the problems of large variations among the same machines. The fourth and perhaps the greatest benefit relates to the development and manufacture of sonographs. With data bus systems, software-driven front panels, and digital displays, the sonograph software can be developed in parallel with the hardware, thus shortening the development cycle. The result is a more sophisticated sonograph, developed in a shorter time at a lower cost.

But even if an upgrade is not faster, a software-driven sonograph has the potential for a better-quality upgrade than a strictly hardware device. This advantage could be lost, however, if the changes in science and technology exceed the capacity of the software to change machine operation. In this case, keeping current for the customer means purchasing a new sonograph.

Conclusions

The technology of medical sonography is changing at an astonishingly rapid rate. One of the primary benefits of this change is the introduction of the microprocessor as an organizer and manager of data in the sonograph, from performing such mundane chores as providing labels and making measurements, to offering a high-level analysis of the signals stored in the sonograph memory. With the small set of computer fundamentals thus far described, we are in a better position to understand the value of a computer within the sonograph or of a small or large computer attached to the sonograph from the outside. Technology has by no means exploited all the possibilities of sonograph evolution along this branch. We can expect a great deal more to come.

References

1. Powis, R.L. Computer based medical education in ultrasound. July/August 1981. Radiology Today 3:16–23.
2. Gillmore, C.M. 1978. Beginner's guide to microprocessors. Blue Ridge Summit, PA: Tab Books.
3. Boyd, A., P. Good, and S. Velt. May 1981. A user's guide to operating systems. Personal Computing: 27.
4. Mazur, K. May 1981. Understanding interpreters and compilers. Personal Computing   :39.
5. Waxman, A. The use of microprocessors in gray scale ultrasound. Santa Clara, CA: Searle Ultrasound (2270 Martin Avenue, Santa Clara, CA 95050).
6. Ophir, J., and N.F. Maklad. April 1979. Digital scan converters in diagnostic ultrasound imaging. Proc IEEE 67:654–664.
7. Lerski, R.A., *et al*. 1979. Computer analysis of ultrasonic signals in diffuse liver disease. Ultrasound Med Biol 5:341–350.
8. Robinson, D.E., and G. Kossoff. July 1979. Computer processing of line mode echogram data. International Congress Series 505. In Proceedings of the Second Meeting of the World Federation for Ultrasound in Medicine and Biology, ed. T. Wagai and R. Omoto.   :11–16.

Chapter 7

How to Scan Faster Than the Eye Can See: Real-Time Systems

We learned about the formation of two-dimensional images in Chapter 2, on B-scanning. To briefly summarize here, to form an image, the sonographer moves the transducer over the body surface, and the returning echoes are transduced into electrical signals that are stored in the scanner memory. The most physically demanding part of this imaging scheme is moving the transducer so that the scan lines used to generate the image are uniformly distributed throughout the image. When enough of the image appears to make a judgement on the quality of the image, the sonographer decides whether or not to keep the image. This decision is based on such items as: the organs depicted; the quality of the scanning; the proper field of view; and the presence of pathology. The result is a series of static images of the body, stored on X-ray film, depicting the body in various cross sections.

Consider a situation, however, in which the physically difficult part of the image-making process is automated. In such a setup the transducer—or more correctly, the ultrasound beam—is moved automatically. We can increase beam movement to a point that image formation is limited by how far the ultrasound must travel in order to return echoes to the transducer. The image is refreshed with each beam sweep, and as the transducer is moved about, the echo signals change with the movement. The echo sources thus change in "real time." The image is still two-dimensional but is rapidly refreshed with each scan of the ultrasound beam. If we increase the scanning rate sufficiently, the scans blend together so smoothly that the motion within the scanning field can be portrayed, while still presenting organ size, shape, position, and texture. Thus, a real-time system is, in actuality, an automated B-scanning process in which the motion of the ultrasound beam is under machine control (Figure 7-1). Positioning the scanning plane, choosing the organs to be scanned, setting time gain compensation (TGC), and recognizing structures, however, are still in the hands of the sonographer.

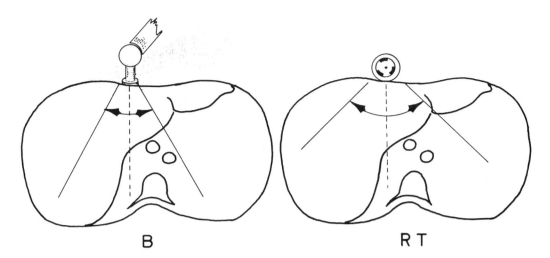

B   R T

7-1   The connection between B-scanning and real-time scanning. *B* represents a single-pass B-scan with a single transducer.
A real-time system *RT* carries out a similar sort of scan, but
transducer movement is under machine control.

Because we are still dealing with a B-scanning process, the basic formation of
signals to be displayed is the same. But as in B-scanning, the direction of the
ultrasound beam must be known by the machine in order to place the trace on the
display correctly. The position information is encoded through techniques specialized for the various methods of moving the ultrasound beam. Once the returning
echo forms a primary signal in the transducer, amplification and detection of the
signal are very much the same as in the B-scanner. Real-time systems can employ
all of the detection schemes that are possible in the B-scanner. Once a video signal
is formed, it can be stored, but only to a limited degree. It is at the transducer and
display levels that static and real-time scanners begin to diverge significantly.

The constantly reconstructed image of a real-time system means that a very
short-term memory can be used. For example, a medium- or short-persistance
phosphor on a cathode ray tube (CRT) forms a stable analog image. But image
information often needs to be inserted in a patient's record (written remarks about
what was in the image are usually inadequate).

A record of the image therefore can be made by placing a camera to the face of
the CRT and taking a photograph. However, details of the image will reproduce
well in the photograph only by holding the transducer still. Moreover, because the
image cannot be seen and photographed at the same time from a single monitor,
what ends up on film is often uncertain.

Early static scanners turned to an analog scan converter to provide a stable
image display that could be immediately evaluated and photographed if desired.
This technological addition to the static B-scanner changed the style of B-scanner
use. But the analog scan converter is not good at rapid-image formation and
selected erasure, abilities that are needed in a real-time sonograph. As a result,

analog scan conversion was never really suited for real-time applications. On the other hand, the digital scan converter was a "natural" for the requirements of real time.

Organization to Move the Beam

From the outside, the most obvious difference between a real-time system and a static B-scanner is the transducer. And among the designs for real-time systems, the outstanding difference is again the transducer. The task is to move the ultrasound beam automatically, and numerous techniques are available to do this. New techniques are being developed by many ultrasound companies. Understanding the essentials of real time will enable the rapid application of these new technologies once they arrive on the market.

The first means of moving an ultrasound beam was simply to move or wobble the transducer in a sector (Figure 7-2). This technique coupled a single transducer with a motor to drive the transducer in a sweeping sector motion. In one early model, the transducer directly contacted the skin, and the real-time image appeared for only the short time it took for the wobbling motion to squeeze the coupling gel out from the transducer-skin interface. Later, placing the transducer inside a housing filled with fluid permitted free movement of the transducer and improved ultrasonic coupling into the tissues. The fluid bath can range in size from a small volume in a plastic cap to a very large water volume with a large transducer placed inside (Figure 7-3). Regardless of size, the task is the same: to have controlled motion of the transducer in the fluid medium, with the ultrasound coupled to the patient through the fluid medium.

The limitations in using a fluid-filled housing are inherent in the transducer movement design itself. For example, transducers placed within a fluid-filled chamber are not easily changed to handle varying patient conditions. In addition, the scanning can be nonuniform near the edges of the scanning field, where the transducer must be slowed, stopped, and then driven in the opposite direction. And as the fluid path between the transducer and the body increases, the scanning sector angle decreases. As a result of this scanning geometry within the fluid path, wobblers have typical scanning angles of 30° to 60°, with only a few reaching 90° or beyond. All of these transducers are grouped under the general heading of mechanical sector scanners.

Among the mechanical sector scanners is the rotating head transducer assembly (Figure 7-2). In this design, one or several transducers are mounted in a cylinder that is rotated using a small servo-controlled motor. The cylinder sits in a fluid-filled chamber to allow controlled rotation of the cylinder and transducers. The fluid-path container or cap is often shaped to match the circular motion of the rotor. The size of the cap is a function of the transducer diameter, the number of transducers, and the distance between the transducers and the cap. Unlike the wobbler, this beam-movement design is constant and uniform, with no inertial

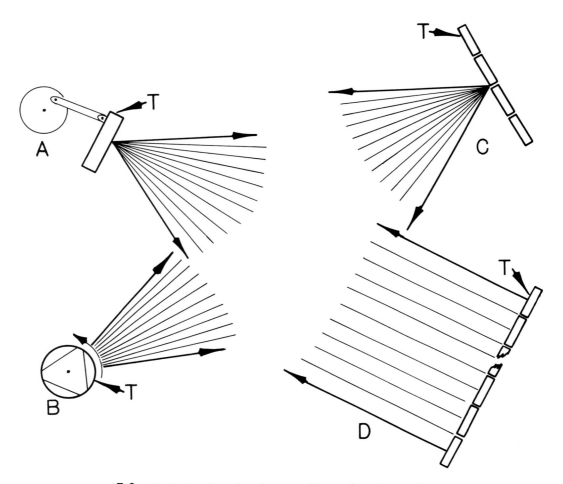

7-2   Methods of moving ultrasound beams in real time. Example A shows a single transducer *T*, driven by a small motor, generally called a wobbler. Example B shows a rotating cylinder with several transducers, generally called a rotating scanhead. Example C shows a sector scan from a phased array. Beam movement here is electronic. Example D shows a linear array of elements, and the beam is electronically scanned down the array.

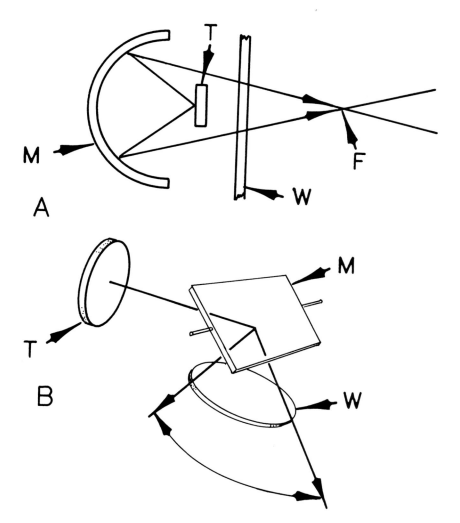

7-3 Use of mirrors and water paths in real-time scanheads. In part A, an unfocused transducer *T* can be placed in front of a mirror *M* to focus the beam *F* through an acoustic window *W*. In Part B, a focused, stationary transducer coupled with a moving mirror can carry out a sector scan through an acoustic window *W*.

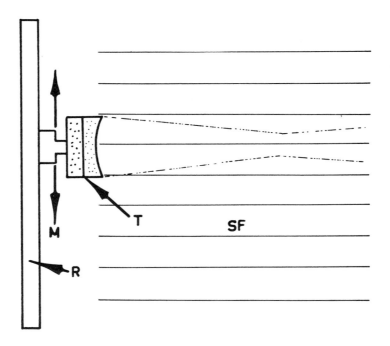

7-4 Single-element linear real-time scanning. Effective, small-parts scanning is possible with a single transducer *T* moved along a single track *R* to produce a linear scanning field *SF*.

problems of starting and stopping the transducer motion. Because of the small distance between the transducer and cap, rotating transducers can have sectors typically larger than wobblers, varying from 90° to 120°. Like the wobbler, however, the transducers are usually fixed focus, and the housing prevents any effective changes in transducers to match scanning problems in the patient.

For both the wobbler and the rotating scanhead, the field of view is a sector (Figure 7-2). But this is not the case in another mechanical scanner, which moves a single transducer laterally in a tracked, linear scan (Figure 7-4). The linear motion produces a rectangular field of view. Because of the physical problems in moving the transducer over large distances, these scanheads are specialized for small-parts scanning, and require fixed, sharply focused transducers moved over short, linear scanning paths.

Another mechanical method of producing a linear scanning field is that of rotating a small transducer in a sector, while the ultrasound beam is directed at a parabolic mirror (Figure 7-5). The transducer sits at the effective focal point for the mirror, which forms a set of parallel beams at the entrance into the body. Because of the problems attendant with making large acoustic mirrors, this scanning technique has also been limited to small-parts and small-area scanning.

So far, we have moved the ultrasound beam by moving the transducer. The goal, however, is to move only the ultrasound beam. Movement is also possible if we form and move a wave front as a source of waves. This is the concept behind the phased-array systems. A wave front is formed from a set of transducer elements

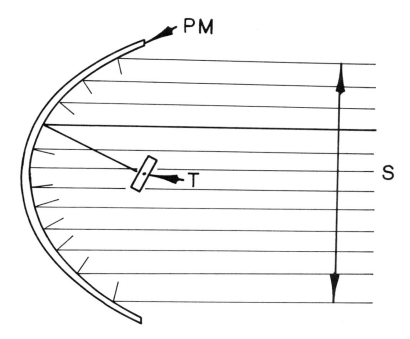

7-5   Single-element linear real-time scanning using a mirror. A linear scanning field *S* can result from placing a rotating transducer *T* at the focal point of the parabolic mirror *PM*. This approach has found utility in small parts and vascular scanning.

that are themselves unfocused. The constructed wave front is usually bent to send the ultrasonic waves to a focal region, and at the same time, is electronically steered in a sector scan. The transducer has no moving parts; the focusing and steering are accomplished by changing the timing among transducer elements. This technique is examined in more detail later in the chapter.

The annular array represents a technological mix of both the phased array and mechanical sector scanner [1]. The individual annular rings are controlled like the phased array to form a curved wave front that can focus to a point. Moving the beam, however, requires moving the whole array, which can be damaging to delicate transducers. To protect the transducer elements, the array is often held stationary and the beam reflected off a plane mirror [2]. The mirror can move in a controlled wobble, or several mirrors can be rotated like a rotating transducer. A standoff between the mirror and array permits larger-diameter arrays to be used than would be possible if the transducer were in direct contact with the skin. These larger diameters can place focal zones longer distances from the transducer, with extended focal zones as well. The concepts behind both the phased and annual array were covered in Chapter 3. The annular array is discussed in more detail later in this chapter.

Timing events, as used in a phased array to form and focus a transducer beam, can also be used in very large linear arrays. The beam, however, is moved in a linear fashion down the array. The result is a combination of the focusing techniques used for phased arrays, with a controlled sequence-switch that moves the beam along the array. The result is a rectangular field of view. Like the phased array, the focal-zone position is often a front-panel control, permitting either regional selections or a more dynamic process that involves automatically moving the focal zone and creating the final image from only the focal-zone positions. This technique is called *dynamic focusing*. Like the phased array, linear arrays are treated in more detail later.

Unlike static B-scanning, timing plays a more central role in real time. The following section looks more closely at the timing architecture of real time.

Timing Considerations in Image Formation

Like the static B-scanner, a real-time system builds a two-dimensional image from a series of individual pulse-listen cycles, storing the acquired data on each cycle. Using the soft-tissue average propagation velocity of 1,540 m/s, the echo transit time is 13 µs (13×10^{-6} s) for each centimeter of tissue depth. Consequently, the maximum time it takes for the most distant echo to reach the transducer in any field of view is:

$$PLT = (13 \times 10^{-6} \text{ s/cm}) \times FOV, \tag{7.1}$$

where PLT is the pulse-listen time, and FOV is the field of view in centimeters. If N is the number of lines of sight that make up a single image frame, then the time for a single frame is:

$$FT = PLT \times N, \tag{7.2}$$

where FT is the time to scan one image frame. The maximum rate at which the image can be renewed, then, is the reciprocal of the frame time FT, and

$$FR = 1/FT, \tag{7.3}$$

where FR is the frame rate in hertz. Clearly, then, the frame rate of any real-time device will be limited by the depth of the field of view and the number of lines used to make one image frame.

Several calculations can show the limitations these equations impose. For example, consider a 10-cm field of view. The total time to obtain echoes from 10 cm deep will be:

$$PLT = (13 \times 10^{-6} \text{ s/cm}) \times 10 \text{ cm} = 130 \times 10^{-6} \text{ s}.$$

If each frame of the real-time image has 120 lines, then the time for one frame will be:

$$FT = 130 \times 10^{-6} \text{ s} \times 120 = 1.56 \times 10^{-2} \text{ s}.$$

The frame rate, FR, will be equal to:

$$FR = 1/(1.56 \times 10^{-2} \text{ sec}) = 64 \text{ Hz}.$$

The highest frame rate possible, then, is 64 Hz. The actual frame rate on the machine can run less than but not faster than that. Calculations for other situations can show that as the field of view or depth increases, the maximum available frame rate decreases.

If, however, we want to keep the frame rate of the device constant and still increase the depth of field, the number of lines that form each image frame has to decrease. And these are precisely the trade-offs that are made when moving to a high scan-density, high-resolution, real-time image. The trade-off becomes even more acute when dynamic focusing is added to a system.

In dynamic focusing, the focal zone is moved to several positions within the field of view, and the image is constructed only from the signals contained in the focal zone. If a machine has four of these dynamic focusing zones, for example, then each line of sight on the display is really made from four pulse-listen cycles, where the focal zone is moved into a new region on each cycle. If we look back at our calculated example, dynamic focusing over four zones would quarter the frame rate to 16 Hz.

Dynamic focusing, then, can provide high-resolution images, but the sacrifice entails a lowered rate of image formation, and, importantly, a lessened ability to depict motion with the real-time system. This shortfall in the resolution of dynamics will be most evident in the large field-of-view, high-resolution, real-time systems. In fact, the degradation in resolving motion is so significant with dynamic focusing that it is not a useful technique for echocardiography.

Experience indicates that a minimum number of scan lines is needed to successfully depict anatomy within a cross section [3]. As a result, a balance exists between the number of scan lines, the frame rate, and the field of view for a real-time system. Most real-time sonographs use 100 lines to 256 lines to form an image. Typical frame rates are 15 Hz to 50 Hz. But at the largest fields of view, the frame rates are at their lowest, limiting the usefulness of real time for fast-moving structures. The heart is such a structure, and motion here requires a fairly high frame rate. In obstetrics, for example, high frame rates are needed to correctly estimate heart rate or to begin to identify heart disease in the neonate. A comparison of numbers might help define some of the useful boundaries of any real-time device.

Consider a heart rate of 80 beats per minute (bpm). The heart is beating every 60 s/80 bpm = 1.33 bps (beats per second). A frame rate of 15 frames per second will divide this motion into 15 parts every second, separated by 66 ms (66×10^{-3} s). Rapid-moving structures such as an opening or closing mitral valve or moving aortic valve will not be completely depicted. And as the heart rate increases, the ability to depict motion will decrease. In contrast, a fetus with a heart rate of 170 beats per minute will have about 2.8 beats every second. A frame rate of 15 frames per second will divide those 2.8 beats into 15 parts. This lets us accurately determine the heart rate, but any detailed characteristics of heart motion will be lost in the slow frame rate. In adult echocardiography, a frame rate of at least 30 frames per second is needed to adequately sample the heart motion. For children or neonates with higher heart rates, the frame rate must be even higher.

It turns out that most of the available real-time machines have a maximum field-of-view depth of close to 20 cm. This could just be a coincidence, but a few calculations will show a common thread of balancing the frame rate against the field-of-view depth. To begin, consider a frame rate that produces a flicker-free display at 30 frames per second, which is easily matched to a standard TV display. The time to form a single frame, which we will call the frame time is:

$$FT = 1/30 \; Hz = 0.033 \text{ s.} \tag{7.4}$$

If the image takes 128 lines to form a single image frame, then the frame time divided by the number of lines (128) will produce the time to make 1 line of sight. The estimate of the number of lines per frame comes from an observation that more than 100 lines are needed to make an image appear complete, but more than 150 lines will produce significant overscanning even in the wider portions of the beam. Also, 128 is 2^7, which is a number that can be generated by simple digital control circuits. Continuing our calculation, the pulse-listen time, PLT, for one line of sight is:

$$PLT = 0.033 \text{ s}/128 \text{ lines} = 2.6 \times 10^{-4} \text{ s.}$$

If we now divide PLT by the transit time for each centimeter of tissue, we get the resulting field of view depth, which is:

$$FOV = 2.6 \times 10^{-4} \text{ s}/13 \times 10^{-6} \text{ s/cm}$$
$$FOV = 20 \text{ cm.}$$

Other factors likely entered the decision as well, such as the typical depth of information portrayed on a static B-scanner. The reasons for the choices may be hard to find, but the connection between the frame rate and the depth of field is solid. Understanding the limits of data gathering can clearly define the limits of machine design.

Image Considerations Unique to Real Time

The typical digital, static B-scanner gathers image data into the scan converter memory at a pulse repetition frequency (PRF) of 1,000 Hz to 2,000 Hz. A PRF of 1000 Hz will produce 2,500 pulse-listen cycles within a 2.5-s scan. The distance traveled by the transducer can be quite small, producing a markedly overscanned image in that several pulse-listen cycles will go into the specific information occupying a given pixel. Within the B-scanner scan converter is "peak value" detection, where the largest value for any pixel is chosen from all the available values. This is called the "compound mode" in some systems. Regardless of name, the technique requires keeping the largest value for all the signals presented to occupy any pixel.

When the B-scanner storage rules are changed to a *last-value mode,* also known as the *survey mode,* the latest value from the last pulse-listen cycle is used to fill the memory location. On the display, the image changes as if the gain in the system were suddenly decreased. The image can be partly restored by increasing either the gain of the receiver or the output from the transmitter some 6 dB to 9 dB. The amount of increase is often a function of how good the peak value selection process is in the scan converter. These altered image qualities can be observed by anyone with a current digital B-scanner that has both a compound and a survey mode.

What does this have to do with real time? In fact, the last-value mode of operation is the normal mode of operation for a real-time system. Each line of sight is a single pulse-listen cycle, and the echo information is stored in memory or brought to the display in a relatively untarnished form. None of the current real-time machines appears to apply any sort of time averaging or overscanning techniques that would permit a peak value to represent any given echo signal. The combined frame rate and line-density requirements of real time provides a major barrier to any sort of peak-value processing. Even in real-time systems using dynamic focusing, each segment of the image is formed from a single pulse-listen cycle.

Both overall image quality and penetration by a real-time system are affected by underscanning. The textural qualities of real-time systems are different from those of the B-scanner, although the ability to separate unlike tissues may not be compromised. For like gains, the ultrasound power output from a real-time system is often higher than the B-scanner, owing to the nature of last-value scanning.

Along with acquiring echo information on a single pass, the real-time transducer is in motion during both transmitting and receiving segments in all the mechanical scanners. Does this motion play a role in image formation? We can determine this by comparing the lateral motion of the ultrasound beam with the axial motion of the ultrasound burst.

Consider a transducer moving through a 90° sector, with a frame rate of 30 frames per second. In addition, the field is composed of 128 lines of sight. The transducer must span the field in the time it takes to form one frame, which is 0.033 s. In the 90° sector, the transducer is moving 90° in 0.033 s, which is 90°/0.033 s = 2727°/s. It takes ultrasound 20×13 μs = 260 μs to traverse 20 cm of tissue. Thus, the beam will move 260×10^{-6} s $\times$ 2727°/s = 0.71° in the time that it takes for an ultrasound burst to leave the transducer, reach 20 cm in the tissue, and return. This timing means that at the 20-cm depth, the transducer axis will have moved 200 mm $\times$ tan (0.71°) = 2.5 mm. This is considerably less than the effective beam width at the same range for most transducers. Thus, transducer motion will not significantly increase any blur in the image. What causes the image to blur in some machines, then? Although there could be any number of causes, transducer motion during image formation is not one of them.

One of the more obvious but least considered aspects of real-time scanning is the fixed angle the beam scans through within the scanning plane. This fixed angle forces an unusual signal mix to form the image of organs or structures. The beam may not always be perpendicular or even close to perpendicular to the boundaries and structures depicted in the image. The result is an uneven presentation of boundaries in any single view. Compared to the static B-scanner, a real-time system does not provide the single-scan adaptability of a single transducer mounted on a flexible scanning arm. On the other hand, the mobility of the real-time transducer can counteract this limitation by increasing the number of views for any single organ or structure.

Along with the incomplete boundaries, a fixed-angle scanning system also has a changing axial resolution that is a function of the incident angle between the beam axis and the interface being examined. In addition, axial resolution is a function of the effective beam width. Thus, linear scanning on nonlinear structures and sector scanning on near-linear structures produces axial resolution and measurement problems near the edge of the image. It is natural and wise to place the beam orthogonal to the surfaces of interest, near the center of the scan field, and at the same time to accept the degraded image at the edges of the field. Examples of the problems in fixed-angle scanning are illustrated in Figures 7-6 and 7-7.

Enhancing the depiction of organ boundaries when the beam is not orthogonal to the interface is the degree of focusing in the transducer. Medium focused transducers, for example, have an increased ability to look at specular reflectors away from 90°. A weakly focused transducer, in contrast, cannot support much deviation from normal before the specular reflector signal drops more than 20 dB in amplitude [3]. Many of the current real-time systems have well-focused transducers that allow larger deviations from the perpendicular, yet still depict boundaries.

In contrast to specular reflection, the scattering that composes most of the tissue texture information is fairly independent of the ultrasound beam direction. As a result, the portrayed tissue texture is a function of both the transducer diameter and the transducer center operating frequency. As the frequency increases, for example, the larger scattering sites become more specular in quality, changing the image texture. Many of the contributors to tissue texture, however, are still quite small, and textural information is still identifiable for tissues regardless of frequency.

Because of the large signal mix commonly presented to a real-time system, the evolution of image quality has been dramatic. An examination of early unfocused linear-array and mechanical wobbler images reveals little appreciation of the gray-scale requirements that are incumbent on current real-time systems. The only truly consistent display of gray scale came from early Kossoff machines. The latest entrants into the marketplace, however, demonstrate a recognition of the essential elements of image formation that will permit real-time systems to compete with the static B-scanner in image quality.

Beyond handling signals within a real-time system is the necessity of managing the image at the display. The human visual process is geared to discriminate between boundaries and, moreover, between boundaries that move [5]. The visual discrimination of a boundary can be enhanced by displaying the echo signals as white on a black background. In this display format, the boundaries appear subjectively larger, and are easy to see when in motion [6]. If the signal- to noise-ratio

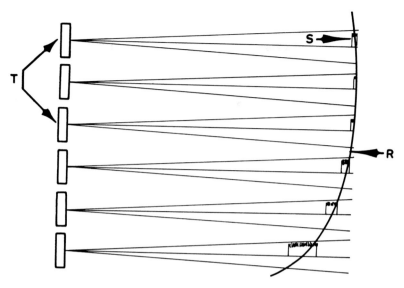

7-6 Problems with beam width and linear scanning. Because of the fixed angle scanning of the linear array, curved interfaces *R* can appear thicker than life because of beam-width integration onto the axial signal *S*, producing, as well, a loss in axial resolution.

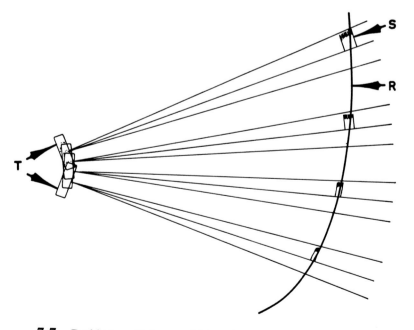

7-7 Problems with beam width and sector scanning. Because of the fixed-angle scanning of the sector scanner, interfaces at an angle with the beam can be thicker than life because of beam-width integration onto the axial signal *S*, producing as well, a loss in axial resolution.

in the image is small, however, freezing the image can result in an apparent loss of resolution. In actuality, the problem is one of discriminating a static boundary in the face of noise. This is like trying to look through a wet, spotted windshield in the rain. Behind the standing visual noise of spots and drops, boundaries and objects in motion can be appreciated, but they essentially disappear when motionless.

On the other hand, displaying black on a white background provides a chance to depict small signals that are barely discernable against the display gray background. As a result, many of the noise problems contained in real-time image formation become more evident. But as the number of grays used to depict the image increases from 16 to 64, the depiction of small signals improves, and the small signals that help create the tissue texture are more readily visualized. The physiology of visual perception and how it relates to displays is discussed further in Chapter 16.

Interfacing the Image to the Outside

Once the scanning transducer beam gathers the image data, it must be displayed. The earliest method of display was an analog cathode ray tube with a phosphor combination that retained the image long enough to prevent an intensity flicker at slow scanning rates but was fast enough to maintain the real-time qualities of the machine display. The CRT trace simply maps the position of the ultrasound beam on the display, refreshing the image at the ultrasound beam scanning rate. Many of the current real-time systems still use this display.

A primary limitation with this sort of display is a lack of compatibility with other equipment. If another display is added to the system, the new display must be a replica of the first, with a common set of beam-intensity and position signals. And the signals that drive these CRTs may not be effective on CRTs of a different design or manufacture. Recording images onto another medium such as a videotape is also not possible because the driving signals for the display do not fit into the videotape-recorder format. Photos are possible provided the transducer is held still and the face of the display CRT photographed. But dynamic organs such as the heart cannot be usefully recorded with a simple camera.

One method of circumventing this limitation in the analog display is to mount a video camera in front of the CRT and hook the camera output to a video display. This technique converts the image-formation rate determined by the real-time frame rate to a standard video format [7]. Now the image can be shown on other standard monitors and recorded onto videotape. The video recording later can be played back through the TV monitor or through another monitor. Further, the images can be replayed as desired, stopped and a single frame examined, or advanced in slow motion. All this added capability results from choosing the right medium to display and store the images.

Between the display CRT that we see and the image formed on the original sonograph display is another layer of technology that must be matched to the sonograph and our visual requirements. The adjustment end point is a good image transfer through the interface to the TV display that removes no diagnostic information [7]. This form of scan conversion is not expensive if strict boundaries are not placed on the information transfer. But, like the sonograph, the video components in this technology layer wear out; consequently, the whole system must be monitored for drift or variations in component functioning that can covertly change gray scale. This is still a successful means of providing scan conversion in machines not designed to do so already, and extends the utility of an initially limited sonograph.

Of course, images can be recorded by mounting a camera on the front panel, using any of the available photo formats. Although a still camera cannot provide explicit information on dynamics, it can be synchronized with cardiac events, using the electrocardiogram to take photos as predetermined portions of the cardiac cycle. A footswitch can also be used with a motorized camera that automatically advances the film with each actuation. This enables events to be rapidly recorded on the display. But the best way to record a real-time image is through a digital scan converter.

Chapter 5 stated that the scan converter changes the analog video signal into a set of binary numbers and that these numbers are then stored in a random access memory. This sequence is unchanged for real time. But the method of entering data into the memory may differ widely from one real-time system to another and from a real-time system to a static B-scanner.

To begin with, automatic scanning imposes a higher rate of data acquisition in a real-time system than in a static B-scanner. This increased data rate puts new demands on the ability of the RAM to acquire digital data. For example, operating with 128 data scan lines and a frame rate of 30 frames per second imposes an overall pulse repetition frequency of 30 frames per second $\times$ 128 lines per frame = 3840 Hz (lines per second). Clearly, scan converters unable to handle a data rate of 4 kHz cannot perform in this real-time system. Some of the early scan converters had trouble keeping up with this data rate, but the new scan converters seem well-equipped to handle it.

Along with the data rate as a controlling factor is the method of placing the data into the memory. The digital scan converter can be designed after the static B-scanner, for example, so that the rays from the scanning transducer are written into memory in columns if the scan is linear and across the memory if the scan is a sector. In other words, data placement is managed the same way as in the static B-scanner.

An alternate method is a dedicated data entry that does not reproduce the ray positions in the scan plane onto the memory. For example, a sector scan need not enter the memory as a sector; it can be placed in memory on a column-by-column basis, where each of the scan-line data streams occupies one column. Reading the data out of the memory is modified to synthesize the final display sector. This kind of memory organization provides some efficiency in data entry time and uses nearly 100% of the available memory in forming the final image on the display.

Except for changes in organization for data entry and retrieval, signal-handling processes after reading out of memory are essentially the same as for any digital scan converter. The digital signals are called up at a standard TV rate, synchronization and control signals are added, and the signals are then passed through a digital-to-analog converter, which puts the image information back into the standard analog TV format. With this standardization, the signal can be placed into another monitor, videotape recorder, or multiformat camera. Moreover, the image can be frozen in the digital memory for detailed examination or front panel photography. And because the image is digitally stored, digitally-based annotation can be added to the image and electronic, digital calipers can measure distances. The amalgamation of these two technologies, the digital scan converters and the real-time sonograph, enables procedures to be performed that neither machine is capable of carrying out separately. More information on the organization and design concepts of the digital scan converter is included in Chapter 5.

More on Phased and Linear Arrays

Despite the almost magical qualities ascribed to the phased array, the device is guided by the same transducer rules that apply to single-element transducers. Like the single-element transducer, the phased array must focus inside its effective near field. The degree of focusing is still a function of the transducer diameter and the range of the focal point from the array. And steering the transducer beam off-normal decreases the beam intensity and increases the side-lobe energy [8]. These effects are a consequence of each transducer element functioning as a single diffraction aperture, and of the whole array acting like a diffraction grating (Figure 7-8). The lobes that result from the summed diffraction patterns are called *grating lobes*. Within the sonograph electronics, echoes resulting from grating lobes are indistinguishable from the on-axis echoes, and as the transducer beam moves farther off-normal, the transducer signal-to-noise ratio decreases. Thus, in certain situations, a phased array is subject to artifacts that are often hard to recognize as such.

Nonetheless, one of the benefits of the electronic control in a phased array is the ability to place the focal zone into specific locations in space. Knowing these locations means that the image can be built from information contained only in the focal-zone locations. This is called *dynamic focusing*.

In forming an image using dynamic focusing, the goal is to form a composite beam that has nearly the same width over the entire field of interest [9]. A look back at equation 3.5, which defines the parameters in the beam width, shows that the half-maximum beam width is a constant so long as the f-number is constant—that is, so long as the ratio of focal length to aperture diameter is constant. Thus, moving the focal point farther from the transducer in dynamic focusing requires increasing the number of elements included in the phased-array transmitting-set.

Given all the positive benefits of the phased and linear array, how do they compare with the features of a mechanical sector scanner? The answer to this

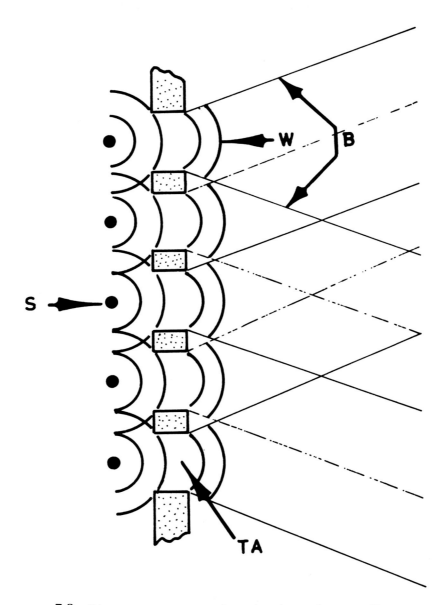

7-8   Linear array as an acoustic grating. A transducer acts like
an acoustic diffraction aperture *TA*, where the source *S* is close
to the aperture. A set of transducers acts like a set of diffracting
apertures, called a diffraction grating. The waves *W* pass through
an aperture spread *B* in a diffraction pattern, forming side lobes
called grating lobes.

question is multifaceted; we will begin with the matter of focusing in both systems. A moving single-element transducer has a beam intensity independent of the direction the beam is pointing, relative to the scan head housing. This is not the case for a phased array [8]. As the phased-array steering angle increases away from normal, the intensity of the beam decreases, reaching a minimum close to 26.5° away from normal. And as the steering off-normal increases, so do the grating lobes. This change in beam quality with scan angle does not occur with single-element transducers.

Within the sonograph is a pulser/receiver that is matched to the transducer. In phased and linear arrays, each array element usually has a separate pulser/receiver that is under central control for focusing and beam steering. And each transducer element and pulser/receiver must be alike. The summing rules for the signals on the receive portion of the cycle must be controlled to obtain focusing that is fixed or dynamic. And all the timing requirements for transmitting, beam steering, focusing on the receive cycle, beam steering on the receive cycle, and selecting the proper array elements must be handled by the machine control circuits. This high level of housekeeping is best handled by a computer and has no equal in single-element, real-time sonographs.

A major concern in many phased and linear arrays is nonsymmetrical focusing. Phased arrays and linear arrays can be focused along the array axis with electronic control, as well as transversely to the axis by applying some sort of physical focusing technique. The result is a beam that has a changing focus along one axis only, parallel to the array length. As a consequence, nonsymmetrical fields form that can confuse a sonographer unprepared for this sort of beam formation. Some phased arrays have solved this problem by using a rectangular array, in which the beam can have reasonable symmetry (Figure 7-9). None of these problems appears in the single element transducer.

One of the most successful means of dealing with beam nonsymmetry is the annular array. By timing the individual rings of the array, focusing that rivals the single-element transducer is possible. Further, by making the array rather large in diameter, focusing can occur far from the transducer. The individual rings also do not have to be the same frequency. For example, the smaller inner rings can be a high frequency, the intermediate rings can be medium frequencies, and the outer rings the lowest frequency. Not only can information be gathered as a function of distance from the transducer, but different frequencies can be used to gather frequency-dependent information from a common region [10]. More important, the transducer frequency can be chosen for the focusing and penetration needed to do the job.

Annular arrays hold potential for other sorts of additions and modifications, such as the theta array, which combines a linear and annular array [11]. This technique is not yet commercially available, but clearly shows how new and advantageous improvements can be realized in hardware.

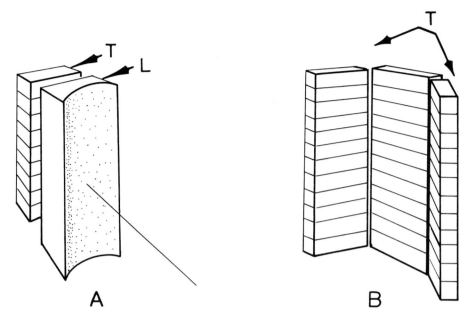

7-9   Lateral focusing in linear arrays. Generally, linear arrays *T* are not focused transversely to the array axis. The array can be focused along this axis with a lens *L,* as shown in Part A. Alternately, three arrays can be combined and controlled to focus the beam transversely, as shown in Part B.

Shortfalls in Real Time

It is commonly held that regardless of the transducer organization, real time does not provide all the information that is available to a modern static B-scanner. In general, we tend to trust real time less than the static scanners in making a final analysis, perhaps because of the documented success with B-scanners or because the sort of signal mix presented by a real-time system is different from, as opposed to less than, the static image presentation. In any case, the technique currently used in many laboratories is to look first and quickly with real time and look in detail with the B-scanner. What, then, are the deficiencies of real time that tend to inhibit its use?

A frequent observation about real time is that a single recorded photo from a real-time system does not tell much about where we are looking in the body. Granted, many of the tissue qualities and anatomical formations produced by real time can give good clues as to where we are looking, but each image carries an ever-present question mark; the field of view is simply too small to make a definitive guess. However, a look at an unmarked, static B-scan image, compounded or not, provides the same sort of uncertainty. The difference between the two is the existence of a standard protocol for B-scanning and the lack of one for real time. The static system always fits into a known set of scanning-plane positions, with known external anatomy and scanning-plane angles. And that information is printed on the film as a standard annotation. As a result, the small sector scans common to single-pass B-scanning are not considered to be as restrictive as real-time images, even though both types may be covering the same scanning area.

Within the field of view, real-time scanning is carried out at a fixed angle, changing the appearance of the image from that common to the B-scanner. As was pointed out earlier in the chapter, fixed-angle scanning changes the ability to depict a boundary. This imposes a need to make the examination dynamic, looking for all the boundaries. The real-time imaging task is to determine size, shape, position, texture, and dynamics of organs and structures within the body. A single picture cannot provide this information. Like the static B-scanner, either a series of photos is needed or a review of the recorded video image.

In addition, fixed-angle scanning affects the distribution of resolution over the image area. When the beam is not perpendicular to the interface being examined, axial and lateral resolution are no longer independent of one another, and axial resolution will become dependent upon the beam width.

Although the architecture of the beam can change the effective axial resolution of a real-time system, changing the transducer to improve the situation is either very difficult or expensive. Mechanically moved transducers usually rest in a fluid medium and cannot be conveniently changed for a scanning task. Additional transducers are expensive because the entire scan head must be changed, and even then the scan heads often do not have the needed focal-zone positions to improve the imaging. Phased arrays and linear arrays are equally as expensive, although they have the capacity to change the focal-point position and depth of focus in the scanning field. But even though a focal-zone position can be changed, the frequency of the transducers cannot. So, the better axial resolution needed in small-parts scanning or small-heart scanning (neonates) is not available to phased arrays. To handle this need, a special type of real-time system has appeared in the form of a small-parts scanner. Small-parts scanners use mechanical scanning of one sort or another to produce the small, stable ultrasound field needed for these scanning techniques. Impressive linear-array technology for high-frequency transducers (10 MHz or above) has appeared in prototype form, but has not yet been produced commercially. For now, mechanical systems hold considerable sway in small-parts scanning.

Although fields of view and transducers have been major challenges for real time, the principle complaint against real time has surrounded the issue of overall image quality. Real-time systems have not generally matched the image quality and information content of the contemporary static B-scanner. The reason for this is clearly the fault of machine design. Real-time users have primarily been interested in determining size, shape, and position, and in gaining a little information on tissue texture and a great deal of information on dynamics. Video signal ranges in most real-time sonographs have typically been 30 dB, have used 16 or fewer gray levels, and have exhibited a preprocessing curve that often assumes the signal mix to be the same as the static B-scanner. The result has been images that fall dramatically short of the quality obtained by the static B-scanner.

But this situation is changing. More equipment manufacturers and equipment designers are aware of the different signal mix inherent to real-time applications and are incorporating some well-established signal processing techniques used in static B-scanners. For example, new designs are increasing the number of pixels used to make the image, are expanding the number of gray levels available in the image, are broadening the dynamic range of the video signals for better small-signal separation, and are increasing the availability of variable pre- and postprocessing for better image analysis. Such improvements have enabled several current machines to compete favorably with the B-scanner quality.

Although real time may have less-than-desired image quality, it offers no lack of information for the sonographer and sonologist. If anything, real-time sonographs provide too much information in a form that is hard to edit. What is required, then, is a means of removing unwanted information and enhancing that which is needed. This is no easy task. Information on scanning-plane positions and angles requires firsthand observation, which imposes a participation requirement on the attending physician. Again, using a specific examination protocol and annotating unusual images is a situation much less difficult to handle.

Recording selected images with a camera is one way of reducing the amount of stored information. But one of the most valuable aspects of real time is the real-time image flow that shows the dynamics of both the examination and the patient. As a result, videotape recording, in which the dynamics of the study can be fully appreciated, is a valuable means of storing real-time information. But videotapes are bulky and not easy to store. This shortfall may be overcome with the newly developed technology of video-discs, which can provide recordings of video signals over extended time periods, with fast, and effective indexing. The current cost of the discs and the time necessary to master them make this technology impractical at present. Still, the discs are less bulky than tapes and more immune to physical punishment. Videodiscs could change real-time image storage significantly.

The problems with real time that we have identified so far—image quality, machine organization, data storage, and physician participation—are fairly obvious to most practitioners. A more insidious and less apparent problem is the illusion that "anybody can scan and be taught to scan with real time." As discussed earlier, the essential difference between the static B-scanner and the real-time system is the movement of the transducer. But being able to move the transducer is not the only requirement for a skilled sonographer. Anatomy must be understood in order to place the automatically scanning transducer in the right place; the image must be made according to the precepts of good imaging, showing the information the physician needs for a diagnosis; the TGC must be set properly to provide information on relative reflectivity; and a high level of understanding of machine function is needed to know when the machine is producing an artifact and when it is telling the truth about what is inside the body. Real time looks easy, and machines have been designed to that end, but the evidence is clear: Real time still requires handling by a skilled sonographer.

In many ways, the real-time sonographer must be more adept than formerly, but in a different segment of the scanning process. It is no longer the movement of the transducer that is so important, but the movement of the scanning plane. All the references and landmarks for scanning are inside the body rather than outside. And these references are often vascular organizations rather than bones and muscles. Well-understood, three-dimensional anatomy is thus needed in the orientation process. And the presentations of pathology need to be recognized immediately in order to alter the scanning protocol for increased or specialized documentation. Real time in the hands of an expert sonographer is a potent diagnostic tool.

Advantages of Real Time

The previous list of drawbacks notwithstanding, real time has added greatly to the effective use of ultrasound in medicine. The machines, for the most part, are low cost, permitting private ownership in offices and clinics. Numerous alternative machine designs are also now available to the buyer. But the advantages of real time involve more than cost.

Perhaps the greatest asset of real time is its relative ease of use. The scanning ultrasound beam is under machine control, removing one of the more difficult aspects of ultrasound applications. Still, an examination of current machines shows a plethora of knobs and buttons, which means that although transducer manipulation may be easier, machine setup is not.

The ability to move the transducer easily and quickly often means a shorter examination time. The static B-scanner can try to compete in this department with the survey mode of operation, but a real-time system is undoubtedly faster. Rapid data acquisition and the easy surveying means that more can be seen in a shorter period of time, increasing the number of patients a department can handle in a day. Thus, the real-time system is not only less expensive to buy, it is less expensive to use because of increased sonographer efficiency.

In addition, with a shortened examination time, the sonographer can spend more time actually examining the patient. A result of this is a heightened understanding of anatomy and pathologies in each individual patient. With anatomical references moved to inside the body, the sonographer must identify structures more quickly and readily than with the static B-scanner, in which a series of static images represent the information being reviewed. The mobility of the real-time transducer assembly in the hands of a skilled sonographer simply allows a faster and more thorough examination of the patient than available using many static B-scanners.

Because scanning is now machine controlled and the transducers are designed to have small contact areas, real time offers the use of smaller windows to image inside the abdomen and thorax. Some of the mechanical sector scanners are quite good at this, using smaller windows than could be utilized by the static B-scanner.

Neonatal head scanning through the frontal fontanel is an excellent example [12]. In the specialized scanning area, real time has clearly enabled an increasing number of patients to be included in the category "successfully examined with ultrasound."

At the same time, the increased use of real time in specialized scanning has resulted in pressure on manufacturers to bring real-time image-making ability up to par with that of the static B-scanner. Manufacturers are responding to this increased demand for performance by making real-time machines with many of the B-scanner data manipulation features as well as improved image quality. As a consequence of expanded use and experience with real time, the ultrasound community is comprehending better what real-time image requirements must be. Within the next few years, real-time systems will surely match the image quality of B-scanners.

Real time has, in addition, increased the utility of a variable preprocessing scheme that was not effective in static B-scanning. In the B-scanner, variable preprocessing meant rescanning the patient to determine if the selected preprocessing curve was the one desired. In real time, the image is always being renewed, so any change in gray-scale definition or allocation can be immediately appreciated. Repeated comparisons of the results using different preprocessing curves adds only a few seconds to the total examination time for the patient, but potentially a great deal of information.

Because real time lets us see the motion of targets as they move, anything foreign to the body that forms echoes and is moving can be seen. This is the case, for example, in performing needle biopsies and amniocentesis. Real time provides a clear opportunity to see where the needle is located, whether or not the site of interest was sampled or not, and what intervening tissues happen to be present. "Safe" amniocentesis is a reality because of real time. And more radiology departments are using "skinny needle" techniques to obtain tissue samples for a histology confirmation of the image and patient presentation. Real time has expanded the use and improved the safety of needle biopsies, even in the central nervous system.

But perhaps the most interesting and exciting effect of real time is an increased willingness on the part of users to try new applications of diagnostic ultrasound. Within the last two years alone, new techniques in the application of ultrasound have been introduced, such as neonatal head scanning to detect anatomy-altering lesions and bleeding into the CNS; surgical applications of real time directly to the organ of interest during a laparotomy or thoracotomy; techniques in adult neurosurgery; and the continuing new looks at old organs to detect previously unseen or hard-to-see lesions. Such aggressive new applications will help to guarantee an even-more-skilled group of real-time users.

Conclusion

A look at the organization of the real time sonograph shows that the machine design is centered on the technology used to move the ultrasound beam automatically. Despite this automatic movement, the sonograph still must know where the ultrasound beam is pointed in space to accurately place the "ray" of information into the digital scan converter memory.

Real time imaging appears real time because the sonograph refreshes the image from 4 to 50 times each second. But a trade-off exists here between the number of lines used to make the image and how often the image can be refreshed. High scanning resolution usually means low frame rates and compromised motion resolution as a result.

The digital scan converter has really given the current real time sonograph its character. The image qualities and capabilities like freeze frame and electronic calipers come from the design and utility of the digital scan converter. Variable preprocessing, variable postprocessing, and displays with 32 or 64 gray levels are making the real time sonograph carry more and more of the features we used to expect only on the static B-scanner.

Real time ultrasound is deceptively fast, which is a quality we often interpret as "simple to use." In truth, the real time sonograph is much harder to use because the user-skill requirements have shifted from transducer manipulation and external anatomy to fast identification of abnormalities and internal anatomy. Picking the image to save and knowing where the scanning plane is pointing based on internal anatomy are the real skills now. Despite these difficulties, real time sonography has broadened and matured ultrasound into reliable, well-accepted form of imaging.

References

1. James, A.E., Jr. *et al.* April 1980, Advances in instrument design and image recording. Radiol Clin Nor Am 18:3–20.
2. Havlice, J.F., and J.C. Taenzer. April 1979. Medical ultrasonic imaging: An overview of principles and instrumentation. Proc IEEE 67:620–641.
3. Winsberg, F. August 1979. Real time scanners: A review. Medical Ultrasound 3:99–106.
4. Kossoff, G. September 1972. Improved techniques in ultrasonic cross sectional echography. Ultrasonics:221–227.
5. Gibbs, J.S., *et al.* 1981. Image perception. In The physical basis of medical imaging, ed. C.M. Coulam, J.J. Erickson, F.D. Rollo, and A.E. James, Jr. New York: Appleton-Century-Crofts.
6. Hering, E. 1964. Outlines of a theory of the light sense. In Achromatic reciprocal interaction among parts of the visual field. Cambridge: Harvard University Press.
7. Maginness, M.G. 1978. Gray scale performance of displays for dynamic ultrasound imaging. JCU 5:329–333.
8. Smith, S.W., *et al.* May 1979. Angular response of piezoelectric elements in phased array ultrasound scanners. IEEE Transactions on Sonics and Ultrasonics: 26:185–191.
9. Ligtvoet, C.M. *et al.* 1977. A dynamically focused multiscan system. In Echocardiology, ed. N. Bom. The Hague: Martinus Nijhoff.
10. Melton, H.E., Jr. and F.L. Thurstone. 1978. Annular array design and logarithmic processing for ultrasonic imaging. Ultrasound Med Biol 4:1–12.
11. Mindl, J., and A. Macovski. 1977. Recent advances in the development of new imaging techniques. In Vol. 1, Recent advances in ultrasound and biomedicine, ed. D.N. White. Forest Grove, OR: Research Studies Press.
12. Johnson, M.L., and C.M. Rumack. April 1980. Ultrasonic evaluation of the neonatal brain. Radiol clin Nor Am: 18.

Chapter 8

Stealing Techniques From the Bats: Doppler and Pulsed-Doppler Techniques

For those of us who have had the chance to live around trains, train whistles carry a romance all their own. The sound of a train whistle shifting down in frequency as it passes is an integral part of that romance. And the romance deepens when we realize that the information about the train's movement is hidden in that downward shift in sound. The same information is hidden in the siren sounds from a fast-moving police car as it passes or the sound of a horn as a car speeds by. This apparent shift in frequency is called the Doppler shift, named for Christian Doppler, the Austrian physicist who first formulated a description of the effect in 1842.

A biological measure of the amount of information that is contained in the Doppler shift can be appreciated in the use of this phenomenon by animals to track a moving prey. The prime user is, of course, the bat, which uses the Doppler shift to compute the intercepting pathway between itself and a flying morsel of food. Observations of bats suggest some limitations in using the technique to determine information about a moving object. Nevertheless, the fact that bats have survived indicates that they have found a practical solution to the problem of finding food while in flight in the dark.

One of the more-extensively studied bats is the Panamanian mustache bat, which captures small flying insects [1]. If we compare some of the characteristics of the bat's application of ultrasound to ours, we can see how successful the bat really is. For example, the bat uses ultrasound in the 50 kHz to 65 kHz range [1]. In air, that frequency produces wavelengths of 6.6 mm to 5 mm, respectively. In comparison, diagnostic ultrasound uses wavelengths of 0.68 mm to 0.3 mm. The mustache bat produces a monotonic burst that ranges in length from 5,000 µs to 30,000 µs [1, 2]. Diagnostic ultrasound bursts are 1 µs to 2 µs long. After the long monotonic burst, the mustache bat chirps down in frequency about 10 kHz, with the chirp lasting some 2,000 to 3,000 µs [3]. We have nothing comparable to this chirp in diagnostic ultrasound. Despite these long wavelengths and long pulse lengths, the bat has an effective resolution of about 1 mm in air—not bad when compared to our 1.5-mm to 3-mm resolution in the body.

Why the long burst and chirp in the bat? The answer is found by observing the bat in flight and measuring central nervous system functions in the bat [2]. The monotonic burst provides a steady transmitted frequency used to determine the Doppler shift in a returning echo. The chirp provides information on the character of the target as a function of frequency. Target range is provided by counting time between transmission of a burst and reception of an echo. Target velocity comes back in the Doppler shift and target character comes back in the echo from the chirp, with the amplitude perhaps changing as a function of the chirp frequency. This is the sort of thing we would like to imitate some day in diagnostic ultrasound.

Excluding the chirp, we can do nearly the same thing in diagnostic ultrasound by a slightly different approach. Instead of flying insects as targets, the targets in the body are moving acoustical interfaces such as heart structures, vessel walls, and red blood cells. The Doppler shift information often can be converted to velocity information, offering a chance to quantify the amount of flow through a vascular structure, as well as providing precise information on the character of the flow. The place to begin is at the basic Doppler effect.

Formation of the Doppler Shift

An understanding of the Doppler shift is based on established events that occur as the waves move out from a source. The starting point for our discussion is a source of sound waves. Further, the source is a point source, which is small relative to the wavelength of the sound it produces (Figure 8-1). If we position the point source within a wave-conducting medium, the waves form a set of successive spheres, each sphere moving away from the source at the natural propagation velocity of the medium. To simplify our geometry a bit, we will look at the source and waves in two dimensions. The waves thus appear as a set of concentric circles rather than spheres moving outward from the source.

The waves can move away from the sound source only at the propagation velocity of the medium. This constraint is central to the Doppler shift, because a predictable Doppler shift in frequency cannot occur in a system without a constant wave velocity.

For example, when the source moves from right to left at the constant velocity, the waves moving in the direction the source is moving are pushed closer together than if the source were stationary (Figure 8-1). This compression of waves derives from the constant wave-propagation velocity inherent in the system. As the source moves through space at a constant velocity, the wave just leaving the surface of the source is pushed closer than normal to the wave that left just in front of it.

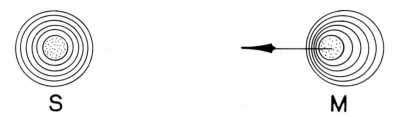

S   M

8-1 Doppler effect from a moving source of waves. In a uniform medium, waves must move with the same velocity in all directions. For a stationary source *S*, the waves form symmetrically around the source. With movement *M*, the waves move out symmetrically from the position the source was in at the instant the wave left the source. Each new wave is displaced in the direction of motion.

This process of moving the wave components spatially closer together increases the frequency, or pitch, of the wave. If a moving source compresses the waves in one direction, then the same waves are pulled apart in the opposite direction. This pulling apart produces a downward shift in frequency. And all this happens at the same time on the same source moving through the medium.

How can this occur? The constant wave velocity keeps the waves from picking up any added velocity that might be supplied by the moving source. That added velocity appears not in faster-moving waves, but in spatial changes in the waves that alter the effective frequency of the traveling wave.

Doppler Equation From Concepts

We need a more formal statement, however, of the events happening during the Doppler shift and of the relationship of the physical parameters that contribute to the shift. The best means of expressing this relationship is through an explanation of the Doppler equation. This could be a rigorous undertaking, but our interest is only in developing the equation conceptually in order to better use the sonograph, rather than entering into a complex discussion of the equation's mathematical derivation. The goal is a clear understanding of what the equation means.

The first observation is that a moving source of waves compresses the waves together in the direction of motion and pulls them apart along a line opposite to that motion. The amount of frequency shift produced in the wave can be measured as the amount of change, *Df*, that the propagated wave experiences. Looking along the direction of motion first, we can conceptualize a small experiment by asking what will happen if the velocity of the source increases? If the wave velocity is still fixed, the increasing source velocity will simply move the waves closer together along the direction of motion, and move the waves farther apart opposite to the direction of motion (Figure 8-1). In other words, the amount of Doppler shift, *Df*, will change in proportion to the velocity of the source. The higher the velocity, the greater the wave distortion and the greater the change in frequency, *Df*. So, the first mathematical statement is the proportionality:

$$Df \propto V. \tag{8.1}$$

A closer look at events, however, shows that the frequency shift is not a constant (Figure 8-1). The wave compression is greatest along the direction of motion and the rarefaction is greatest along the same line, but opposite to the direction of motion. In between these two extremes are all the remaining changes in pitch. Clearly, the amount of Doppler frequency shift seen depends upon the position from which we happen to be looking at the source. Thus, one more factor must be included, that of the position used to observe the source of waves. This position factor is expressed as the angle between one line drawn from our observation point to the sound source and another line extending from the sound source in the direction of motion. This angle is called the Doppler look angle, θ.

Tracking the change in frequency, *Df*, as a function of look angle shows that the maximum change is at 0° and 180°. Further, at 90°, the Doppler shift, *Df*, is 0. If we graph these observations, the resulting values begin to look like a cosine function of the look angle (Figure 8-1). This is indeed the case, and the angle can now enter the proportionality. The change in frequency is directly proportional to cosine θ and the proportion now looks like:

$$Df \propto V \cos \theta. \tag{8.2}$$

But considering all the other constants, what would happen if the velocity of propagation were to increase? If the waves were to move away from the source more quickly, they could not compress together as closely as before with the same velocity. The ability to compress becomes less as the velocity of propagation increases. The result is an inverse relationship between the velocity of propagation and the frequency shift. Thus, the wave propagation velocity can enter the proportionality as:

$$Df \propto (V \cos \theta)/c, \tag{8.3}$$

where *c* is the propagation velocity of sound.

The only remaining thing to be considered is the frequency of sound. Does changing the frequency of the emitted sound have any effect on the Doppler shift magnitude? The amount of spatial compression obtained from a moving source is a constant, a function only of the source velocity and the propagation velocity. But increasing the sound frequency means this spatial change of wave components becomes a larger fraction of the spatial separation of waves. Thus, the amount of frequency shift in the emitted sound will depend upon how close the waves are to begin with, or, in other words, the frequency. Thus, the change in frequency, *Df*,

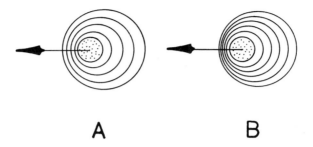

A   **B**

8-2 Changing Doppler effect with frequency. Both sources *A* and *B* are moving at the same velocity. Source *B*, however, has a higher frequency, resulting in a higher Doppler shift for the same velocity.

is going to be greater at higher frequencies than at lower frequencies because the spatial displacement takes up a larger and larger fraction of the wave separation (Figure 8-2). The proportionality now looks like:

$$Df \propto FV (\cos \Theta)/c, \qquad (8.4)$$

where *F* is the frequency of the sound when the source is at rest.

At this point, we have only a proportionality; an equation is necessary for any quantification. Although all the physical parameters of the event are here, they need a constant in order to convert the proportionality into an equation. For ultrasound, the Doppler shift is the sum of the Doppler effect from a moving receiver (the reflecting object intercepting the transmitted waves) and a moving source (the reflected waves act as if the echo source were a moving source). While the calculation can be found in any number of physics texts [4], we are interested only in the outcome, which is the number 2. Thus, the Doppler equation is:

$$Df = 2 F V (\cos \Theta)/c \qquad (8.5)$$

The equation contains all the parameters that can change in an apparent Doppler shift. In summary, increasing the sound frequency, the velocity of the source, or the look angle changes the Doppler shift accordingly. Increasing the propagation velocity of the sound decreases the Doppler shift.

The equation will appear later in this text in regard to predictions of events and in Doppler applications. Users should take time to know and understand this equation.

Making and Receiving Ultrasound for Doppler

Producing ultrasound for Doppler applications is slightly different from production for imaging. The difference lies in the Doppler requirement to specify the actual frequency being transmitted and to fix the relative phase of the transmitted wave.

Transduction occurs, as before, with a transducer that is piezoelectric. But now the transducer is excited by applying an electrical field that oscillates at the desired transmitting frequency (Figure 8-3). The phase and frequency of this transmitted ultrasound will be compared with the returning echoes to determine what changes in these two parameters occurred in the tissues. Consequently, the transmission process should not introduce any sort of phase or frequency distortion. In other words, the transducer should respond to the exciting voltage in a high-fidelity manner.

In addition, the returning echoes need to be received and transduced into voltages that are useful inside the machine (Figure 8-3). As in the transmitting process, the received echoes need to be transduced with no shift in phase or frequency. Doppler detection also needs high-fidelity reception.

Transmission of ultrasound depends upon both the exciting voltage and the natural resonant frequency of the transducer. If the transducer rings at a frequency slightly different from the exciting voltage, the difference can appear in the Doppler output as noise. Agreement between the transmitted frequency and the natural resonant frequency is needed. With an ability to transmit and receive ultrasound, we are now ready to process the Doppler information.

CW Doppler Organization

One of the earliest and still-useful forms of Doppler in ultrasound is the so-called continuous wave, or CW Doppler. After a few cycles, detecting a Doppler shift is independent of pulse length, and the transmitter can be turned on all the time; hence the term *continuous* to describe the transmitter being continuously on.

If the transmitter is always on, the returning ultrasound cannot be received by the transmitting transducer. To receive the echoes, then, two transducers are used in a single housing for simultaneous transmitting and receiving. These transducers are often unfocused and canted slightly toward one another to form an overlapping region for the two beam patterns [5]. Within this region, the echoes generated in the transmitting beam can be detected by the receiving transducer.

The continuously transmitting source can provide an easy reference for frequency changes in the returning echoes. The received echoes and the transmission frequency are compared for any frequency shifts within the received ultrasound

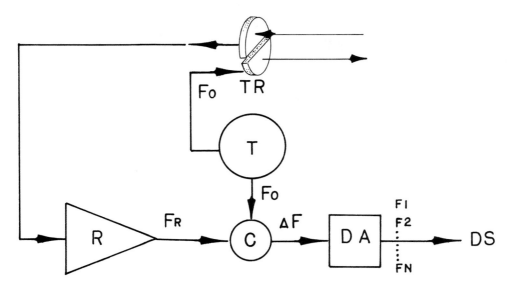

8-3 Organization of a CW Doppler. The CW Doppler transducer, *TR,* has two parts, one for constant transmission, the other for constant reception. *T* is the transmitter; *R* is the receiver, with an output of the received frequency, *FR: C* is a comparator that compares the transmitted frequency, *Fo,* with *FR;* ΔF is the difference, which is the Doppler frequency shift; *DA* is the Doppler analyzer; F_1 to *FN* are the frequency components; *DS* is the display.

signals. In addition, the returning signals could be tested for shifts in phase that would yield directional information about the echo sources. The simplest machine has only Doppler information, but a more complex device could add directional detection as well.

The primary information derived from the sonograph is the Doppler shift frequency, *Df.* This frequency shift varies directly with the echo-source velocity. Because of the typical velocities found in the body and the ultrasound frequencies used, the Doppler shift falls within the human audio spectrum. This convenient frequency range permits the Doppler shift to be run directly to a speaker for audio evaluation. In addition, the audio frequency can be converted to a voltage, smoothed, and fed to a chart recorder to record the frequency shift as a function of time [5]. This sort of record can be used to document the motion of fast-moving echo sources that are difficult to sort out by Doppler audio alone, such as fetal heart or fetal chest-wall motion.

Within the CW Doppler system, however, it is uncertain where the echo sources are located. The CW system offers sensitivity but does not offer an accurate determination of just where the echo sources are located within the beam. In addition, different echo sources might have motions in opposite directions at the same time within the same beam, confusing the audio and subsequent record.

Even more critical is the inability to limit a Doppler interrogation to a single small region of interest.

Extending CW Doppler Capabilities

The primary function of a CW Doppler system is to detect and display (audio output) the Doppler shift, detected in signals returning to the transducer. The direction of flow is not a priority. When direction is a concern, however, the CW Doppler system can be extended to include direction. The task is to detect and display the direction of motion of echo sources as either moving toward or away from the transducer. Detecting direction is often carried out by examining the phase of the returning signals using a circuit called a quadrature phase detector. The output has two channels; one is for motion toward and the other for motion away from the transducer. The two channels can then be fed into separate speakers, one for movement toward the transducer and the other for movement away from the transducer. The modified signals can also be displayed on a strip-chart recorder according to direction, upright for motion toward the transducer and down for motion away.

Another way of extending Doppler capabilities is to use the Doppler signal to detect only the presence of flow. In this technique, a Doppler transducer is attached to an articulated arm with position sensors in the articulations, as in the standard B-scanner arm (Figure 8-4). These arm signals are used to position a trace on a cathode ray tube (CRT) display to match the position of the transducer. The electron beam in the CRT is turned on when a Doppler signal is present and is turned off when a Doppler signal is absent. The transducer is moved in a series of linear scans over a vascular compartment. As the transducer is moved over the compartment, the region of flow is represented on the screen. This process "paints" an image of the compartment lumen that contains flow. The technique is called flow imaging or Doppler imaging; these terms are also used in reference to the combination of real-time imaging with Doppler. A better term would be *Doppler arteriography*.

Doppler devices can also be improved by adding analyzers that determine frequency components present in the Doppler shift signals (Figure 8-3). These components can be used to help provide information on the character of red blood cell (RBC) motion occurring within a vascular compartment or other moving echo sources. The output from these analyzers is brought to displays or strip-chart recorders for visual inspection.

But for all the capabilities of the modified CW Doppler, it still lacks an ability to provide unique spatial information. This added capability will come from combining pulse-echo techniques with Doppler analysis.

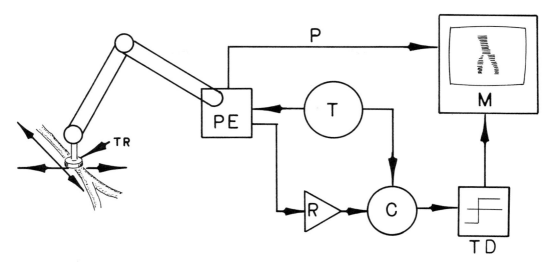

8-4 Organization of a Doppler image device. This device is designed to image blood flow in a vascular compartment. *TR* is the transducer; *PE* is the position encoder; *P* is position information for the display; *T* is the transmitter; *R* is the receiver; *C* is the frequency comparator; *TD* is a threshold detector (Doppler signals above a set amplitude are displayed); *M* is the monitor display.

Pulsed-Doppler Concepts

CW Doppler systems offer some spatial data but do not provide precise information about the range of echo sources; they only offer lateral position information. As a result, vessels next to one another that fall into the transducer beam at the same time produce superimposed Doppler signals at the Doppler output. Repositioning the beam can sometimes improve this situation, but human anatomy is often not that cooperative. To separate vascular compartments more discretely, the sampling process must become more positional, which means applying an echo-ranging technique.

Combining echo ranging with Doppler analysis produces a pulsed-Doppler system (Figure 8-5). In this design, a burst of coherent ultrasound is transmitted into the tissues. As the burst moves through interfaces, both moving and stationary, the frequency of the reflecting energy is shifted up or down as a result of interface motion. Still, Doppler analysis has no inherent positional information; consequently, range-gating is used. This technique involves transmitting a burst of ultrasound and counting time until echoes arrive from a region of interest, and then opening the receiver and Doppler analyzer. After being on for a short time, the receiver and analyzer are turned off again. Thus, by listening to echoes from

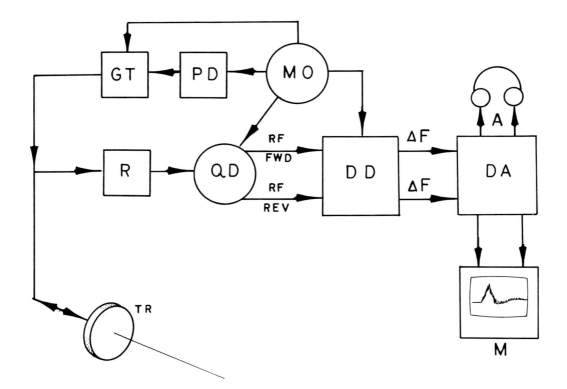

8-5 Organization of a coherent pulsed-Doppler device. The pulsed-Doppler uses the same transducer for transmitting and receiving, sending out bursts of ultrasound and analyzing the echoes for frequency shifts. *TR* is the transducer; *GT* is the gated transmitter; *PD* is the pulse repetition frequency decrement counter, stepping down the master oscillator frequency; *MO* is the master oscillator; *R* is the rf receiver; *QD* is the quadrature detector, separating the signal into two channels, forward and reverse; *DD* is the Doppler detector; Δ*F* is the Doppler shift frequency, *DA* is the Doppler analyzer; *A* is the audio signals for speakers or headphones; *M* is the monitor display.

a specific time epoch, a specific region of space can be examined for any interface motion.

In many pulsed-Doppler systems, the echo amplitude, phase, and frequency information are all processed from the returning echoes [5]. From a comparison of phase information, the relative motion of the echo source toward or away from the transducer can be determined. Further, by looking at the amount of frequency shift, an echo-source velocity evaluation is possible. If the motion is connected to other events, such as the cardiac cycle, motion processes may need to be observed over a long time period. The Doppler analysis will address, then, the frequencies present in the sampling region and how these frequencies change over time. Positional information about the moving echo sources is obtained from the range-gating technique. All of these data must be fitted into an understandable display. The final device is a coherent pulsed-Doppler system (Figure 8-5).

A Coherent Pulsed-Doppler System

In order to determine the presence of phase information in the returning echoes, the system must have an internal reference [6]. This reference is provided by a circuit called the master oscillator. The oscillator normally operates at the center operating frequency of the transducer. It provides a steady oscillating electrical signal that will be used at several locations in the sonograph.

The master oscillator feeds a signal to the transducer through a gated transmitter. This transmitter is a simple electronic window that admits a prescribed number of electrical oscillations to the transducer. But the phase of these signals must always be the same. To keep this phase steady, the pulse repetition frequency (PRF) is determined by subdividing the master oscillator frequency. This PRF control signal sets the start and stop times for the gated transmitter. The result is a master oscillator that always feeds the transducer at the same phase and frequency. Once the burst of energy leaves the transducer, the system is ready to receive echoes and to process the resulting signals.

In the sequence of events, the transmitted energy is shifted in frequency as a result of interface motion and returns to the transducer for conversion into an electrical signal. As in the pulse-echo system, the first amplifier is a radio frequency (rf) amplifier (Figure 8-6). It has the same requirements for stability and low noise as any ultrasound amplifier, but has the additional requirement of not shifting the phase of the returning signal during amplification. In addition, time-gain compensation (TGC) may be applied at this point in the signal stream, and the amplifier must be able to respond to the TGC voltages in a predictable manner.

From the rf amplifier on, the pulsed-Doppler system changes character dramatically, compared to the usual echo-ranging system (see Chapter 2). The next signal processing is a determination of the direction of motion. This detection occurs within a circuit called a quadrature phase detector. Although this circuit has a single input, it has a dual output, with one output representing motion toward the transducer and the other output representing motion away from the transducer. This separation is usually made at the rf level; the two channels are still Doppler shifted rf, but are 90° out of phase with one another [6].

With signals separated according to the direction of motion, a second detection is applied that separates the Doppler shift from the rf signal. This primary Doppler detection occurs in both channels, and the output is an audio signal. The form of the audio can be simple or complex, depending upon the character of the motion detected by the system. If many Doppler shifts are present, then the audio can be complex. At this stage, the detection processes need to be linear and produce no significant noise in handling the signal.

With the Doppler shift at the audio level, we can now apply the first form of Doppler analysis, which is the human auditory system. The audio signals are brought to a set of speakers through a pair of amplifiers that maintain the forward and reverse channel separation. This analytical approach can be rather successful, but is subjective and difficult to teach to others. Furthermore, the ability to differentiate specific frequencies and their amplitudes is limited to a very small segment of our population with perfect analytical pitch. Clearly, additional analysis is needed that is far less subjective and produces results that can be recorded.

Secondary Doppler analysis is provided by electronic circuits that separate out the frequency components within the Doppler signal. For example, listening to Doppler signals can indicate the presence of high frequencies, suggesting increased velocities in the sample volume, but exact values cannot be determined by listening only. The Doppler analyzer, however, can evaluate the returning signals for their signal complexities and convert this information into a form for display. The methods for analysis are described in more detail later in the discussion.

Deciding the format in which to display Doppler analyzer information depends upon the quality of the information provided by the Doppler analyzer and what information we want to extract from the data. For example, frequency as a function of time would be useful for many analyses we might wish to conduct.

We have reviewed the general organization of a coherent pulsed-Doppler system. With this organization in hand, let us look at some of the machine functions in more detail.

Defining the Sample Volume

The purpose of using a pulsed-Doppler system is to gather Doppler information from only a limited space. This region is called the sample volume (Figure 8-6). It is positioned by the event timing within the receiver/analyzer portion of the system. In the machine, time and depth have the same meaning because the average velocity of propagation is constant. Thus, we can position the sample volume by keeping the receiver section turned off after the ultrasound leaves the transducer, and turning the receiver on after waiting a proper amount of time. The receiver is left on for only a short time, then turned off again. Exactly when the receiver is

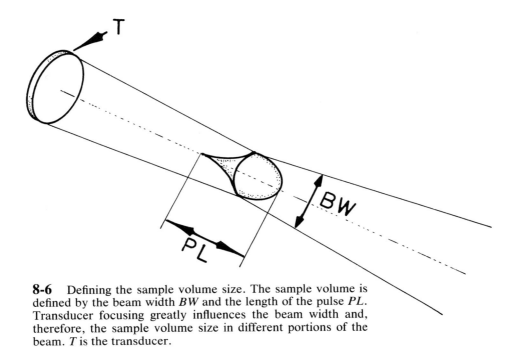

8-6   Defining the sample volume size. The sample volume is defined by the beam width *BW* and the length of the pulse *PL*. Transducer focusing greatly influences the beam width and, therefore, the sample volume size in different portions of the beam. *T* is the transducer.

turned on determines, in part, the sample volume range. How long the receiver is left on determines the length of the sample volume. Defining the sample volume, however, does not end here.

In the tissue, the sample volume length is directly determined by the pulse length [6]. Because the master oscillator drives the transducer, the length of the transmitter gating determines effective sample volume length. The gating, on the other hand, can be short, spanning only 1 or 2 cycles, or much larger, spanning 5 or 6 cycles. The gating duration is chosen both for the capabilities of the transducer to start and stop vibration and for the lowest frequency shift (representing the lowest velocity at any given look angle) to be displayed in the system. For example, the bat deals both with lower transmitted frequencies and very small target velocities that are typical of insects being hunted. As a result, bats use very long monotonic bursts that offer long sampling times to improve both low-velocity determinations and overall Doppler accuracy [2].

As we might expect, the lateral sample volume dimension is determined by the beam width (Figure 8-6). As a result, the sample volume changes dimensions as it responds to both the changing beam width and the burst duration. Because of this beam-width dependence, numbers quoted by manufacturers about sample volume dimensions must be qualified by the point in the beam where these numbers apply. Unspecified numbers should be understood to be only at the focal point of the transducer beam, increasing in either direction away from the focal point. Once more, knowing the beam profile for the transducer provides useful details about overall machine function.

Doppler Analysis

The output from a Doppler detector is a mix of audio frequencies that result from a mix of velocities present within the sample volume. The function of the Doppler analyzer is to determine those frequencies present and, if possible, the relative amplitude of each frequency component. Further, we would like to see how these frequencies change over time. The final output should thus show both the frequency content and how the frequencies change over time.

If a known range of frequencies is present, one method of analog analysis is to apply a set of filters to the signal mix, with each filter passing only a narrow range of frequencies. By putting many of these filter channels together, the range of expected frequencies can be spanned by any number of channels (Figure 8-7). For example, a set of 32 channels could divide the frequency range into 32 segments. Within any segment, all the frequencies are present as if they were one. This technique is called analog multifilter analysis. The output from the multifilter system is a plot of frequency as a function of time, with the relative amplitudes for each division expressed in gray scale (Figure 8-8). This technique was first applied to voice frequency analysis and was later extended into Doppler ultrasound.

Another more frequently used analytical technique is called the zero crossing detector. This circuit simply counts the number of times an audio signal crosses zero (nodes) and emits a pulse for each of these crossings [6]. If the audio frequency increases, the number of crossings per unit time also increases, bringing these output pulses closer together. The spacings can be translated into a relative frequency statement, ultimately relating the zero crossings to the frequencies present in the Doppler signals. Each zero-crossing event can be expressed as a dot on the display, with a Y-axis position related to the separation between spikes. The result is a plot of frequency as a function of time in a form called a time interval histogram, even though this is not a real histogram. Nevertheless, the frequencies present in the Doppler signals can be expressed on a display or a recording. Unlike the multifilter analyzer, however, the time-interval histogram has no information on relative frequency amplitude, a feature that has some importance in ongoing Doppler analysis.

Although the zero-crossing detector and time-interval histogram provide a great deal of information on the Doppler frequencies present, they are still limited in their overall portrayal of events in the Doppler shifted signal. For example, the zero-crossing detector cannot determine if a zero-crossing event is due to a Doppler signal or to a noise spike. This means the detector is quite noise sensitive, placing an unusual dependence upon noise qualities present in the circuits leading up to the Doppler analyzer. In addition, the zero-crossing detector cannot read a very complex wave form for all the frequencies present [6]. Large amplitude portions of the signal mix will swamp out smaller, often diagnostically important signals. Thus, the zero-crossing detector and time-interval histogram prove to be good qualitative evaluators of changing frequency content, but inadequate quantitative

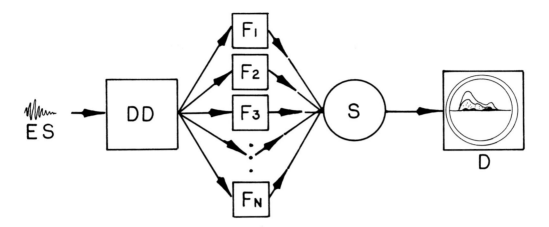

8-7 Doppler signal multifilter analysis. Complex Doppler audio signals can be analyzed by applying a set of filters with different frequency passbands. *ES* is the echo signal; *DD* is the Doppler detector; F_1 to *FN* are the individual filters and frequencies; *S* is a signal processor to bring the components together for display; *D* is the display.

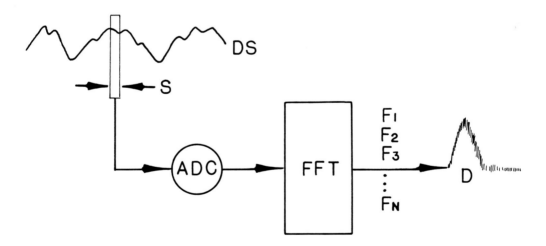

8-8 Doppler signal fast Fourier transform analysis. The fast Fourier transform analysis begins by sampling the Doppler signal *DS*, for a small period *S*. The sample is converted to binary numbers by an analog-to-digital converter, *ADC*, and sent to the *FFT* device. Out of the FFT are the frequency components, F_1 to *FN*, which are displayed, *D*.

estimators of the individual frequencies present. Also, careful analysis of complex signal mixes clearly shows that the zero-crossing detector responds in a nonaveraging manner, which means that a smooth output from the zero-crossing detector cannot be used for even an average value of the Doppler frequencies present. Without reliable averaging, the ability to quantitate flow vanishes.

If these known problems are associated with the zero-crossing detector, why has it been around so long and why does it still appear in many of the Doppler systems now on the market? The answer relates to the qualitative output from the circuits. The zero-crossing detector is simple to design and make and provides a good qualitative look at changes in the frequencies present in the Doppler signals, even if the frequencies cannot be quantified. As in the case of the analog scan converter, however, the arrival of a digital device that can do the same thing better has displaced the analog technique from its primary position. The new technique is called the fast Fourier transformation, or FFT.

At the heart of the fast Fourier transform device is a digital computer that examines the input signal for its frequency components by applying a very fast Fourier analysis routine (Figure 8-8). But the digital computer can analyze only digital signals, so the first item needed to apply this technique is a very fast analog-to-digital converter that samples a portion of the Doppler signal (for example, about 10 ms), and converts that signal mix into a set of binary numbers to determine the frequencies present in sequence. The result is a presentation of the discrete frequencies and the amplitude of each frequency component. (A detailed explanation of Fourier components of waves was provided in Chapter 1.) The discrete digitally-based information out of the FFT means that sophisticated mathematics and statistical routines can be applied to the output data on a nearly real-time basis. Unlike the zero-crossing detector, the results can be quantified because of the well-characterized digital routines. Once more, digitalization is bringing about a small revolution in another aspect of diagnostic ultrasound.

With these analytical techniques available, the data from the analyzer need to be effectively displayed.

Displaying Doppler Information

A large amount of information is contained in an analog Doppler signal. Because most displays are two-dimensional, only a limited amount of information can be shown at any one time (Figure 8-9). The task of choosing what information to show is a function of evaluating the questions asked to determine if they are answerable by the analyzer. For example, changes in the frequency spectral content can be asked of the zero-crossing detector, but we can ask nothing about the amplitudes of the individual frequency components. Any conclusions are limited by the effective output from the Doppler analyzer.

If, however, we seek information about the way the frequencies change during the cardiac cycle, then a valuable display can be the frequency components as a

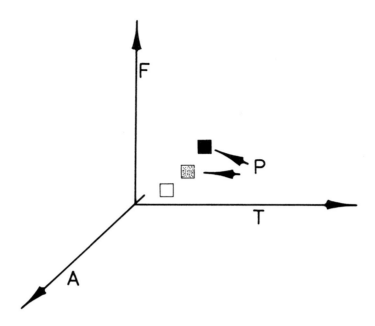

8-9 Information in a Doppler spectral display. Frequency components are shown as individual picture elements (pixels), *P*, positioned according to frequency along the Y-axis, *F*. The X-axis is time, *T*, and the relative amplitude (A) of each component is shown as a level of gray scale.

function of time. Further, the direction of flow can be indicated by the component position relative to a zero line, with "up" being motion toward the transducer and "down" being motion away from the transducer. This sort of display provides information on the form of the frequency change over time, the frequency components present over time, and the direction of motion, all in a single recording.

Another form of display that might be of interest involves displaying the frequencies present and their amplitudes. The frequency mix, however, is often a function of time. For example, flow in a vessel is variable through the heart cycle, and frequencies present will be a function of when the Doppler is sampling during the cardiac cycle. Clearly, displays of frequency and amplitude need to be synchronized in specific times within the cardiac cycle.

Another form of display combines segments of each of the first two display forms. In it, the frequencies are shown as a function of time, but each component amplitude is displayed as a gray-level intensity. The result is information displayed on three axes, one for frequency (Y-axis), one for time (X-axis), and one for amplitude (gray scale) (Figure 8-10).

It is often necessary to see positional information at the same time the Doppler information arrives in order to correlate the Doppler signal with the vascular compartment being examined. Under normal circumstances, this is not an easy mix of information to display. But, by combining an M-mode display with Doppler

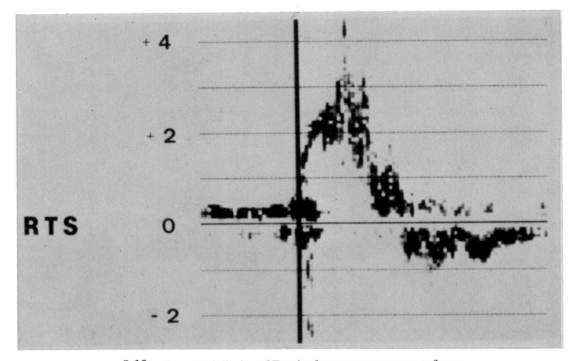

8-10   A spectral display of Fourier frequency components from
the ascending aorta. The basic form of a spectral display shows
Fourier frequency components on the Y-axis and time on the
X-axis. The amplitude of the frequency components appears as
gray scale intensity. This is a recording of flow in the ascending
aorta, viewed from the suprasternal notch. A close examination
clearly shows the pixels that make up this digital display.

information, an unusual and valuable display format is possible (Figure 8-11). This
format is called an M/Q display and derives its name from the combination of M-
mode with flow (designated Q) that appears on the display. The M-mode format
provides motion and position information along with a line on the M-mode trace
that indicates the sample volume position. This format is used primarily for echocardiography, but could extend into other areas [7].

Still, M-mode is not the only means of showing positional information to place
the sample volume. For example, an A-mode trace can be used to place the sample
volume if the sonographer can read anatomical information from an A-mode
display. Although reading an A-mode display is not difficult, the technique is not
currently taught in most educational programs and a new Doppler user must acquire
the skill to use a device with an A-mode trace to show position. Many of the early
pulsed-Doppler devices showed only an A-mode trace and a position of the sample
volume within this trace.

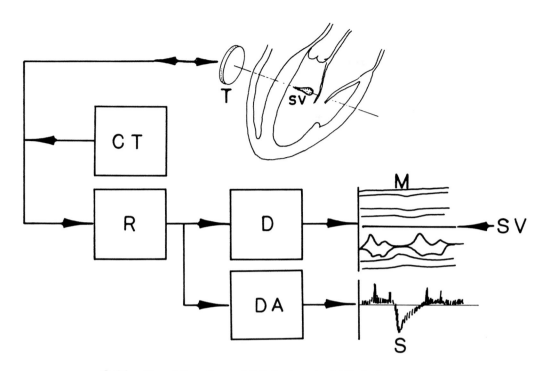

8-11   Signal flow for an M/Q device. An M/Q device is organized to process the same echo signal for both frequency and amplitude, requiring no time sharing between imaging, *M,* and Doppler analysis, *S. SV* is the sample volume; *T* is the transducer; *CT* is the common transmitter; *R* is the rf receiver; *D* is the amplitude detector; *DA* is the Doppler analyzer; the *SV* line shows the sample volume location on the M-mode display.

Duplex Imaging: Imaging Plus Doppler

The task for the Doppler device is to detect motion within the body. But although numerous body components move internally, not all are worth examining with Doppler. For example, valve leaflets in the heart have specific motion that is best examined with M-mode or a real-time two-dimensional image, rather than Doppler. Other moving structures in the body that might be of interest, however, are the red blood cells. They move a great deal, often in telltale patterns in the presence of disease, both in the vessels and in the heart. In both the vessels and the heart, however, it is not easy to place a sample volume into a specific compartment, especially if Doppler sounds are used alone to decide the sample volume location. A solution is to combine imaging and Doppler information at the same time to offer anatomical information about organ and vessel architecture and flow information carried by the RBC. This is the essence of duplex imaging.

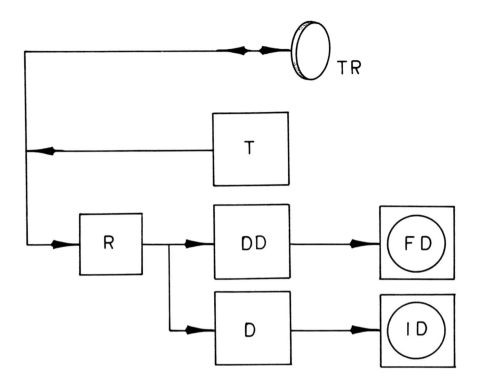

8-12 Signal flow for a true duplex imager. In true Duplex imaging, the image and flow information are processed simultaneously and displayed simultaneously. *TR* is the transducer; *T* is the transmitter; *R* is the receiver; *DD* is the Doppler detector; *FD* is the flow display; *D* is the amplitude detector; and *ID* is the image display.

Combining imaging and Doppler information by extracting both imaging and Doppler data from the same echo signal is a true duplex system (Figure 8-12). An imaging sonograph and a Doppler sonograph really require different sorts of data from the same signal, however. The requirements on the signal to draw off that information are different as well. For example, to maintain adequate axial resolution in an image, an imaging system requires a short duration pulse that is not necessarily coherent. In contrast, the Doppler system prefers longer pulses that are coherent, and these longer pulses degrade the axial resolution (Figure 8-13). As a result, using Doppler bursts for imaging degrades the image resolution and creates a sampling problem when gathering image information with a sweeping beam and Doppler with a steady beam. A solution is to use two different systems with two different transducers and simply intermesh the pulse-listen cycles from each mode. This is clearly not a true duplex operation. If the two systems were used in true duplex, they would be operating simultaneously and very likely interfering with one another. Currently, true duplex appears only with M/Q mode and A-mode displays [7].

Because of the complex and often insoluble problems associated with true duplex operation in real-time imaging, most systems currently on the market combine

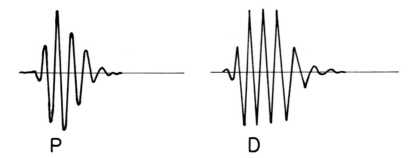

8-13   The character of pulses for Doppler and imaging. The pulse for a pulse-echo system *P* is as short as possible and has a steady rise and fall. The pulse for a pulsed-Doppler system *D* rises rapidly and maintains several cycles of constant amplitude and frequency before decaying. The Doppler pulse is generally much longer than the imaging pulse.

imaging and Doppler into a modified duplex system. It is still duplex because both imaging and Doppler data are gathered from the same imaging plane, but the two operations are interlaced in a pattern that permits nearly optimum operation of both systems. In some systems, the two-dimensional real-time image is used to locate the anatomy of interest, and then the imaging is turned off while the Doppler portion of the machine operates. Other systems automatically switch between the real-time image and the Doppler function, with the real time updating at a low but still effective rate. In both approaches, the task is to use the real-time image not as a diagnostic instrument but as a positional tool for the Doppler sample volume.

In duplex imaging, the division of labor at the transducer level becomes an area of concern. An early and still-used approach is the dual transducer technique, which uses separate transducers for imaging and Doppler. In this configuration, an outboard transducer is connected to the imaging transducer through a mechanical coupler and encoder that establishes a rigid mounting for the Doppler transducer and position information that can be relayed back to the sample volume indicator on the image [6]. The task is to place the Doppler sample volume in the same plane as the imaging system, so that the anatomy seen on the imaging display can be used to position the sample volume accurately. Early duplex systems used this technique but often had registration problems in which the sample volume drifted outside the imaging plane. Some of the newest systems use this technique with some success and appear to have solved these registration problems.

Another technique that removes some of these registration problems is to use the same transducer(s) for imaging and Doppler. In mechanical scanning systems, this arrangement sets the sample volume squarely in the imaging plane. This sort of system requires a steady hand because the sample volume position is indicated on a frozen two-dimensional image. Although this might appear to be a problem, user experience clearly indicates that it is not. Even inexperienced sonographers seem to have steady hands.

Registration between transducers is not the only concern for pulsed-Doppler users. Other physical limitations placed on Doppler analysis also deserve mention and are described in the next section.

Physical Limits on Doppler Analysis

The primary target for Doppler application in the body is the red blood cell. This is a very small target with a size of 7 μ to 10 μ. The small size insures that a true scattering process is involved in the RBC–ultrasound interaction. With such a small target and complete scattering of energy in all directions, the amount of energy that can reach the transducer is usually very low. As a result, the Doppler signals used for analysis are typically 20 dB or more below the specular echoes that result from vessel boundaries [6]. Thus, an imaging system that sets the vessel boundaries as large echoes may not present any indication of scattering signals from the vascular compartment, but these small signals are picked up by the Doppler transducer, amplified, and analyzed for Doppler shifts. Such small signal levels not only limit the range of Doppler signals that are possible from vessels, but also limit the useful depth at which Doppler can be used. Typically, we can use imaging much deeper in the tissues than Doppler.

Like a pulsed echo-ranging system, the pulsed-Doppler system must change its pulse repetition frequency as a function of depth. Because ultrasound takes 6.5 μs to traverse 1 cm of tissue, the time taken to retrieve echoes from deeper tissues is longer. Thus, for most Doppler systems, the pulse repetition frequency is decreased as the depth is increased. This pulse repetition frequency will determine the highest Doppler shift that can be accurately sampled by the Doppler system.

Basic sampling theory tells us that if we want to accurately represent a wave by sampling its value over time, we must sample it by not less than twice its frequency (Figure 8-14). For example, if we wished to sample a 2,000-Hz signal in order to follow its cyclic changes, we would have to sample it at 4,000 Hz. If we sample it at less than 4,000 Hz, then the accuracy of the representation is lost and the output from the sampling process begins to make the 2,000-Hz signal look much lower in frequency. This process is called aliasing; in it, a high-frequency wave (2,000 Hz in this case) appears to be a much-lower-frequency wave because of a failure to sample the wave properly.

Applying this knowledge to the sampling process used in pulsed Doppler sets an upper limit on the Doppler shift that can be accurately represented in a pulsed-Doppler device. The system is in fact sampling at the pulse repetition frequency and this frequency sets the limit. From this theory comes the general rule in pulsed Doppler that the highest Doppler frequency that can be sampled without aliasing in the Doppler system is one-half the pulse repetition frequency. Expressed as an equation, it is:

$$Fmax = PRF/2, \qquad (8.6)$$

where *Fmax* is the maximum Doppler shift, and *PRF* is the pulse repetition frequency of the system. Calculating an example shows that a system operating at 4.6 kHz PRF could accurately display a maximum Doppler shift of 2.3 kHz. This maximum frequency that can be sampled accurately is known as the Nyquist limit, after the mathematician who developed this sampling theorem.

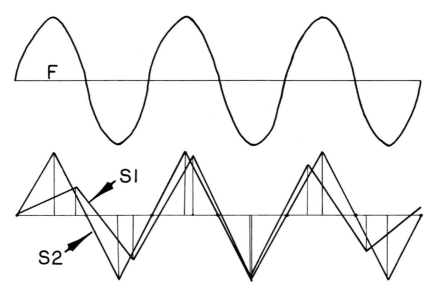

8-14   Concept of the Nyquist limit. To sample frequency *F* accurately, requires a sampling frequency not less than 2 F. *S1* is the result of sampling at 0.75 F, which represents *F* poorly. *S2* is the result of sampling at 2 F, which is the Nyquist limit for the sampling frequency.

An upper limit on the upper-Doppler shift frequency that can be accurately depicted suggests a possible lower limit on the Doppler frequency as well. The lower limit is determined by the duration of the sampling time. If a system uses an FFT with a sampling duration of 10 ms, for example, then the lowest frequency that can be detected is ¹⁄₁₀ ms, or 100 Hz. Only between these two limits—the Nyquist limit and the sampling duration—can the Doppler shifts be accurately depicted by a pulsed-Doppler system.

Along with the PRF, the formation and shape of the sample volume also influences the output obtained from a pulsed-Doppler system. For example, one of the indicators of disturbed flow in a vascular compartment is the appearance of an abrupt increase in Doppler frequency components, called spectral broadening. The added frequencies result from RBC motion that is confused and multidirectional. Given the right conditions, this sort of output can occur in normal flow situations if the architecture of the flow and sample volume interact properly (Figure 8-15).

If the sample volume is very small relative to the flow, for example, the impulse signal resulting from the small sample volume will have high-frequency components as the sample volume shapes the resulting audio output. This process introduces new Fourier components to the resulting audio, and these components will appear as spectral broadening in the analyzed audio, making the flow appear disturbed when it is not.

Spectral broadening can also occur when the architecture of the flow is complex but not disturbed relative to the sample volume size. The complex flow can generate flow gradients within the sample volume, making the output spectrum broad once

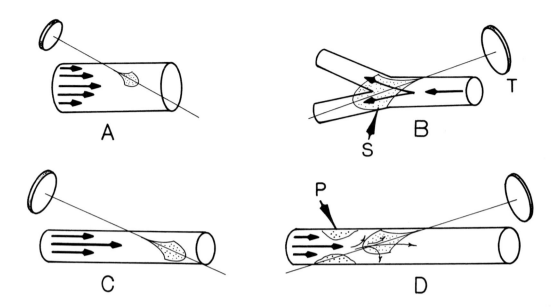

8-15   Sources of Doppler spectral broadening. Part A: Spectral broadening from sampling the gradient at the edge of a flow velocity pattern. Part B: Broadening from complex flow divisions within the sample volume. Part C: Broadening from high-velocity flows intercepting a small sample volume, creating a modulated Doppler signal. Part D: Broadening from disturbed or turbulent flow caused by disease.

again. As before, we have the appearance of abnormality when none exists.

Spectral broadening can occur, furthermore, when the flow is divided into two or more channels within the sample volume. The multidirectional flow appears as variable velocities to the analyzer, and the audio output appears with an increased spectral content, and thus, effective spectral broadening. As before, the situation is normal and the broadening is an artifact of the flow–sample volume interaction. Of course, spectral broadening can also happen with true flow disturbances. The trick is knowing which is which.

Along with the architecture of the flow within a sample volume, the shape of the sample volume can also influence events. The sample volume changes shape as a function of depth because the beam width changes with depth. For this reason, many Doppler transducers are only moderately or even weakly focused. With a fairly steady beam width, the sample volume will change little with changing depth.

It is evident that trying to carry out a Doppler analysis is not always as easy as it appears. However, by knowing what errors can creep into the analysis and the sorts of limitations that are part of the sampling process, the role of the overall Doppler analysis can be transformed from one that is qualitative to one that is quantitative.

Quantifying the Doppler Results

Within the organization of the pulsed-Doppler system, nothing has opened the door to quantification so much as the use of digitally-based FFT systems. As noted earlier, FFT devices take the analog signal arriving from the Doppler detector, convert samples of this signal into digital numbers, and analyze these numbers for the frequency components present in the Doppler signal at that time. The use of digital Doppler devices permits the use of averaging and weighted-averaging techniques that would be difficult at best and all but impossible in the analog world. Recently, however, an analog Doppler analyzer has been developed that appears to be a good averaging device [8]. The remaining analyzers that are successful calculators of Doppler frequencies are digital.

But going digital means placing a limitation on the number of frequency divisions (or bins, as they are often called) that are used for the display. This limitation means that the continuum of frequencies that makes up the spectrum of analog signals must be divided into a finite set of values. Like the digitalization that limited the number of gray levels available to a digital scan converter, digitalization of the Doppler signal limits the number of frequencies that can be displayed. Because the FFT runs on binary numbers, the number of divisions rests with the number of bits used to portray the frequencies present in a sample of the Doppler signal. For example, a 6-bit system can have 64 values, a 7-bit system can have 128 values, and an 8-bit system can have 256 values. Many of the systems now available will take the number of bits available and apply that number to both forward and reverse flow, leaving only half as many for each direction of flow. Thus, a 256-sample system will have 128 bins for forward flow and 128 bins for reverse flow. The number of frequencies that go into each bin can be calculated by dividing the Doppler frequency range by the number of sampling values. For example, a system that goes from 4,000 Hz to −4,000 Hz, with a total span of 8,000 Hz with 128 frequency bins, means that each bin spans 62.5 Hz.

Because of the stability and analytical accuracy of a digital system, quantification is possible. This quantification will depend upon the Doppler equation and an understanding of how it works.

From the Doppler analyzer come the frequency components of the Doppler signal. From the individual frequency components, an average frequency can be calculated. This average can be placed in the Doppler equation, and the equation solved for velocity. For example, the transposed Doppler equation looks like:

$$V = Df\, c/2\, F \cos \Theta \qquad (8.7)$$

where V is the average velocity, Df is the average Doppler shift frequency, c is the propagation velocity, F is the transmitted ultrasound frequency, and Θ is the look angle. If we do not have a true representation of the flow and cannot calculate the average velocity, the same equation can still be used to determine the range of velocities present by making the calculation based on the range of frequencies from the analyzer.

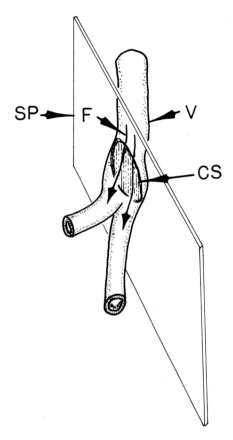

8-16   Oblique angle errors in duplex imaging. If a scanning plane *SP* intercepts a vessel *V* at an angle, the image cross section *CS* may suggest that flow *F* is in the scanning plane when it is not.

Within the Doppler equation, however, are several factors that may not be determined accurately enough to permit highly accurate quantification. The transmitted center ultrasound frequency, for instance, may not be what we think it is. But most systems are designed to maintain this parameter very closely. Even so, the look angle, Θ, can be a great problem. This angle may not be accurately determined or even determinable. Some of the systems that rely upon an accurate determination of cos Θ get around the uncertainty by looking at close to 0°, which permits larger error in the look-angle determination and has little influence on the results.

A determined average velocity coupled with an accurate measurement of the flow compartment diameter permits a direct calculation of flow. For example:

$$Q = V A \qquad (8.8)$$

where Q is the average flow (volume/unit time), V is the average velocity, and A is the area of the flow compartment cross section. Values derived from this technique can be compared to values found with invasive techniques or direct measurements tabulated by physiologists.

Within this framework of collected measurements and values is the requirement to know the angle, Θ, with some confidence. This requires knowing that the vascular compartment is contained in and parallel to the scanning plane. Missing this geometry means that a vascular compartment might be accurately determined within the scan plane but not parallel to it because the vessel intersects the plane obliquely (Figure 8-16). Determining whether or not this condition exists will require a good real-time image to evaluate the anatomy properly. With the foregoing knowledge of Doppler science and Doppler analysis limitations, let us look at some of the current areas of application.

Areas of Doppler Application

An early application of Doppler was to determine fetal viability by locating and depicting fetal heart motion [9]. In addition, Doppler was used to locate the placenta and umbilical insertion at the placenta in order to determine if the placenta was positioned properly. All this is possible without a pulsed-Doppler system or additional imaging. The Doppler systems for this purpose were and still are CW and are designed and constructed simply.

As we learned earlier, pulsed Doppler can lead to quantification techniques. A prime area for this application is in umbilical blood flow and its relation to intrauterine growth retardation [10, 11]. The successful application of Doppler in this area is based on the use both of real time to locate the umbilical artery accurately, as well as a Doppler analyzer with true averaging. All the digital FFT systems have the potential for averaging, and one analog system recently described in the literature can average.

Another area of application is in the detection and analysis of flow through the carotid artery [12]. In this application, the vessels (i.e., the common, internal, and external carotid arteries) are all close to the body surface and can be easily examined with high-frequency Doppler techniques. These vessels can be scanned using CW and pulsed-Doppler systems, with and without additional imaging from a real-time system. Because some vascular diseases are echogenic and can be seen either in or on the edge of a vessel lumen, and real-time image is useful in rapidly surveying the arteries for disease. When the vascular disease is not visible with ultrasound, only the Doppler can provide ultrasonic information on compromised flow. In addition, the vascular anatomy can often be extraordinary, requiring some visual landmarks to correctly place the sample volume in the vessels. The goal is to determine the presence of any vascular disease and the degree of vascular compromise associated with that disease.

These Doppler techniques can be extended to other vascular compartments that can be visualized with real time and examined with Doppler [13]. As noted earlier, the Doppler echoes are much smaller than echoes from larger reflectors, and the depth of the vessel from the transducer becomes a controlling factor in obtaining Doppler signals from deep structures. Often the window to the vessel places the Doppler transducer axis perpendicular to the direction of flow, preventing a good interrogation of flow using the Doppler technique. Aggressively seeking different acoustical windows could improve some of these limitations. When a good angle and signal-to-noise levels are possible, the only real limitation to the use of Doppler is the imagination.

An example of a flow-dependent area with good Doppler potential is the heart [14]. Here the flow through valves can be evaluated in terms of adequate opening of the valves and a water-tight seal when the valves close. Thus, incompetent valves can be evaluated by examining flow during the open portion of the valve cycle and any evidence of flow when the valve is closed. Because the degree of disturbance in flow is associated with disease, Doppler can be used to evaluate both the presence and degree of valvular disease without the use of cardiac catheterization.

Still, a heart can fail for reasons other than valve disease. A heart can suffer from distributed disease or segmental disease that can contribute to heart failure. Individuals suffering from this sort of decreased heart function have cardiac outputs determined by cardiac catheterization, provided the patient can withstand the operation. Although this invasive technique supplies solid information, it does not lend itself to the observance of trends in the patient or to making a first evaluation of cardiac output to decide if further measurements are needed. Here the application of quantifiable Doppler ultrasound could yield reliable results without major risk to the patient. The cardiac stroke volume can be determined by examining the velocity of flow in the aorta. The flow is viewed from the suprasternal notch [15]. The ascending aorta can be measured from a parasternal view, using real time, an M-mode, or an A-mode device. These separately determined parameters can be combined to calculate the amount of blood pumped on each ventricular contraction. The cardiac output is calculated by multiplying the stroke volume times the heart rate. Although these techniques may not readily yield absolute values that are close to real, they can show trends in cardiac output that could prove useful to the overall cardiac picture of the patient.

In any of these applications, we are looking at the movement of RBCs through vascular compartments in the heart and distant vessels. New uses of Doppler that extend to other vascular compartments and vascular beds, such as trying to detect breast cancer by variations in blood flow patterns in the tumor [16], will depend upon what questions we ask of the local physiology. It is physiology that we rely upon to provide deviations from the normal patterns of flow; and the output is generally different from the images we are used to seeing. Time, education, and experience are all mechanisms of understanding that will provide the opportunity to use Doppler to its full potential.

Conclusion

Although the application of Doppler in ultrasound is not new, it is not as widely used as other forms of ultrasound. Our discussion began with the use of echolocation by bats to find prey and progressed, ultimately, to the organization of duplex imaging, a technique combining real-time imaging with pulsed Doppler. A firm grasp of the Doppler equation, which we developed from conceptual origins, is essential to understanding the pulsed Doppler system. The equation showed that the Doppler shift is proportional to the transmitted frequency, the velocity of the target, and the cosine of the look angle, and inversely proportional to the velocity of ultrasound propagation. By controlling the parameters of this equation, the Doppler device can detect the presence of flow disturbance and eventually be used in quantification techniques. These techniques depend upon an accurate estimation of the Doppler shift components, which are provided by new fast Fourier transformation (FFT) methods. The FFT digital process will markedly extend the use and reliability of Doppler ultrasound, and is already giving us a new view of vascular physiology.

References

1. Simmons, J.A., M.B. Fenton, and M.J. O'Farrell. January 1979. Echolocation and pursuit of prey by bats. Science 203:16–21.
2. Suga, N., and P.H-S. Jen. October 1976. Disproportionate tonotopic representation for processing CF-FM sonar signals in the mustache bat audio cortex. Science 194:542–544.
3. O'Neill, W.E., and N. Suga. January 1979. Target range-sensitive neurons in the auditory cortex of the mustache bat. Science 203:69–73.
4. Halliday, D., and R. Resnik. 1960. Physics for students of science and engineering. 2nd ed. New York: John Wiley & Sons, 1960.
5. Waxham, R.D., April/May 1980. Doppler ultrasound. Radiology Today.
6. Baker, D.W., and R.E. Daigle. Noninvasive ultrasonic flowmetry. In Cardiovascular flow dynamics and measurements, Chap. 3., N.H.C. Hwang and N.A. Normann. University Park Press, Baltimore, 1977.
7. Brandistini, M.A., and F.K. Forster. Blood flow imaging using a discrete-time frequency meter. In 1978 Ultrasonics Symposium Proceedings. IEEE: 348–352.
8. Gill, R.W.. 1979. Performance of the mean frequency Doppler modulator. Ultrasound Med Biol 5:127–247.
9. Brown, R.E. November 1971. Doppler ultrasound in obstetrics. JAMA 218:1395–1399.
10. Gill, R.W., W.J. Garrett, P.S. Warren, B.J. Trudinger, and G. Kossoff. 22–27 July 1979. Monitoring blood flow in the fetal umbilical vein. In Proceedings of the Second World Meeting of the World Federation for Ultrasound in Medicine and Biology, Miyazaki, Japan: 201–205.
11. Gill, R.W., B.J. Trudinger, W.J. Garrett, G. Kossoff, and P.S. Warren. March 1981. Fetal umbilical venous flow measured *in utero* by pulsed Doppler and B-mode ultrasound. Am J Obstet Gynecol 139:720–725.

12. Phillips, D.J., W.M. Blackshear, Jr., D.W. Baker, and D.E. Strandness. January–February 1978. Ultrasound duplex scanning in peripheral vascular disease. Radiology/Nuclear Medicine: 6–10.

13. Clifford, P.C., R. Skidmore, J.P. Woodcock, D.R. Bird, R.J. Lusby, and R.N. Baird. February–March 1981. Arterial grafts imaged using Doppler and real-time ultrasound. Vascular Diagnosis and Surgery: 43–57.

14. Baker, D.W., G. Lorch, and S. Rubenstein. 1977. Pulsed doppler echography. In Echocardiology, 201–221. The Hague: Martinus Nijhoff.

15. Light, L.H. 1977. Aortic blood velocity measurements by transcutaneous aortovelography and its clinical applications. In Echocardiology. Martinus Nijhoff, The Hague: 233–243.

16. Halliwell, M. February 1981. Doppler ultrasound shows promise for breast cancer detection. Radiology/Nuclear Medicine: 12–22.

PART TWO

Extracting Information from the Images

Chapter 9

Effects of Tissue
on Ultrasound

A major capability of the technology of gray-scale ultrasound is its ability to display tissue texture. In general, tissue texture is a pattern comprising dots of various size, shape, position, and intensity, formed by the interaction of several factors, both internal and external to the sonograph. Moreover, the patterns appear different among different sorts of tissue. Although not all gray-scale sonographs portray tissue texture in the same way, the patterns are sufficiently repeatable that local and diffuse changes in tissue quality change the ultrasonic tissue texture in identifiable ways. These textural changes are then used clinically. The primary mechanisms for such changes are complex and are modeled using rather complicated mathematics. They represent one-half of the tissue-ultrasound interaction, the influence of the tissue on ultrasound.

The tissue texture contained in an image is best seen on single-pass scans of organs, but still appears in many compound scans that store only peak values. Some examples of different textures are shown in Figure 9-1, 9-2, and 9-3. Near the top of the image is a fine texture that increases in size laterally and axially, proceeding to the more distant portions of the scan. Dot size, shape, separation, repeated patterns, and component amplitudes all contribute to the image appearance. Two processes play a significant part in the overall textural qualities of the image. The first process is the simple return of echoes from distributed macro- and microanatomy. The second process is a phase-sensitive process called speckling, formed by the interference patterns of all the echoes arriving at the transducer at the same time [1, 2]. The speckling process is connected with the same anatomy as simple reflection, but in a less direct way. Most of the models of speckling treat it as a random process [3]; however, this view is more a reflection of our inability to be specific about the reflection and wave-summing events. As we shall see, real-time imaging with multiple transducers offers ample evidence that speckling may be hard to describe, but it is not random.

How do we begin to fit the pieces of this puzzle together in order to use tissue texture effectively? This chapter outlines a practical model to be used to predict some of the tissue-induced behavior of ultrasound. In addition, it offers some realistic rules for tissue-texture applications. Our step-by-step model includes enough complications to cover many of the tissue-ultrasound events, and yet is

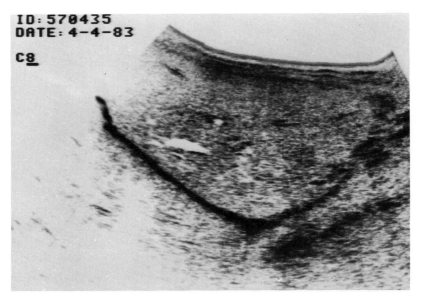

9-1 Typical texture of a liver in full view. The image of a liver shows a changing texture as a function of depth. The anterior texture contains many small echo signals that vanish with increasing range from the transducer.

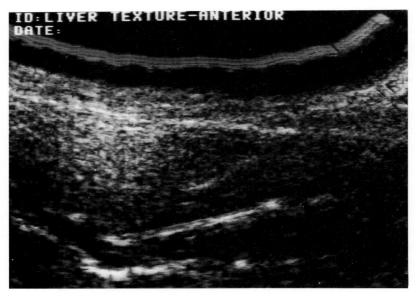

9-2 Anterior tissue texture. The portions of a scan closer to a transducer includes very small echo signals that contribute to the image texture.

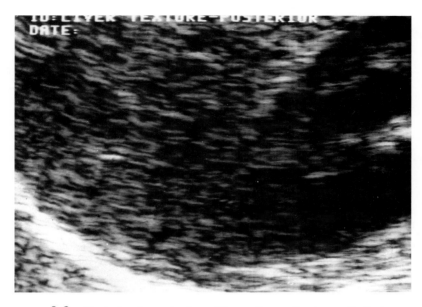

9-3   Posterior tissue texture. The portions of an image farther from the transducer do not have the small echo signals that add a fine quality to the texture. Only the larger echo signals remain in the more distant portions of the image, producing a coarser texture.

simple enough to convey some understanding of the textural presentations of static B-scanning, real time, and M-mode.

Before launching into a discussion of our model, some facts about ultrasound waves and reflection are reviewed briefly below.

Waves and Reflection

The basic ultrasound wave is a compressional or longitudinal wave. To propagate, the wave needs a carrying medium with particles that can move within some elastic limits. The longitudinal motion of the medium forms regions of compression and rarefaction. The medium returns to the resting condition after the wave passes. The transition into these regional changes in density is generally smooth, but abrupt changes are possible with rapidly changing wave fronts or waves that exceed the elastic limits of the medium. Operating within the elastic limits ensures that any material displacement will return to a normal resting state after the mechanical energy passes.

Traveling waves operating within the elastic limits of the medium will add together in a simple manner called superposition. The waves can pass through the same space at the same time, adding to form a new wave that is the sum of all the traveling parts. The waves continue on, unaltered by their simultaneous occupation

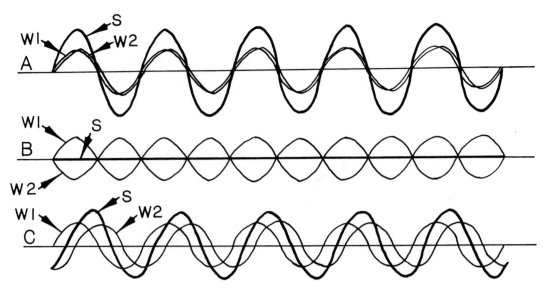

9-4   The phasic summation of waves. The superposition of waves permits waves of equal strength but different phase to add together, producing a result varying from the sum of the individual amplitudes to zero. Part A: Waves *W1* and *W2* have equal amplitude and are in phase, forming the sum *S*. Part B: Waves *W1* and *W2* are equal in amplitude but 180° out of phase, producing the summary wave *S*. Part C: Waves *W1* and *W2* are out of phase by 90°, forming a new wave *S* that is out of phase with both the component waves and is smaller than the sum shown in Part A.

of the same space. The resulting wave is a function of the frequency, phase, and amplitude of each component wave. For example, two waves with the same frequency and amplitude can sum to a new wave twice as large, or to zero or to some value between these extremes, depending upon the phase or timing between the waves (Figure 9-4). These wave events occur in both transverse and longitudinal waves.

The mechanics of wave reflection, on the other hand, are a function of the wavelength and the lateral size of the reflecting interface. If the lateral dimensions of the interface are very large relative to the wavelength, the reflection follows the same rules as does the reflection of light off a mirror: the angle of incidence is equal to the angle of reflection. How much energy is reflected at the interface is proportional to the difference in acoustical impedance across the interface. In addition, the intensity of the reflected wave is proportional to the square of the difference in impedance. The specular reflection process is largely independent of the ultrasound frequency; thus, specular reflectors will remain so with increasing frequency. On the other hand, specular reflectors at a high frequency may not be so at a lower frequency, and scatters at a low frequency can be more specular at higher frequencies.

If the dimensions of the interface are less than or close to the ultrasound wavelength, the reflection mechanics follow the rules of scattering [4]. The term

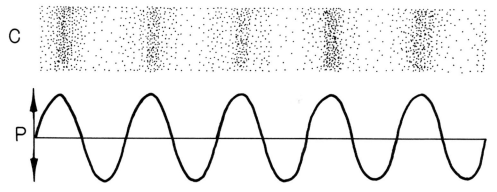

9-5 Relationship between a compressional wave and regional pressure. A compressional wave can be viewed as a set of rhythmic changes in density and pressure. *C* shows changes in density for a compressional wave. *P* shows the change in relative pressure corresponding to the changes in density.

scattering indicates the way the ultrasound energy is dispersed by the interface. The energy is literally "scattered" in all directions.

Very small particles can individually intercept only a small portion of the advancing wave front, and that small portion of intercepted energy is scattered away. Because the small amount of dispersed energy is spread in all directions, only a small portion is actually reflected back to the transducer. As a result, the echo from a single scatterer may be too small to appear on a display. But as the number of scatterers increases, the scatterers' effect on the advancing ultrasound energy increases, and the amount of ultrasound scattered back to the transducer increases.

If a scattering body has a size close to the wavelength of an ultrasound wave, the character of the reflection will change, becoming more specular as the frequency increases [3]. Even very small scatterers have this property, so the amount of energy reflected back to a transducer from small distributed scatterers will increase in proportion to the third of fourth power of frequency. As a result, a small change in ultrasound frequency can often produce a large change in the relative reflectivity of scattering objects.

An essential factor in the mechanics of ultrasonic interference is the phase shift that is imposed on the reflected wave at some interfaces. If the change in acoustical impedance is from a lower to a higher value, for example, the reflected wave is phase-shifted 180°, and the wave is effectively inverted. In a transverse wave, this is easy to understand, but in a longitudinal wave, what does inversion mean? If a longitudinal wave is represented as a pressure over distance, then a sine wave of pressure around an ambient pressure line will represent events within the longitudinal wave (Figure 9-5). A 180° phase shift means that a region in space that should be in compression is now in rarefaction and vice versa. On the other hand, if the impedance change is from the higher to a lower value, the reflected wave is not phase-shifted at all. These phase relationships at the acoustical interfaces are independent of frequency.

Although reflection phase shifts are independent of frequency, this independence may not hold true for the propagation velocity [5]. When the propagation velocity of a wave becomes a function of frequency, complex waves can change shape as they pass through a material. If the velocity change is large for a small change in frequency, waves that started traveling together will separate according to frequency as they propagate through the medium. This mechanism is called dispersion. Although dispersion is not a major factor in most soft-tissue propagation of ultrasound, it can subtly and unpredictably influence events at a transducer.

With the foregoing science in hand, we are ready to look at the events in tissue attenuation.

Tissue Attenuation Model

A Homogeneous Medium

The echoes received by the transducer cause a range of voltages out of the transducer in which the largest signal can be in excess of 100 dB above the smallest (Figure 9-6). This range of signals represents everything from the largest echo from a specular reflector close to the transducer to the smallest echo still visible above the noise. This impressive signal range evolves from the frequency-dependent attenuation imposed on the ultrasound as it travels through the tissues. Because of the typical transmitting powers, these voltages often span values from 1 V to 10 μV. As we learned in Chapter 2, the input voltages are defined by the transmit-receive (TR) switch that sits between the transducer and the first radio frequency (rf) amplifier in the receiver. It is this fixed window that echo-signal voltages out of transducer must fit within (Figure 9-7). The echo amplitudes that return to the transducer are controlled by the transmitter voltage that sets transmitted power. Because of this relationship, the echo signals are fitted into the TR switch window by properly setting the transmitted ultrasound energy. In sonographs with a fixed transmitter output and a variable receiver gain, the transmitting voltage and the TR switch are matched by design and measurement during manufacture. In sonographs with a fixed receiver gain, the echo signals are fitted into the TR switch window by changing the transducer energy output. Two tissue-ultrasound interaction processes are included in this huge range of signals: first, the attenuation imposed on the ultrasound beam by the tissue; and second, the variation in reflectivity among reflectors. We will look at them separately, then recombine them to form a more complete grasp of the events within the tissues.

A common attenuation rate ascribed to biological soft tissue is 1 dB/cm/MHz. This attenuation rate is usually determined by measuring the change in a transmitted signal amplitude as ultrasound passes one way through a piece of tissue. By sweeping the ultrasound frequency over values of, say, 1 MHz to 10 MHz, the dependence upon frequency also can be determined [6]. In most biological tissue, the frequency dependence is close to linear for the frequencies typical of diagnostic

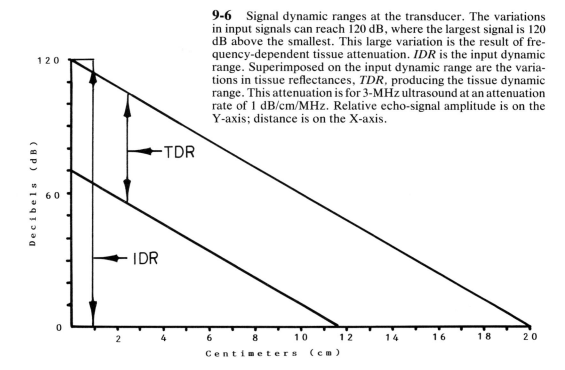

9-6 Signal dynamic ranges at the transducer. The variations in input signals can reach 120 dB, where the largest signal is 120 dB above the smallest. This large variation is the result of frequency-dependent tissue attenuation. *IDR* is the input dynamic range. Superimposed on the input dynamic range are the variations in tissue reflectances, *TDR*, producing the tissue dynamic range. This attenuation is for 3-MHz ultrasound at an attenuation rate of 1 dB/cm/MHz. Relative echo-signal amplitude is on the Y-axis; distance is on the X-axis.

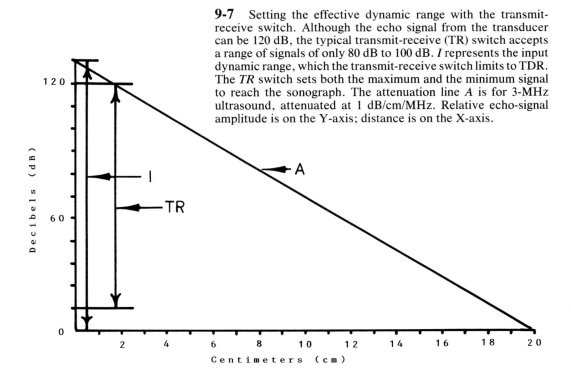

9-7 Setting the effective dynamic range with the transmit-receive switch. Although the echo signal from the transducer can be 120 dB, the typical transmit-receive (TR) switch accepts a range of signals of only 80 dB to 100 dB. *I* represents the input dynamic range, which the transmit-receive switch limits to TDR. The *TR* switch sets both the maximum and the minimum signal to reach the sonograph. The attenuation line *A* is for 3-MHz ultrasound, attenuated at 1 dB/cm/MHz. Relative echo-signal amplitude is on the Y-axis; distance is on the X-axis.

ultrasound [7]. The attenuation rate per unit distance can be calculated by multiplying the attenuation rate by the frequency of ultrasound in megahertz. For example, a 3-MHz ultrasound wave will be attenuated:

$$3 \text{ MHz} \times 1 \text{ dB/cm/MHz} = 3 \text{ dB/cm}. \tag{9.1}$$

The following mental exercise will help us to conceptualize what this attenuation means to the sonograph. Consider an attenuating medium that removes energy from the ultrasound beam at 1 dB/cm/MHz. Within the medium is a perfect reflector that returns 100% of the incident energy. Moreover, the reflector is movable. The sonograph has a 100-dB dynamic range into the receiver, and the ultrasonic output from the transducer is controllable to match the echo signals to the TR switch dynamic range. The transducer is operating at 3 MHz; because this is a thought experiment, it is the only frequency present. By setting the echo signal to the highest amplitude out of the TR switch with the perfect reflector right next to the transducer. As the reflector is moved away from the transducer, the echo signal decreases in amplitude until it finally vanishes from the display. At what range does it vanish? And how might we make that determination without moving the reflector? To calculate that value, we need to examine what is happening to the signal within the medium.

If we simply calculate the vanishing point from the known dynamic range of the TR switch, the result looks like:

$$100 \text{ dB}/3 \text{ dB/cm} = 33.3 \text{ cm}. \tag{9.2}$$

Unfortunately, the experiment will show that the signal vanished at one-half that distance. What was wrong with our reasoning? Our error lies in forgetting that the sonograph is an echo-ranging device. The ultrasound must leave the transducer and return. Within the medium, the ultrasound intensity drops 3 dB/cm going to the reflector and another 3 dB/cm on the return trip. Within the medium, it is the signal returning to the transducer that goes to 0, not the ultrasound penetrating to the reflector. In fact, at a range of 16.7 cm, the reflected ultrasound is still 50 dB above the smallest signal (Figure 9-8). These 50 dB of ultrasound signal strength will be lost on the return trip.

The events can be viewed from two different vantage points: the decrease in echo-signal amplitude can be though of as either a one-way trip at 2 dB/cm/MHz and a dynamic range of 100 dB, or as a two-way trip at 1 dB/cm/MHz. The results can be summarized into a single equation:

$$DR = 2 \, aFZ, \tag{9.3}$$

where DR is the total signal dynamic range in dB, a is the attenuation rate (one way) in dB/cm/MHz, F is the ultrasound frequency in MHz, and Z is the range from the transducer in cm. Because most sonographs show range as if it were a one-way trip, we get used to thinking in only a one-way tissue-attenuation rate. It will be easier to use the 100-dB dynamic range and an attenuation rate of $2a$, which is an attenuation rate of 2 dB/cm/MHz. In whatever manner we think of these events, the sonograph TR switch dynamic range will have a powerful influence on the effective imaging penetration at any given frequency in diagnostic ultrasound.

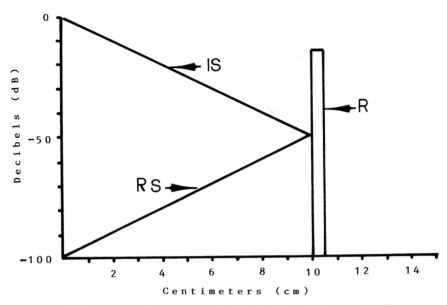

9-8   Attenuation on transmitted and reflected ultrasound. The attenuation occurs on both the incident ultrasound, *IS,* and the reflected ultrasound, *RS. R* is a perfect reflector just out of range as the reflected ultrasound produces a signal 100 dB below the maximum signal. Relative echo-signal level is on the Y-axis; distance is on the X-axis for 5-MHz ultrasound, attenuated at 1 dB/cm/MHz.

It is also worthwhile to change the signal referencing. Because we are using units of decibels, the signals can be referenced against either the smallest signal or the largest signal. Because of individual variations among machines in terms of the smallest signal that can be presented, a reference against the largest signal is a better choice. The Y-axis, then, will have units of decibels, with the largest signal set at 0 dB, and smaller values represented as −dB values below this reference (Figure 9-9).

A Nonhomogeneous Medium

Up to this point in the discussion, the medium has been homogeneous, with no regional changes in attenuation. The ultrasound beam has also been uniform over distance. In practice, neither of these assumptions is true. When these two variables are later factored into the tissue-attenuation model, some commonly seen but seldom explained events become clear.

Examine, first, the situation where an ultrasound beam encounters a region of less-than-normal attenuation (Figure 9-10). The ultrasound beam is still uniform, so the only influence on the beam strength is the tissue attenuation. Events will be mapped as before by looking at the change in echo-signal amplitude from an ideal reflector as the signals pass through the TR switch. Within the medium is a

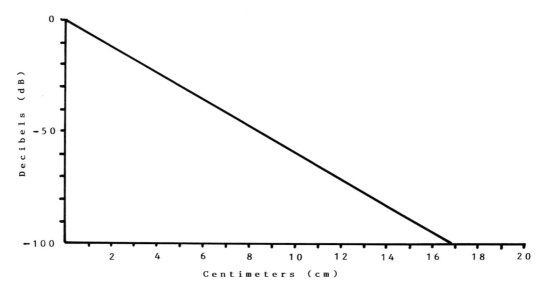

9-9   The attenuation profile for a perfect reflector in a uniform medium. The attenuation profile comes from moving a perfect reflector from the face of a transducer until the echo signal disappears. The line represents the echo-signal amplitude at each distance from the reflector. Relative echo-signal amplitude is on the Y-axis; distance is on the X-axis for 3 MHz-ultrasound, attenuated at 1 dB/cm/MHz.

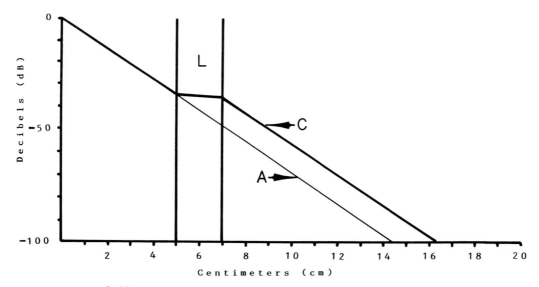

9-10   Changes in the attenuation profile with a low attenuator. The presence of a low attenuating material *L* displaces the attenuation profile beyond the structure from the expected line *A* to the new profile *C*. Signal amplitudes posterior to a low attenuating structure will appear larger than expected. Relative echo-signal amplitude is on the Y-axis; distance is on the X-axis for 3.5-MHz ultrasound, attenuated at 1 dB/cm/MHz in the surrounding material and 0.01 dB/cm/MHz for *L*.

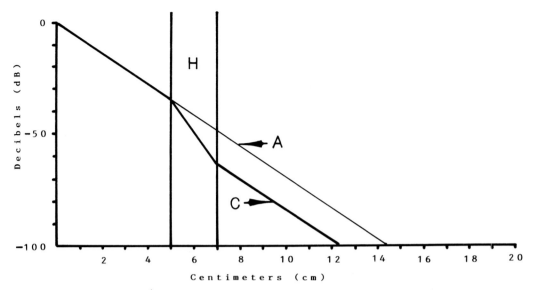

9-11 Changes in the attenuation profile with a high attenuator. The presence of a high attenuating material *H* displaces the attenuation profile beyond the structure downward from the expected line *A* to the new profile *C*. Signals posterior to a high attenuating structure will appear lower than expected. Relative echo-signal amplitude is on the Y-axis; distance is on the X-axis for 3.5-MHz ultrasound, attenuated at 1 dB/cm/MHz in the surrounding material and 2.0 dB/cm/MHz for *H*.

2-cm layer of material with an attenuation rate 0.01 times less than the normal 1 dB/cm/MHz, positioned at a 5-cm range. As before, we will use a 3-MHz ultrasound frequency.

The signals start falling from the 0 dB starting point at a rate of 6 dB/cm (2 dB/cm/MHz × 3.0 MHz) for 5 cm. A signal from this range will be down 30 dB (Figure 9-10). At the new medium interface, the attenuation rate changes to 0.06 dB/cm, so in the 2-cm distance, the signal will decrease another 0.12 dB. Beyond the low attenuating material, the normal attenuation resumes. It is as if the decreasing signal line were broken and displayed 2 cm deeper. In this case, the penetration effectively increased 2 cm. As the intervening material increases its attenuation rate, the penetration range comes closer to the transducer, finally conforming to the homogeneous medium penetration.

The intervening layer with the lower-than-normal attenuation rate has increased the signals posterior to the layer 12 dB above normal, that is, 12 dB above what we would expect if the attenuation had been uniform (Figure 9-10). This is none other than our old friend acoustical enhancement, seen posterior to low attenuating structures such as cysts, vessels, and fluid-filled organs like the kidney.

On the other side of the coin is a region in which the attenuation rate is higher than normal (Figure 9-11). Let us assume the same geometry as before, but now the 2-cm interval has an attenuation rate of 2 dB/cm/MHz. As before, the first 5 cm reduces the signal by 30 dB. Through the 2-cm layer, the attenuation rate doubles to 12 dB/cm, and the 2-cm distance will decrease the signal 24 dB. Beyond

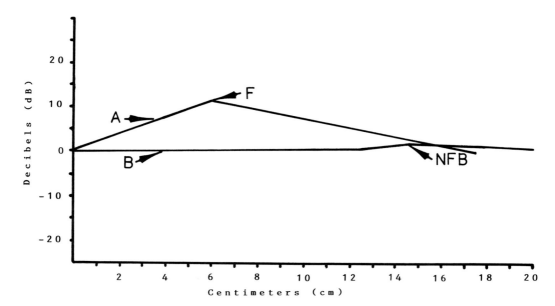

9-12 Changes in echo-signal amplitude with focusing. *A* is a 3.5-MHz, 16-mm diameter transducer, focused at 6 cm. The focusing process causes the echo signals from like echo sources to increase in amplitude as they approach the focus of the transducer *F*. Beyond the focal point, the broadening beam produces a decreasing echo-signal amplitude. An unfocused transducer with the same diameter and frequency, *B,* shows a small increase in the echo-signal amplitude at the boundary between the near field and the far field, *NFB*. Relative echo-signal amplitude is on the Y-axis; distance is on the X-axis.

the 2-cm layer, the normal attenuation rate resumes, but with a signal 12 dB lower than normal. The result is decreased penetration and a signal level beyond the intervening layer that is 12 dB smaller than expected. This is, in fact, the acoustical shadowing seen behind lesions and structures that have a higher-than-normal attenuation rate.

Transducer Focusing Effects

The tissue attenuation model so far has postulated a uniform ultrasound field from the transducer. The beam profile supplied by a transducer or sonograph manufacturer clearly shows that focused transducers do not treat like reflectors alike. Depending upon the degree of focus, the response of a focused transducer to the same target can vary as much as 20 dB from the transducer face to the most intense portion of the focus, and typical values hover around 15 dB for B-scanning transducers and 10 dB for some of the real-time transducers (Figure 9-12). The amount of variation in the ultrasound beam will change the apparent tissue-attenuation rate.

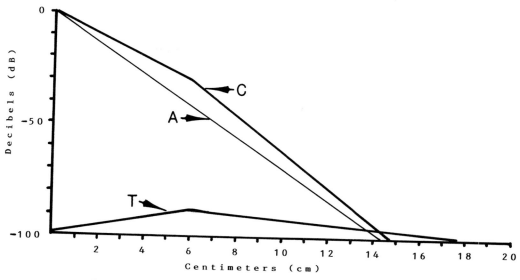

9-13   Combining the tissue attenuation with transducer focusing. A 3.5-MHz, 16-mm diameter transducer focused at 6 cm,
T, combines with the 3.5-MHz attenuation profile *A* to produce
a combined echo-signal attenuation profile *C*. In this new profile,
the attenuation rate into the focal point is less than the attenuation out of the focal point. Relative echo-signal amplitude is
on the Y-axis; distance is on the X-axis.

Using the ultrasound beam profile envelope expressed in decibels, the ultrasound
focusing effects can be factored into the tissue-attenuation rate model by simple
addition. Figure 9-13 shows the attenuation profile produced by 15 dB of focusing
in a 3-MHz transducer, with the focal point 6 cm from the transducer. The combined effect of focusing and attenuation causes two attenuation rates, a slower-
than-normal rate into the focal point, and a faster-than-normal rate out of the focal
point. Despite the transducer focusing, the maximum penetration is not substantially changed. Increasing the degree of focusing will not extend penetration any
farther (Figure 9-14). In fact, penetration will often decrease for a tightly focused,
short–focal length transducer with a very rapid beam spread following the focal
zone.

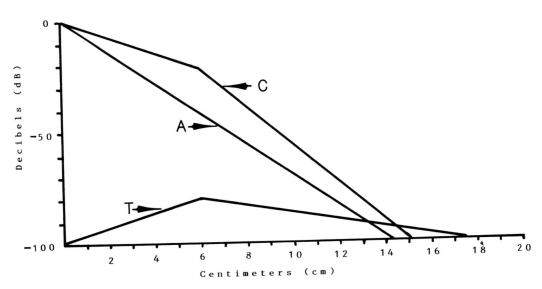

9-14 Combining the tissue attenuation with increased transducer focusing. A 3.5-MHz, 19-mm diameter transducer *T*, focused at 6 cm, with a gain of 20 dB into the focus, combines with the 3.5-MHz attenuation profile *A* to produce a combined effect *C*. The increased focusing decreases the rate of attenuation into the focal point and increases the slope of the attenuation profile beyond the focal point. In addition, the increased focusing produces only a marginal change in effective penetration. Relative echo-signal amplitude is on the Y-axis; distance is on the X-axis.

The combined effect of attenuation and focusing can be dramatically changed by regions having changes in attenuation rate. For example, Figure 9-15 shows the effect of a low attenuating layer in front of the transducer focal point. The combined effect of a focusing transducer beam and a region of low attenuation is a sharp change in the attenuation profile within the "cystic" structure. In the clinical situation, this sort of uneven intensity can cause distributed interfaces not visible in the anterior portion of the cyst to become so in the posterior portion, with acoustical enhancement still present posterior to the low attenuating structure.

If the cyst appears after the focal point, (Figure 9-16) the defocusing ultrasound beam experiences less of a change through the cyst than when the cyst was in front of the focal point. As a result, the field within the cyst is more uniform, which can assist in accurately portraying any interior complexities that the cyst might contain.

A similar sort of beam-profile wrinkling occurs when a layer of higher-than-normal attenuation is encountered. Examples of these profiles are shown in Figures 9-17 and 9-18.

We now need to factor in the variations among echo sources.

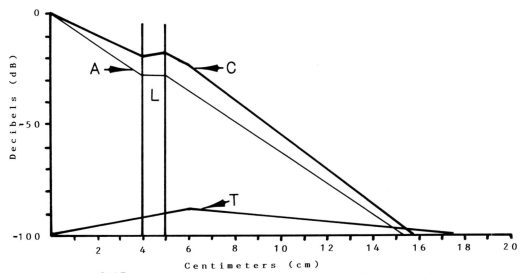

9-15   Combining tissue attenuation, transducer focusing, and a low attenuating material. The transducer in Figure 9-12 now encounters a low attenuating material *L,* located in front of the transducer focal point. The transducer profile *T* combines with the attenuation line *A* to produce the combined effect *C.* The increase in echo-signal level posterior to a low attenuating medium is called acoustical enhancement. Relative echo-signal level is on the Y-axis; distance is on the X-axis; the attenuation rate is 1 dB/cm/MHz; *L* is 0.01 dB/cm/MHz.

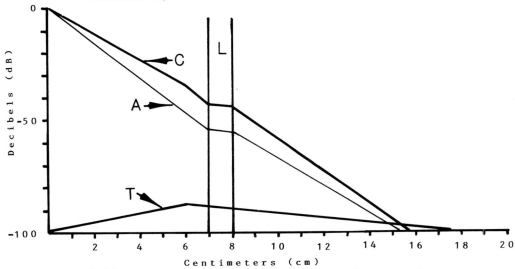

9-16   Combining tissue attenuation, transducer focusing, and a repositioned low attenuating material. The transducer in Figure 9-12 now encounters a low attenuating material *L* posterior to the focal point. The transducer profile *T* combines with the tissue attenuation profile *A* to produce the combined effect *C.* The effective penetration is independent of the low attenuator position, but the distortion to the attenuation profile is much less posterior to the focal point. Relative echo-signal amplitude is on the Y-axis; distance is on the X-axis; the attenuation rate is 1 dB/cm/MHz; *L* is 0.01 dB/cm/MHz.

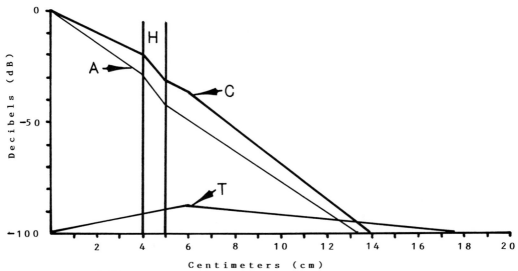

9-17   Combining tissue attenuation, transducer focusing, and a high attenuating material. The transducer in Figure 9-12 now encounters a high attenuating material *H* anterior to the transducer focal point. The transducer profile *T* combines with the tissue attenuation profile *A* to produce the combined effect *C*. The decrease in echo-signal amplitude posterior to a high attenuating material is called shadowing. Relative echo-signal level is on the Y-axis; distance is on the X-axis; the attenuation rate is 1 dB/cm/MHz; *H* is 2 dB/cm/MHz.

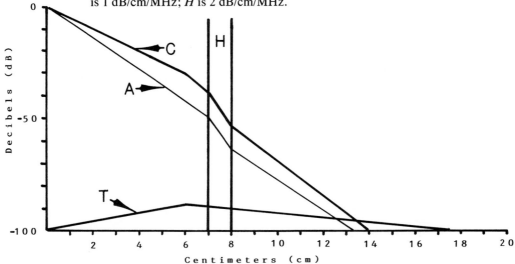

9-18   Combining tissue attenuation, transducer focusing, and a repositioned high attenuating material. The transducer in Figure 9-12 now encounters a high attenuating material *H* posterior to the focal point. The transducer profile *T* combines with the tissue attenuation profile *A* to produce the combined effect *C*. The effective penetration is independent of the high attenuator position, but the distortion to the attenuation profile is much less beyond the focal point. Relative echo-signal amplitude is on the Y-axis; distance is on the X-axis; the attenuation rate is 1 dB/cm/MHz; *H* is 2 dB/cm/MHz.

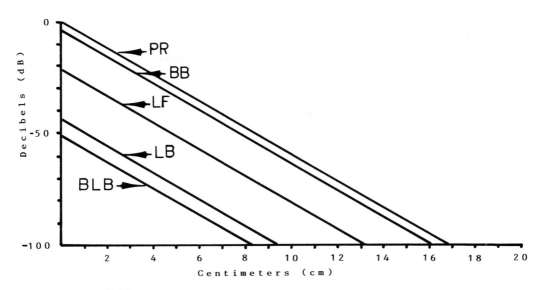

9-19   Reflectivity of different biological interfaces relative to a perfect reflector *PR*. Biological interfaces range from just under 4 dB below a perfect reflector to as far as 51 dB below. The ability to see a particular type of interface at far distances is a function of the signal the interface presents to the sonograph. The brain-bone interface *BB* is just under 4 dB below a perfect reflector and will produce effective echo signals much deeper than a softer interface of liver and fat *LF*. The liver blood interface *LB* resides some 44 dB below a perfect reflector, and the blood-brain interface *BLB* is 51 dB below a perfect reflector. The lower the reflectivity, the greater the difficulty in seeing the tissue echo signals at long distances. Relative echo-signal amplitude is on the Y-axis; distance is on the X-axis; attenuation normalized to 1 dB/cm/MHz; 3-MHz ultrasound.

Variations Among Reflectors

Superimposed on the normal tissue attenuation is the variation among signals due to changes in reflectivity at the interfaces encountered by the ultrasound. Comparing measured acoustical impedances and calculating the reflectivity of various interface combinations can provide an estimate of the range of biological echoes we can expect to see in the tissues. The calculations consider only specular reflection values. Scattering and interference will produce signals even smaller. These values can be compared to a perfect reflector, as in Figure 9-19.

Probably the most perfect reflector to appear in normal scanning is an air-tissue interface. The next brightest reflector is the bone–soft tissue interface. This echo is only about 3.7 dB below a perfect reflector. At the same time, a blood-brain interface is over 50 dB below a perfect reflector. Thus, variations among specular reflectors can take on values ranging over 46 dB, and scattering can extend the range of the lower signals farther still.

The obvious question is: Can we see these variations over all depths? The answer is no. Figure 9-19 shows why. First, the maximum specular reflector, only 3.7 dB below a perfect reflector, is brought to the top of the TR switch window by increasing the transmitter output. Some 46 dB below that are the smallest specular reflectors. They will vanish at 9 cm; thus, beyond the 9-cm demarcation, the dynamic range of the signals among reflectors decreases. The medium specular reflectors 20 dB below the maximum will vanish at 13 cm. Where does the useful penetration stop? How much variation among signals is needed to offer information of value? If the variation is 10 dB, then the useful penetration for any frequency can be calculated from the relationship:

$$DR - S = 2\ aFZ, \tag{9.4}$$

where DR is the TR switch dynamic range, S is the minimum signal dynamic range needed for information, a is the attenuation rate, F is the ultrasound frequency in megahertz, and Z is the effective range for the sonograph. For example, if 10 dB is the minimum signal variation acceptable for 3-MHz imaging, and the TR switch dynamic range is 100 dB, then the effective penetration will be:

$$100\ -\ 10\ dB/6\ dB/cm\ =\ 15\ cm. \tag{9.5}$$

These are only the top 10 dB. If signals as low as 46 dB below maximum contribute to the total image appearance, then even under ideal conditions, the image visual qualities will change beyond 9 cm.

If the transmitting energy were lower than required, this textural change would begin even earlier in the image. For example, a transmitter output decreased 20 dB will cause the maximum specular reflector to vanish at just over 13 cm, the medium specular reflectors to vanish at about 10 cm, and the smallest echoes to vanish at almost 6 cm (Figure 9-20). Clearly, to use the sonograph to full potential, it must be run using its full dynamic range.

In Chapter 3, on transducers, we learned that a damped transducer is not a single-frequency source, but transmits a wide range of frequencies. Often the band width will exceed 40% of the natural resonant frequency of the transducer. Because the attenuation rate is frequency-dependent, a 3-MHz transducer with a 40% band width will run out of 3-MHz energy at close to 17 cm on the display and 2.4 MHz (lower frequency limit 6 dB below maximum) energy at 20 cm (Figure 9-21). The upper frequency limit at 3.6 MHz will vanish at close to 13 cm. Because of the lower frequency components in the transmitted ultrasound, useful signals appear out to display depths of 20 cm for typical real-time and static B-scanning.

With a grasp of these facts, we are ready to build a more complex model of events, beginning at single-body scattering.

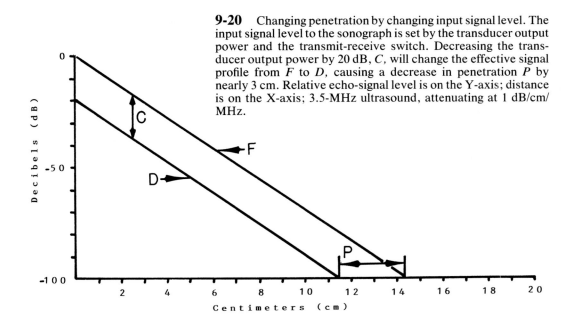

9-20 Changing penetration by changing input signal level. The input signal level to the sonograph is set by the transducer output power and the transmit-receive switch. Decreasing the transducer output power by 20 dB, *C,* will change the effective signal profile from *F* to *D,* causing a decrease in penetration *P* by nearly 3 cm. Relative echo-signal level is on the Y-axis; distance is on the X-axis; 3.5-MHz ultrasound, attenuating at 1 dB/cm/MHz.

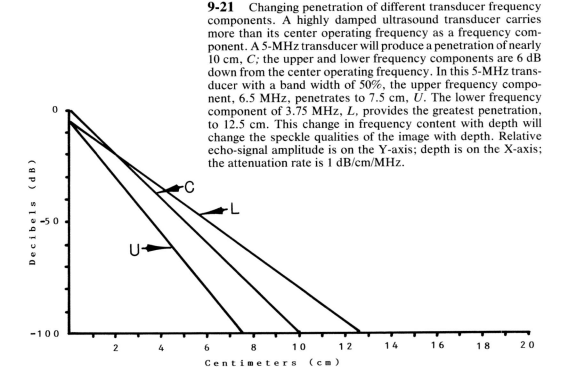

9-21 Changing penetration of different transducer frequency components. A highly damped ultrasound transducer carries more than its center operating frequency as a frequency component. A 5-MHz transducer will produce a penetration of nearly 10 cm, *C;* the upper and lower frequency components are 6 dB down from the center operating frequency. In this 5-MHz transducer with a band width of 50%, the upper frequency component, 6.5 MHz, penetrates to 7.5 cm, *U.* The lower frequency component of 3.75 MHz, *L,* provides the greatest penetration, to 12.5 cm. This change in frequency content with depth will change the speckle qualities of the image with depth. Relative echo-signal amplitude is on the Y-axis; depth is on the X-axis; the attenuation rate is 1 dB/cm/MHz.

Single-Body Scattering Model

Despite the amount of image information that depends upon scattering, the scattering process is discussed little in the ultrasound community. A major reason for this lack of discussion is the sheer complexity of the "multibody, variable compressibility, nonhomogeneous scattering problem." Scattering can be described conceptually, but it is mathematically staggering. The task in this discussion, then, is to formulate a descriptive model of events. We will do this by using analogies and the wave science described in Chapter 1. The single-body scattering situation will be the starting point.

Let us place ourselves in a darkened room with a small hole in one wall to let a shaft of light enter the room. The air is free of any contamination, so the boundaries of the shaft are invisible, unless we place an eye in the light. A human eye will be a sensor detecting any light that deviates from the projecting shaft. Within the shaft is a small, reflecting spherical object. The object is larger than any of the wavelengths of the component waves (this is white light comprising many component colors), but smaller than our visual acuity from a distance. Placed within the shaft of light, the object becomes visible from nearly anywhere in the room. Observations made at a constant distance from the scattering body but at different angles show that the body is always visible at any angle.

The object is visible because it is affecting a portion of the incident light, deviating it from its normal path as part of the light shaft. The object is spreading the intercepted light around the room, and this light is perceived by the eye. This is the fundamental event of scattering. Waves traveling along in a given direction interact with an object and are suddenly sent out in all directions. But careful measurements show that the spreading is not always even.

If the object is now made smaller and smaller, the ability to see the object begins to decrease because the amount of light it intercepts is decreased. At the same time, the variations in brightness from different locations become less until the brightness is independent of the observer's angular position. Consider now a similar situation with a mechanical wave.

Our mechanical wave model includes, like the shaft of light, a set of planar mechanical waves, continuously moving through a homogeneous medium, with a fixed velocity of propagation. Within the medium is a small, hard, scattering object. It is spherical in shape and therefore symmetrical; scattering will be the same regardless of the direction in which the waves strike the object. Instead of using an eye to sense the mechanical wave, we will move a small transducer around the object, measuring any deviations of the primary waves from the normal propagation path.

Let us begin with a very low-frequency wave, with a wavelength much longer than the dimensions of the scattering body. From the wave point of view, the scattering body is very small, intercepting little of the traveling energy. The energy that is intercepted is spread rather uniformly in all directions, with a slightly larger amount of energy returning toward the oncoming wave [3]. An example of what the energy distribution looks like is shown in Figure 9-22.

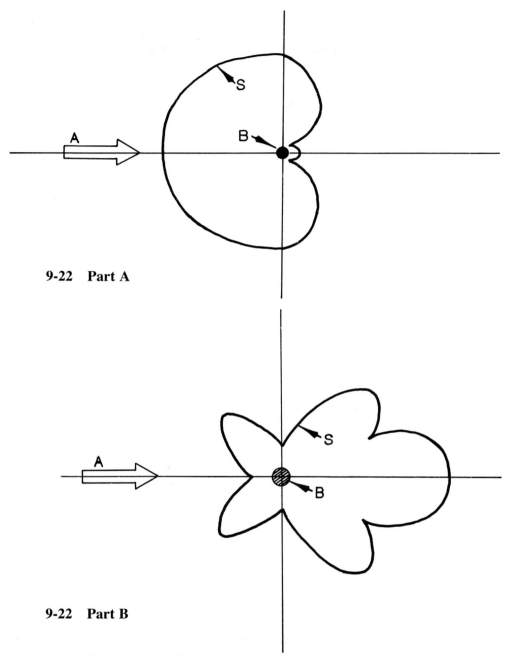

9-22   Part A

9-22   Part B

9-22   Intensity profiles from small scattering bodies. When a scattering body is small compared to the wavelength of ultrasound, the incident ultrasound *A* will be scattered from the body *B* in an almost uniform manner, as shown in Part A. The relative intensity of the scattered wave is shown by the distance of the curve *S* from the scattering body. In Part B, increasing the size of the scattering body will cause the scattering intensity to change shape, with increasing amounts of energy scattered forward.

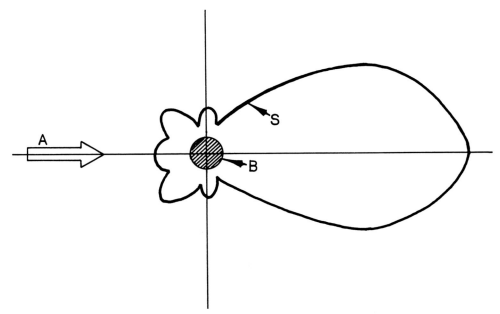

9-23   Scattering from a relatively large body. Incident ultrasound *A* will have a very nonuniform scattering intensity when
it encounters a scattering body much larger than a wavelength.
In this instance, more than 50% of the scattered energy is scattered forward in the direction of the traveling incident ultrasound. This forward scattering can interact with the incident-
traveling ultrasound to produce unpredictable interference patterns, affecting image speckle.

Increasing the wave frequency until the wave length is much smaller than the
scattering body dimensions changes how the wave interacts with the scattering
body. Now a greater portion of the wave front is intercepted. The distribution of
scattered energy is nonuniform, with fully 50% of the scattered energy traveling
in the same direction as the original wave front, but shifted in phase [3]. The
remaining scattered energy is distributed around the scattering body, with regions
of high and low energy. This pattern of scattered energy is shown in Figure 9-23.
The forward scattered energy will interact with the ongoing primary waves, setting
up a destructive interference pattern and potentially a shadow [3].

How large does the scattering object appear to the wave? This parameter is
called the scattering cross section [3]. This cross section is equal to the area of the
incident wave that contains the same amount of energy as is scattered away.
Calculations show that for very small scattering bodies, the scattering cross section
will be a power function of the scattering body diameter, ranging from the fourth
to the sixth power. The larger scattering bodies, however, will present a scattering
cross section equal to twice the cross-sectional area of the sphere. Calculations
and measurements clearly show that a scattering body acts as if it could influence
waves over a larger region than the scattering body physically occupies.

Between these two dimensional extremes is a region of activity in which the scattering body as a dimension close to the wavelength of the traveling wave. Here a variety of scattering and interference phenomena occur. The size of the scattering body even permits diffraction events along with scattering. The result is a complicated scattering pattern with strong energy lobes in specific directions, as well as a strong forward energy lobe that can produce shadowing. This form of resonant scattering produces some complicated results.

Because scattering removes energy from an ongoing wave, its effects are often seen first as a form of attenuation. The ability of scattering to remove energy depends upon the number of scattering bodies along the propagation path, and the dimensional relationship between the scattering body size and the wavelength. Our scattering model will approximate the ultrasound-tissue situation as we next assemble all the factors to form a yet more complex model.

A More Complex Tissue-Ultrasound Model

The background for a more complex model is the normal macro- and microanatomy of the tissue. Echoes arise at acoustical interfaces where the tissue changes acoustical impedance abruptly. These changes occur at organ boundaries, internal structures, and segments of the vascular tree. In addition, tissue organization into cellular aggregates with surrounding connective tissue can provide regularly spaced scattering bodies with consistent diameters. In between the aggregates of cells is extracellular water in various states of binding to proteins and connective tissue [8]. The organization for each tissue type is consistent enough to permit the science of histology, but complex enough to challenge a simple mathematical model of events. It will not, however, bar the way to a descriptive model.

The reflection events portrayed in an image are not acquired from all regions of space at the same time. At any given moment, the electrical signals out of the transducer come from the region of space defined by the ultrasound beam on transmission and the directiveness of the transducer on reception. The receiving directivity of the transducer looks like the transmitting beam width, demonstrating what is called transmit-receive reciprocity [9]. In this manner, the transducer will receive those echoes that originate within the effective beam geometry, including any side lobes produced by the transducer. But the imaging transducer is normally pulsed rather than operating in a continuous wave (CW) mode, which places an axial limit on the physical size of the ultrasound wave set. Thus, the instantaneous volume of space seen by the transducer will be an "event cell" defined by the beam width and pulse length (Figure 9-24). This definition looks very much like the sample volume in a pulsed-Doppler system. The definitions are, in fact, the same, with the volume of space defined by what the transducer "sees" at any given time. And just as in Doppler applications, the event cell will change with the effective pulse length (defined by transducer damping) and the geometry of the beam (defined by beam focusing).

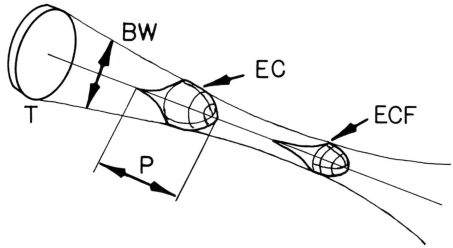

9-24 Definition of the event cell for speckling and interference. The volume of space from which echo signals can arise is defined by the pulse length *P* and the beam width *BW*. As a result, the event cell outside the focus *EC* is larger than the event cell at the focus *ECF*. *T* is the transducer.

The transducer is a phase-sensitive detector of the compressional waves that strike it. This sensitivity can best be seen in a simple experiment in which two reflecting interfaces are positioned some distance from the transducer but located in the ultrasound beam at the same time [2]. One interface has a transition of low to high impedance, and the other has a transition of high to low impedance. The magnitude of the acoustical impedance change for both is the same. One interface will return an echo that is 180° out of phase with the other, but of the same amplitude. If the travel time is the same for both echoes, they will sum together at the transducer as 0, and the two interfaces will vanish from the sonograph display (Figure 9-25). Increasing transmitted power or increasing transmitted frequency will have no effect on the result. Despite the presence of the two interfaces in the ultrasound beam, they cannot be seen by the ultrasound system. If, however, the transducer should be moved slightly so that the exact timing between the echoes is lost and one arrives before the other, the transducer will finally see a portion of the arriving energy (Figure 9-25). Clearly, the appearance of an echo signal on the sonograph display will depend upon the time-dependent sum of all the echo magnitudes arriving at any instant.

Until now, we have examined rather special situations in scattering and reflection to gain an understanding of some of the principles involved. How can we begin to think about the more complicated problem of biological tissue? To begin with, except for microcalcification, the scattering body is seldom a hard sphere. It is soft and compliant, transmitting some of the primary waves through the structure, as well as scattering and diffracting a portion of the incident energy. Thus, the echo produced by any given scattering body is a function not only of its own primary characteristics, but also the characteristics of its neighboring body. The size, separation, and regularity of the scattering bodies will all influence the final result.

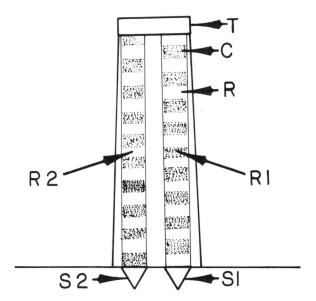

9-25 The transducer as a phase-sensitive device. The transducer *T* is illuminating two identical echo sources, *S1* and *S2*. *S1* represents a change from a low to a high acoustical impedance; *S2* represents a change from a high to a low acoustical impedance. *S1* will cause a 180° phase shift in the reflected wave at the interface, represented by *R1*. *R2* represents a reflected wave that did not experience a phase shift. Bringing the two reflected waves to the transducer at the same time lets the transducer sum the two waves together, producing no net response in the transducer. *C* is a compression region; *R* is a rarefaction.

A method of determining the influence of internal scattering body organizations is a classic scattering measurement technique. A sample of biological tissue is mounted in an ultrasound-propagating medium, an ultrasound source is located on one side of the material, and a receiving transducer is located on the other side [6]. Then the receiving transducer is moved along an arc around the material as the first transducer transmits ultrasound. The result is a map of the ultrasonic energy scattered off the internal organization of acoustical interfaces in the tissue. The nature of the scattering provides information on the size, separation, and regularity of the scattering sources within. Scattering along the direction of the primary wave is called forward scattering. In fact, all the energy forward of a plane perpendicular to the beam axis is forward-scattered energy (Figure 9-26). All the energy scattered to the other side of the plane is called back-scattered energy. A variant form of this experiment is to use a pulse-gated sonograph and a single transducer. The biological sample is mounted as before, but now the back-scattered energy to the transducer is considered, while the tissue sample is rotated within the suspending medium. In both experimental forms, the goal is to gain information on the nature of the biological scattering bodies.

If the scattering bodies within a tissue such as liver are randomly oriented, then the back-scattered energy will be independent of the incident ultrasound direction.

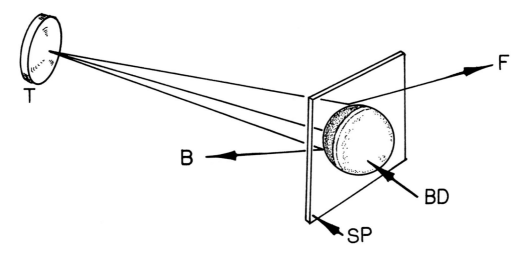

9-26 Physical geometry of a scattering process. Forward and back scattering are defined by which side of a scattering plane *SP* the scattered energy travels into. *F* is forward scattering; *B* is back scattering; *BD* is the scattering body; *T* is the transducer.

The results, however, demonstrate a strong dependence upon the direction of the incident energy [10]. This angular dependence results from a diffraction mechanism superimposed on the normal scattering events and suggests an internal organization that is a semiregular matrix of scattering bodies with a separation close to typical wavelengths used in diagnostic ultrasound. This is consistent with the histological organization of tissue that can be observed with a light microscope. The frequency dependence of back scattering from freshly excised liver suggests that the scattering bodies are less than 30 μ in diameter [10]. Further, the separation and scattering body sizes vary from one organ to another.

If the size and separation of the tissue-scattering bodies can change the apparent texture of an organ, then textural information is a function of external forces that influence the scattering body architecture. For example, a compliant tissue such as fat will change texture as a function of the transducer pressure on the tissue. The external force changes the spatial organization of the scattering components of fat. As a result, nonuniform pressure applied during a B-scan will change the appearance of fat in the image. The same pressure dependence can be seen easily in real time as the scan-head pressure varies during the scan.

But factors within the sonograph also change the appearance of texture, often unpredictably. Because we ask so little about signal processing within the typical sonograph, parameters within the sonograph that can influence image texture are poorly understood. For example, peak detection used in a digital scan converter will produce a tissue texture that is different from the same tissue scanned in a survey mode. The difference results from storing a peak value from a signal mix versus the last value presented for that pixel. Thus, the size and separation of textural components can change with different signal processing into the scan converter memory.

The textural components that contribute to the overall image characteristics include dot size, shape, separation, and intensity variations among signals. If the gray-scale assignment either as preprocessing or postprocessing is altered, the appearance of the texture will also change (Figure 9-27). This can be demonstrated easily in real-time systems with "selectable" preprocessing and in B-scanners with variable postprocessing. The shape of any signal compression before the scan converter input will change the signal dot size and the intensity variations among echo signals. The number of gray levels available to the sonograph for presentation will influence the ability to display variations among signals, and sonographs with 32 or more gray levels will better depict subtle textural changes. Because the range of signal amplitudes within a texture pattern comes from small specular echoes down to very small interference-created echoes, the gray-scale variation among signals displayed by the sonograph will change the display pattern. Further, the manner in which the tissue signal dynamic range is derived, either by compression or suppression, will change the textural patterns again. By ensuring the proper operation of the sonograph through an aggressive quality assurance program, variations in these sonograph parameters can be detected and removed, yielding a stable texture presentation.

Tissue texture, then, is a combination of primary echo formation and spatial interference patterns. The echo sources for the interference patterns are derived from the interfaces and scattering bodies located within the event cell. The pattern is a function of how much energy is scattered forward and the amount of interference caused by this scattered energy. In addition, interfaces separated by multiples of one-half wavelengths can cause constructive and destructive interference if they are simultaneously contained in the event cell. As a result, some continuous structures can appear discontinuous [2]. It is this sort of interference process that produces dots with a lateral size less than the beam width and an axial size less than the pulse duration.

Despite this myriad of influences on the speckle and texture formation in an image, real-time imaging clearly shows a texture stability that is hard to appreciate in the static B-scanner. The displayed texture of a material changes little in a real-time image because the transducer or transducers do not significantly change from one frame to the next and the scanning is mechanically or electronically controlled. Further, the scanning angle is fixed from the scan head, forming a consistent movement of the beam in the tissues. The texture is a function of the tissue organization and the events within the sonograph. When the sonograph is stable, so is the texture, which makes texture a function of events within the tissues, both normal and pathological.

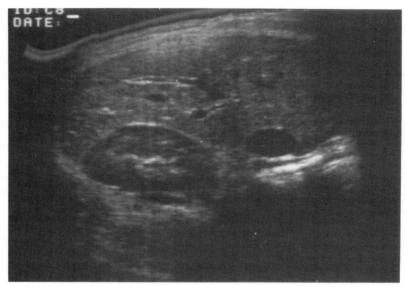

9-27   Part A

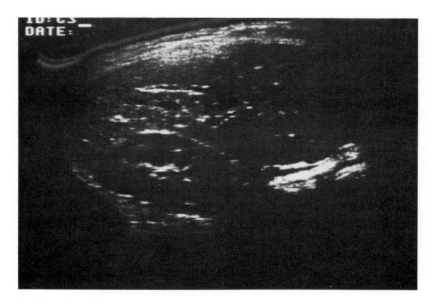

9-27   Part B

9-27   Effects of postprocessing gray-scale assignments. Part A: A linear postprocessing assignment of scan converter values to gray-scale intensity. Part B: A nonlinear postprocessing assignment of scan converter values to gray-scale intensity. This postprocessing curve enhances midrange values.

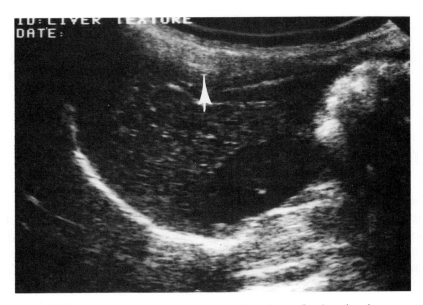

9-28   Change in image texture with a loss of echo signals. When the smaller echo signals suddenly leave the image, a sharp transition in tissue texture occurs (arrow).

To be sure, the textural presentation is not the same from the top to the bottom of a scan for the same tissue. A close examination of the image often shows abrupt transitions between textural qualities (Figure 9-28). These transitions are often obviously coincident with the loss of small contributing signals, displayed on a small number of gray-scale steps. Along with signals lost, the architecture of the event cell changes, following the beam width with increasing range. In addition, all the frequencies within the event cell contribute to the final texture, and as the frequency mix changes with depth, the texture changes with it. In summary, then, contributing to the variation in texture with depth are: a dynamic range among echoes that cannot be carried over the whole image; an event cell that is changing because of beam focusing; and a changing frequency mix in the ultrasound pulse with increasing depth. Even the uniformity of the event cell is disturbed by the scattering events. Depending upon how nonhomogeneous the tissue happens to be, the intensity organization of the ultrasound beam can be quite distorted, as measurements through tissue have demonstrated [11]. These are events hard to predict mathematically, but they occur with such repetition that subtle variations in tissue are still easily detected.

One of the best methods of determining the ability of a sonograph to portray tissue texture is to scan a tissue-equivalent phantom. Tissue-equivalent phantoms are made of an attenuating gel containing small carbon-scattering bodies randomly distributed in the gel [12]. The phantom can have cysts and sequential pins at different depths. The cysts are filled with low attenuating material, causing a subtle acoustical enhancement beyond the structure. Solid structures are filled with material attenuating higher than normal, causing shadowing. Within the phantom, vertical and horizontal pins show lateral resolution and transducer focal-point position. The scattering bodies are selected for size and distribution to mimic a liver texture presentation. A number of sonograph performance factors can be measured using the phantom; these factors are discussed in more detail in Chapters 11 and 12.

Texture and Speckle in M-mode

Because most applications of diagnostic ultrasound use the same types of transducers, texture and speckle are present in each application, but are not always as obvious as in the two-dimensional image. A good example of texture and speckle effects in a different form is the M-mode display. However, not all M-mode displays are the same, so, textural information does not look exactly the same for all M-mode displays.

Forming an M-mode Display

An M-mode display is a time-motion study of acoustical interfaces. Because the motion is examined over time, the technique is often called a time-motion, or TM, display. Along with the time-dependent position of echo sources, signal amplitude can also be part of this study. This information is often carried in the intensity variations on the display.

The first step in forming an M-mode display is to convert the A-mode information about echo signal amplitudes into a B-mode format. This connection is shown in Figure 9-29. Now, however, the amplitude information appears as gray-scale intensities for the B-mode dots that compose the display. The dots result from modulating the electron beam current in the CRT. This form of modulation is often called Z-axis modulation, with X-axis and Y-axis modulation related to the electron beam position on the cathode ray tube (CRT) face. Like the A-mode display, the electron beam is first set into a repeated, unidirectional trace, but in a vertical direction (Figure 9-30). The electron beam is modulated intermittently in response to the presence of an echo signal. At the same time, the trace is moved horizontally at a steady pace. The result is echo-signal range on the Y-axis, time on the X-axis, and echo presence on the Z-axis. The result is a time-motion study as shown in Figure 9-30.

The time-motion information can be transferred to a hard copy by moving a light-sensitive recording paper past a fixed B-mode trace on a CRT (Figure 9-30). This device is called a strip-chart recorder because the recording paper moves or strips past a special display CRT. Standard strip-chart speeds include 15 mm/s, 25 mm/s, 50 mm/s, and 100 mm/s. Higher speeds are often used to observe fast events or in situations where small time intervals need to be accurately studied, such as high heart rates in distressed neonates, or systolic time interval studies in adults.

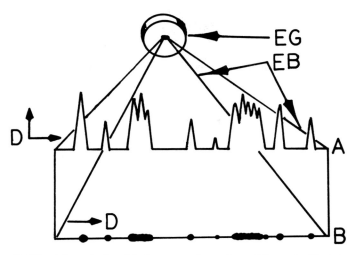

9-29   The relationship between A-mode and B-mode. Part A: An A-mode consists of both X and Y motion of the electron beam *EB*, to form the echo signals. Part B: B-mode, however, has motion in one direction only, but brightness modulates the electron beam to produce an equivalent set of echo signals as dots.

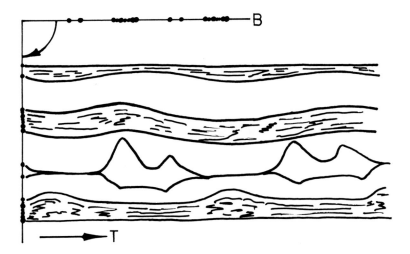

9-30   The connection between B-mode and M-mode. A B-mode trace *B* consists of a series of dots for each echo signal. Rotating this B-mode trace through 90° and moving the trace over time *T* will produce the T/M or M-mode presentation.

By adjusting the recording speed, general or very specific motion qualities can be recorded and studied in detail.

The signals presented to the CRT often are not the video signals coming from the sonograph director. Because the primary intent in M-mode is to record the motion history of moving organs and interfaces, echo-amplitude information has not always been included in the display. Between the raw video and the CRT display are circuits that alter the signal for display, retaining motion and position information, but at the same time, removing amplitude information. At its simplest, this display form detects the presence of an echo signal above a certain level and responds by emitting a pulse with a fixed width and amplitude. The resulting display is much like a bistable, two-dimensional image. It is difficult to separate the large and small signals from one another. In addition, the normal variations in both echo-signal amplitude and width due to different anatomical structures, different ultrasound-tissue interactions, and speckle formation are lost in the display. In pathological situations, motion alone may not be enough to determine which interfaces the transducer happens to be "seeing."

To provide some display weighting for relative echo-signal amplitudes, the simple bistable M-mode is modified so that the amplitude of the pulse is constant for any signal above a threshold value, but so that the width of the pulse is changed in response to the video signal amplitude. The display is still bistable in that all the Z-axis signals have either the same amplitude or a zero value (Figure 9-31). Nevertheless, some sense of echo-signal amplitude is present in the pulse-width modulation. At first glance, the results look like gray scale. A careful examination shows, however, that the gray scale is an illusion created by the spacing and width of constant-intensity lines. Because of the aesthetic qualities of this record, this is the most commonly used M-mode display today.

Pulse-width modulated M-mode comes in more than one form. In early M-mode displays, a method of "softening" the M-mode record was to sample a fixed frequency, square-wave oscillator in proportion to the amplitude of the echo signal (Figure 9-31). Thus, a small signal might sample one or two oscillations, whereas a larger signal would sample five or six. The resulting record has a constant overall intensity, with the large amplitude signals appearing as a set of parallel moving lines at constant intensity. Because we tend to think of each signal as a single interface, it appears on the M-mode record that groups of constantly spaced interfaces are moving together. Despite the display, it is an illusion; the lines are not echo signals but pulse-modulation signals. Still, the leading edge of the echo signals is hard to determine, creating uncertainty during measurements.

One method of decreasing this uncertainty is to provide a clear distinction between the leading echo-signal edge and the remainder of the signal. This distinction comes about by using a relatively long pulse-width modulated signal for the beginning of the echo signal, then switching to a series of smaller width signals for the remainder of the echo signal (Figure 9-31). The large initial signal comes from a pulse-width modulation circuit that responds to voltages above a predetermined amplitude by putting out a fixed width pulse of constant amplitude. The remaining smaller signals are obtained by adding unfiltered, detected video signals (half-wave or full-wave rectified) to the pulse-width modulator output. The result

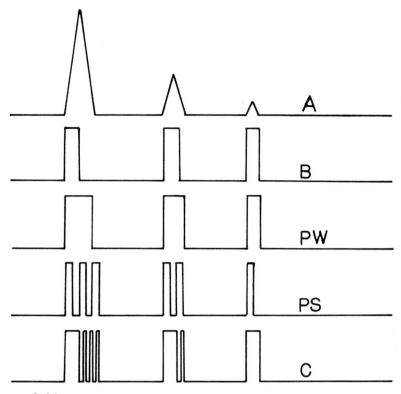

9-31 Modulating the M-mode signal. M-mode signals are not normally modulated to represent echo-signal size in a gray-scale manner. Gray-scale M-mode requires a modulation of both the electron beam intensity and the electron beam size. *A* represents the type of modulating signal used to produce gray-scale M-mode. *B* shows a bistable equivalent for the same signals. *PW* shows how the pulse width can be modulated to represent echo-signal amplitude. *PS* shows how a sample of a high-frequency pulse can be used to show echo-signal amplitude by increasing the number of displayed cycles. *C* shows a combination of pulse sample and pulse-width modulation.

is a dark line indicating the leading edge of the echo signal followed by a series of smaller, less-intense lines for the duration of the echo signal. The duration of these softer signals represents the amplitude of the original echo signal. Because the leading edge in smaller signals represents parts of the same echo signals, the echo signal will move like parallel tracks over the M-mode record. Once again, the parallel moving lines appear to be small interfaces separated by fractions of a millimeter, all tracking together. And once more we are dealing with an illusion, generated by the method of signal handling. We should expect signal separation not to be less than the known axial resolution of the sonograph, which is effectively three wavelengths. Despite the "soft"-appearing record with this technique, this is not a gray-scale M-mode.

If a pulse-width modulated M-mode is not gray scale, what, then, is a gray-scale M-mode display? The gray-scale display modulates its component-dot intensities in response to echo-signal amplitudes (Figure 9-31). In addition, as the echo signals change width, so do the component dots. The result is a visual intensity weighting that is a function of both the echo-signal amplitude and width, accurately representing events in the echo signals. The dot width representing the echo signal can change in only one direction, which is along the Y-axis. On the X-axis is time, which can depict how the signal amplitude changed over time. These are the components that will contribute to the resulting image: signal amplitude in gray scale and gray intensity along the Z-axis, signal width along the Y-axis, and variations in both size and intensity along the X-axis.

Forming M-mode Texture

In the formation of any textural pattern, the factors contributing to the pattern include the mix of dot sizes, the mix of dot intensities, and the spatial distribution among various dots. In bistable and pulse-width modulated M-mode displays, the intensity for all the pattern elements is the same, leaving element size and spatial distributions as the contributing factors. In a gray-scale M-mode display, dot intensity can change with signal amplitude, which adds to the character of the pattern formation. A typical textural pattern for pulse-width modulated M-mode is shown in Figure 9-32. A contrasting textural pattern is also shown in Figure 9-32 for a gray-scale M-mode display.

In both cases, the pattern is a result of changing anatomy within the myocardium, along with macroanatomy reorganization during contraction. Small separations of interfaces within the dimensions of the event cell blink into and out of visibility, as the phase relationship of the received echoes changes over time. Often flow characteristics of the right ventricular outflow tract change the pattern of nonstructural echoes in the right ventricular portion of the M-mode (Figure 9-32). Changes in the character of the contraction of the heart are evident in the textural changes. Out of habit, we look past these clues to cardiac events, inquiring only of information about dynamics. With an awareness of events contributing to the textural presentation, the correlation between cardiac events, both normal and abnormal, can be carefully constructed, increasing the utility of M-mode echocardiography.

Conclusion

The starting point to understanding the formation of tissue texture in a grey scale image is understanding the way tissue changes ultrasound as the mechanical wave travels through the tissue. Because we are used to seeing the image as a one-way process, the two-way travel for the echo is easy to forget. Using two-way calculations, we are able to predict how ultrasound will lose energy in the tissue.

The energy loss along with the differences in reflectivity for different acoustic interfaces produces a very large range of signals out of the transducer. This range is reduced by the transmit-receive switch in the sonograph, which ultimately determines the effective penetration into the tissue.

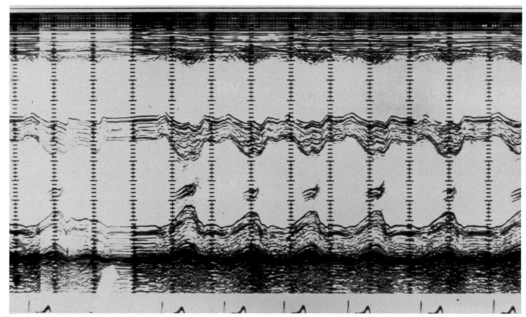

9-32   Part A

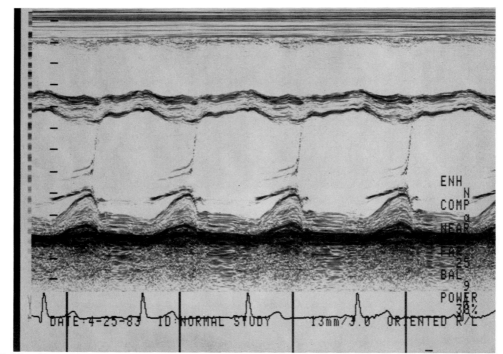

9-32   Part B

9-32   Examples of pulse-width modulated and gray scale M-mode. A) An example of pulse-width modulated M-mode where the width of the echo-signal represents amplitude. B) An example of gray scale M-mode with echo-signal strength appearing as gray scale. Courtesy of Advanced Technology Laboratories, Bellevue, Washington.

The image texture that supplies so much tissue information comes from two primary sources: primary echoes from the macro- and microanatomy of the tissue, and phase-dependent speckle formation. At any given moment in a pulse-listen cycle, the textural pattern is a result of all the echoes received from the event cell, with boundaries defined by the pulse length and the beam width. Thus, as the event cell changes shape and its strength attenuated by the tissue, the image tissue texture changes in a systematic way over the image. And despite the complexity of the formation, we can still see the variations in texture that indicate disease.

References

1. Flax, S.W., G.H. Glover, and N.J. Pelc. 1981. Textural variations in B-mode ultrasonography: A Stochastic Model. Ultrasonic Imaging 3:235–257.
2. Entrekin, R., and H.E. Melton. 1979. Real time speckle reduction in B-mode images. 1979. Ultrasonics Symposium Proceedings. IEEE.
3. Nicholas, D. 1977. An introduction to the theory of acoustic scattering in biological tissues. In Recent advances in ultrasound in biomedicine, vol. 1, ed. D.N. White. Forest Grove, OR: Research Studies Press.
4. Waag, R.C., R.M. Lerner, P.P.K. Lee, and R. Gramiak. 1977. Ultrasonic diffraction characterization of tissue. In Recent advances in ultrasound in biomedicine, vol. 1, ed. D.N. White. Forest Grove, OR: Research Studies Press.
5. Rose, J.L., and B.B. Goldberg. 1979. Basic physics in diagnostic ultrasound, 16. New York: John Wiley & Sons.
6. Lele, P.P. and N. Senapati. 1977. The frequency spectra of energy backscattered and attenuated by normal and abnormal tissue. In Recent advances in ultrasound in biomedicine, vol. 1, ed. D.N. White. Forest Grove, OR: Research Studies Press.
7. Rose, J.L., and B.B. Goldberg. 1979. Basic physics in diagnostic ultrasound, 33. New York: John Wiley & Sons.
8. Bloom, W., and D.W. Fawcett. 1968. A textbook of histology, 131. Philadelphia: W.B. Saunders Co.
9. Wells, P.N.T. 1969. Physical principles of ultrasonic diagnosis. New York: Academic Press.
10. Reid, J.M., and K.K. Shung. 1979. Quantitative measurements of scattering of ultrasound by heart and liver. In Ultrasonic tissue characterization II, ed. M. Linzer, 153–156. National Bureau of Standards, Spec. Publ. 525. Washington, D.C.: U.S. Government Printing Office.
11. Banjavic, R.A., E.L. Zagzebski, E.L. Madsen, and R.E. Jutila. 1978. Ultrasonic beam sensitivity profile changes in mammalian tissue. In Ultrasound in medicine, vol. 4, ed. D. White and E.A. Lyons, 515–518. New York: Plenum Press.
12. Burlew, M.M., E.L. Madsen, J.A. Zagzebski, R.A. Banjavic, and S.W. Sum. February 1980. A new tissue-equivalent material. Radiology 134:517–520.
13. Nicholas, D. 1977. Orientation and frequency dependence of backscattered energy and its clinical application. In Recent advances in ultrasound in biomedicine, vol. 1, ed. D.N. White. Forest Grove, OR: Research Studies Press.

Chapter 10

Bioeffects of Ultrasound on Tissue

Chapter 9 discussed the fact that tissue interacts with traveling ultrasonic waves, altering both the energy content and the shape of the waves over time and distance. The interaction, it turns out, is two way, that is, the tissue not only causes changes in the traveling ultrasonic wave but the wave also causes modifications within the tissue. Because we are just now learning about the bioeffects of ultrasound and the research observations are still incomplete, this chapter does not attempt to summarize those observations in detail. Rather, it discusses the fundamentals of bioeffects, while also including some current observations, as a starting point for readers who wish to study the subject in greater depth in other publications.

Wave Formation

It is often suggested that one way of understanding the interaction of ultrasound on biological tissues is to consider a cork on the surface of a body of water where relatively large surface waves are traveling. To understand the effects of the wave on the cork, we need only watch how the wave and the cork interact. In this simple model, we find that the cork simply moves up and down, experiencing a cyclic motion as the surface waves pass, and the cork remains unchanged. The wave motion moves the cork as if it were only a small component of the wave itself. We can measure the size relationship by comparing the size of the cork to the size of the wave passing through. In this instance, we are dealing with a very large wave relative to the size of the cork, and the cork hardly "notices" the presence of the wave.

But is this the way tissue "sees" ultrasound? The formation of longitudinal waves, as opposed to that of large-surface transverse waves, includes regions of compression and rarefaction involving much smaller particles than would normally be expected for large-surface transverse waves.

Within these regions of compression and rarefaction the molecules of the material compress more closely together and alternately pull farther apart. The density of the material in these regions thus increases or decreases; at the same time, regional temperatures increase with compression and decrease with rarefactions.

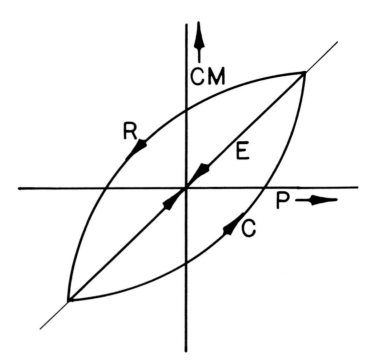

10-1   Tissue compression and pressure relationships. In a per-fectly elastic medium, applying a pressure *P* results in a linear change in material compression *CM,* and changes move along the line *E*. In a nonelastic material, compression will occur along a curve *C* and rarefaction along a curve *R*. The area between the two curves represents energy loss in the compression-rare-faction cycle.

This sort of wave formation, of course, is heavily dependent upon the material carrying the waves. If the material has a high acoustic impedance (the product of density and propagation velocity), it is more difficult to form the waves. And along with the propagation of waves come a number of other events that also influence the distribution of energy and waves within the tissue.

Because of the viscous properties of biological tissue, the compression and rarefaction process does not undergo a linear change in which the energy in both the compression and rarefaction is fully recovered, as shown in Figure 10-1. As a result of this nonlinearity, energy is coupled into the tissue in the form of heat, representing an irrecoverable loss of energy from the ultrasonic wave. This process is generally called *absorption*.

Energy is also systematically lost from the ultrasound beam when small bodies interact with the ultrasonic wave, scattering and diffracting the wave in a variety of directions. This energy loss from scattering and diffraction is coupled to absorp-tion. Together, absorption and energy loss from scattering are called *attenuation*. Absorption, however, produces local tissue heating, whereas scattering simply removes energy from the beam to be dissipated in regions outside of the normal ongoing pathway. Regardless of the mechanism, ultrasound loses energy as it travels, forming an energy gradient along the path of travel. This energy gradient plays a role later in our consideration of the forces exerted on tissue components by a traveling ultrasonic wave.

The expression of events within tissue depends uniquely upon the amount of energy placed into the tissue and the way in which energy is carried through the tissues. At the same time, the amount of energy present is not expressed in a single format. Several methods are available for expressing the energy traveling through tissue per unit time. However, these different methods can be confusing for inexperienced practitioners. The following section of this chapter thus delineates ways of expressing the amount of energy passing through a region of tissue.

Expressions of Intensity

We begin with a direct measurement of all the energy transmitted by the transducer. This direct measurement is called the *total temporal average power*. It is measured in a variety of ways, the most common method employing a force-balance technique that translates the force exerted by the ultrasonic field into the total amount of energy coming from the transducer. The setup is shown in Figure 10-2. This is a temporal average, or time average, because of the nature of the measurement process itself. The transducer is mounted in a water column and pointed toward an absorbing material that is fixed to a force balance pan. The pressure exerted by the ultrasound field is measured by the force balance, and the force is converted to a representative energy based on a known force-energy relationship. Because

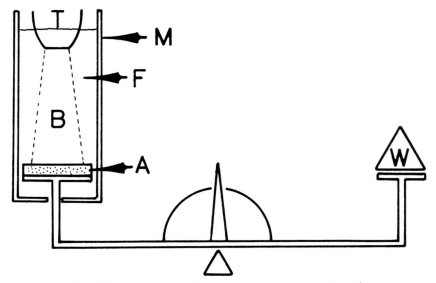

10-2 Model for measuring total power from a transducer. Total power from a transducer can be measured with a force balance. A container *M* holds a fluid *F* and one limb of a force balance. The beam *B* from transducer *T*, exerts a force on the absorbing material *A*. *W* is a counter weight on the force balance to counter the radiation force.

this is a measurement over time, we are in fact dealing with power, that is, the amount or rate of energy delivered to force balance. The unit for this measurement is the watt, and because we are averaging over a pulsatile delivery of energy, the effective units are milliwatts.

The power-averaging process assumes that although the system is operating with a short burst of energy, average power is spread over the total time period of the pulse-listen cycle. For example, if we have a peak power of 10 W, turned on for 2μ at a pulse repetition frequency of 1,000 Hz, we will have a total of:

$$10 \text{ W} \times 2 \times 10^{-6} \text{ s} = 20 \times 10^{-6} \text{ watt-seconds.} \qquad (10.1)$$

Distributing these watt-seconds over a millisecond (1/1,000 Hz) produces a total average power of:

$$20 \times 10^{-6}/10^{-3} = 20 \text{ mW.} \qquad (10.2)$$

It is evident that although peak power can be high for very short time periods, the average power can be quite low when we distribute this energy over a complete pulse-listen cycle.

Because the ultrasound transducer produces the ultrasound field, we are interested in the way the energy moves across a representative area in the field, producing the basic units for all the various levels of intensities expressed as *energy per unit time per unit area*. These units are converted to *milliwatts per square centimeter* (mW/cm²). From this basic assumption, we can examine the various intensities, both determined emperically and calculated from the initial measurements of total power.

One of the primary means of expressing intensity is the *spatial average time average,* or SATA intensity. This intensity averaging technique assumes that the total energy produced by the transducer passes through the profile of the ultrasound beam. Thus, the intensity at any point may be calculated by distributing the energy evenly over the beam cross section. The first requirement, then, is to define the effective beam width. For this calculation, two effective beam widths are used, depending who is doing the calculation. The first is the 10-dB width of the beam, and second the 20-dB width of the beam. The 20-dB width is slightly larger than the 10-dB width and produces a lower calculated SATA intensity. Most calculations, however, are based on the 10-dB beam width [1].

A sample calculation of a SATA intensity would look like this: Consider a total average power of 10 mW and a 10-dB beam width at the focal point of 4mm. A calculated SATA intensity would be:

$$SATA = 10 \text{ mW}/(4\pi r^2) = 10 \text{ mW}/(4\pi \, 0.16 \text{ cm}^2); \text{ thus}$$
$$SATA = 4.97 \text{ mW/cm}^2. \qquad (10.3)$$

A second intensity expression is the *spatial peak time average,* or SPTA intensity. This is more commonly used form of intensity when examining the bioeffects of ultrasound [1], and is frequently employed in publications on bioeffects from the AIUM, for example [2]. This average intensity is based on determining or estimating the spatial peak intensity and averaging this intensity over time. The intensity profile across the beam of a transducer is not uniform, but varies from a maximum at the central position to a much-lower value at the periphery, as shown

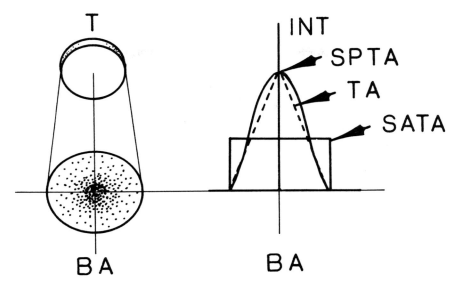

10-3   Approximating transverse beam intensity. An ultrasound beam is not uniform in transverse intensity, but decreases outward from the beam axis *BA*. The *SATA* intensity assumes a uniform beam intensity, whereas the *SPTA* assumes a nonuniform intensity, *INT*. Connecting the *SATA* and *SPTA* intensities assumes a triangular approximation *TA*, for the intensity profile.

in Figure 10-3. This profile of intensity is often approximated by a triangle, with the base of the triangle spanning the 10-dB skirts of the beam. The SPTA value is calculated from the SATA intensity. In general, for medium-focused transducers, the SPTA value is equal to three to five times the SATA calculation because of the shape of the lateral beam intensity. For example, our calculated SATA intensity of 5 mW/cm^2 could be translated to 15 mW/cm^2 SPTA.

Another means of expressing an average intensity is the *spatial peak pulse average,* or SPPA intensity. This intensity expression uses several different factors to determine the amount of energy contained in each transmitted pulse. The first calculation in determining the SPPA intensity is the *duty ratio,* which is a specification of how long the transmitter is transmitting throughout the whole duty cycle. The duty ratio is determined by multiplying the duration of the acoustic pulse by the pulse repetition frequency [1]. The next calculation is the *mean power* within the transmitted pulse. This number is computed by taking the temporal average power output (the total power output) and dividing it by the duty ratio. This calculation provides the mean power within the pulse. Then, by distributing the mean intensity within the pulse over the beam geometry, we have the *spatial peak pulse average.* As in the previous case, where the SPTA was three to five times higher than the SATA, the pulse intensity averaged over the whole beam width can be scaled to the spatial peak value with a number ranging from 3 to 5.

All these calculations include systems both continuous-wave and pulsed. A continuous-wave (CW) system will generally have higher intensities because the system transmitter is always turned on. In the continuous-wave system, the power oscillates between zero and two times the root mean square, or RMS value [1].

Calculation of a peak power then in a CW system is a matter of scaling the average power by a factor of 2.

These intensities are not the only intensities used to express the amount of energy released or contained in an ultrasound beam. Numerous other intensities exist, but the four discussed above are those utilized by a majority of the publications on the subject and cover most of the typical problems in calculating or determining the energy emitted from a transducer. A good overview of measurements and specifications appears in reference [1].

Forces Exerted by Ultrasound

One of the first measurements made to determine the output power from an ultrasound transducer is to calculate the radiation force exerted by the transducer on a small force balance. The calibration of this force balance is postulated on a numerical relationship between the radiated energy and the radiation force, with 1 W of energy producing a 0.067-gm force [1]. As the ultrasound passes through the tissue, the tissue removes energy, producing a radiation force gradient along the ultrasound beam axis, as shown in Figure 10-4. This radiation force could produce a number of effects within the tissue [3].

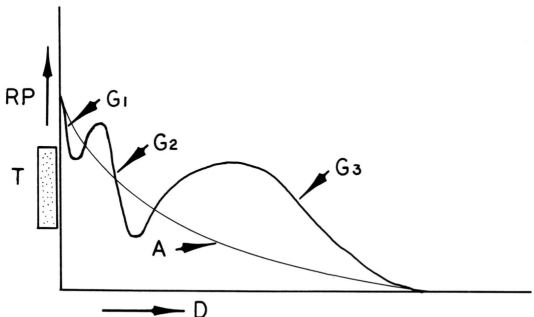

10-4   Large pressure gradients in an ultrasound pressure field. Microstreaming can occur where large pressure gradients occur in the ultrasound field. Superimposing a pressure field on tissue attenuation forms several regions with steep gradients, *G1, G2,* and *G3*. *RP* is the relative pressure, *T* is the transducer, *D* is distance from the transducer, and *A* is the attenuation curve for the tissue.

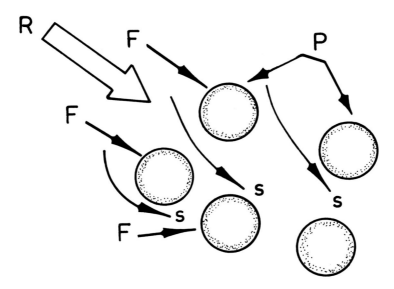

10-5 Applying stokes forces to tissue particles. An energy gradient produces a radiation force *R* that develops Stokes forces *F* on individual particle P. The Stokes forces arise from the medium flowing past the particles *s,* as if the particles were falling through the medium.

One of the primary forces exerted secondary to a radiation force is the *Stokes force* [3]. Stokes forces are expended upon the particles suspended in a propagating medium carrying ultrasonic waves (Figure 10-5), and generally act to move, displace, and potentially distort the particles. They also exert forces on the tissue organization and cell groupings within an organ.

As the ultrasound wave front passes through the tissue, the tissue alters the shape of the front producing a steep leading edge and a much-softer trailing edge, as shown in Figure 10-6. This sort of wave front distortion produces *Oseen forces,* which generate very localized force gradients [3]. Tissues experiencing Oseen forces can be distorted as well because the force gradient extending from the leading edge to the trailing edge of a wave front changes the organization of a biological tissue.

Another set of forces that can appear in tissues are the *Bernoulli forces* [3]. Because of the energy gradient down the axis of the beam, fluids and materials can be transpsorted, forming into small regions of microstreaming. Within the microstreams, the local pressure is lower than the surrounding static regions, producing a pressure gradient on the tissue particles that tends to push the particles toward the center of the microstreaming, as shown in Figure 10-7. Microstreaming has been witnessed in a number of situations in normal tissue.

Another mechanism that can begin to affect biological tissue is *molecular fatigue,* which results from repeated vibration as the ultrasonic waves continually pass through [3]. Perhaps the tissue components most subject to molecular fatigue are the single bonds formed in large macromolecules. Bond failure would cause the larger molecules to separate into smaller components, losing biological activity in the process.

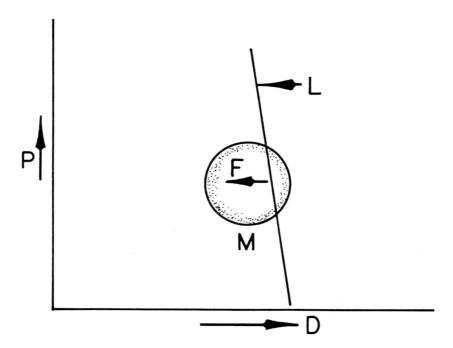

10-6   Developing Oseen forces within the tissue. As a wave front travels through a medium, the medium distorts the wave front, making it increasingly steep. The leading edge *L* forms a demarcation for short-range pressure gradients, producing a force *F* on particle *M*. *P* is pressure; *D* is distance.

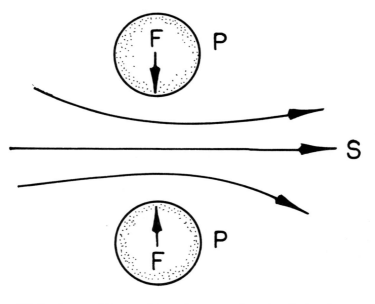

10-7   Bernoulli forces from microstreaming. A radiation force gradient can produce microstreaming *S*, which produces a lateral force *F* on the particles *P*, because the pressure within the stream is less than the surrounding static material.

For medium- and higher-energy ultrasound, localized heating is a normal event [3]. Local heating, in turn, can set up regional convention currents, but more importantly, heating can interact directly with the tissue to cause local lesions. Most of the biological effects of ultrasound observed in medium and high energy levels have been repeated by physically creating localized heating, indicating that local-tissue heating is a primary tissue-damage mechanism at medium and high intensities [3].

Vulnerable Portions of the Cell

Early examinations of the cell using a light microscope revealed what was thought to be a simple organism consisting of a few organelles suspended in a clear medium. Electronmicrography now indicates that a much more complex situation is occurring within the cell than first believed. In addition, physical chemistry shows that many of the cellular processes pivot on a combination of physical and chemical events that are potentially sensitive to mechanical disruption, causing a break down of normal cell function [4]. Let us look at some of the areas within the cell that may be sensitive to forces exerted by an ultrasonic wave and that may contribute to an altered cell function. A schematic cell with components is shown in Figure 10-8.

The Cell Wall

The cell wall is a bilipid membrane, 75Å to 100Å thick, and held together by chemical forces normally found within liquid crystals [4]. Connected to the wall inside and outside the cell, and passing through, are large macromolecules and specialized proteins [5]. The lipid bilayer of the membrane is a result of hydrophobic bonds, produced by the inability of the lipids to mix with the surrounding water. The cell wall is stable but flexible, and is easily disrupted by regional forces that can alter its ability to attach to other cells or to maintain its own integrity to ions inside and outside the cell.

Endoplasmic Reticulum

Many cells perform functions that produce specialized proteins, then exuding these proteins into the outside environment. An example of such a cell is the mucosal cell found in many of the tubes and tracts within the body. The organelle within the cell that regularly makes and packages these proteins is the endoplasmic reticulum. This organelle is made of a lipid bilayer, often in conjunction with RNA particles for protein synthesis. In addition, the endoplasmic reticulum is often continuous with the outside cell wall. Forces that could disrupt the outside cell

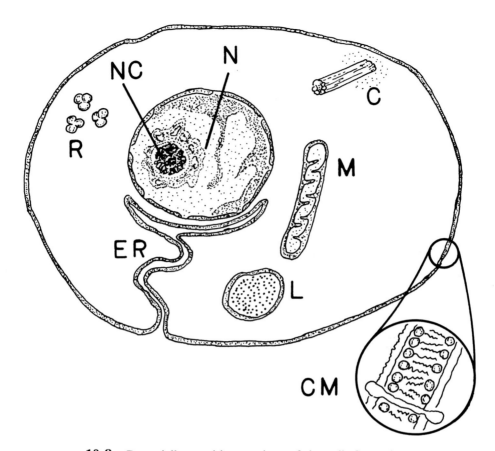

10-8   Potentially sensitive portions of the cell. Several portions of a cell involve either a stable, fine structure or mechanical events that could be disrupted by mechanical waves. *CM* is the cell membrane; *L* is the lysosome; *M* is the mitochondrion; *C* is the centriole; *R* is the free ribosome; *ER* is the endoplasmic reticulum; *NC* is the nucleolus; *N* is the nucleus.

wall could also alter the organization of the endoplasmic reticulum, changing its ability to manufacture and package cellular proteins for body functions.

Cellular Skeleton

Early observers of the cell's organization could neither recognize nor depict the internal cellular organization of microfibrils and microfibers. It is known that the interior of the cell is not a simple cytoplasm with organelles floating around disorganized in space, but is a highly structured interior, dependent upon the distribution of microfibrils [5]. These microfibrils form a cellular skeleton, both affording places for cellular organelles to become passively attached and providing the shape and structure of the cell itself. Mechanical waves that pass through the cell with large pressure gradients across the cell may alter this cellular organization.

The Nucleus

Another potential site for mechanical disruption is the cell nucleus, surrounded by a nuclear membrane containing small openings, called fenestrations, through which messenger RNA travels [5, 6]. The nuclear material represents memory for all of the cell functions, information that must reach the cytoplasm through the nuclear membrane. This nuclear membrane may be as sensitive to mechanical waves as the cell wall.

In addition, the DNA within the nucleus may experience external forces that disrupt the connection of messenger RNA to the exposed portions of the DNA during message transcription.

The Centrioles

Cell reproduction requires a duplication and redistribution of DNA [6]. At the end of replication, the DNA molecules are physically separated into two daughter cells, with the correct number of chromosomes in each of the new daughter cells. The mechanical process of separating the chromosomes into appropriate daughter-cell regions in a mitotic or dividing cell is carried out by the centrioles [6]. These structures consist of small tubes of contracting proteins that are stationed at opposite sides of the cell at division, and are attached to DNA molecules that are being divided. In the last stages of mitosis, these structures physically pull the DNA into opposite poles of the cell. If the physical movement is disrupted during cell division by forces in an ultrasonic wave, the result could be an uneven or disjunctive separation of DNA molecules.

Mitochondria

Mitochondria are the energy sources within the cell, converting oxygen and energy molecules into carbon dioxide and energy. This chemical conversion of energy is dependent upon the physical organization of the electron transport chain within the walls of the mitochondrion [3]. Disruption of either the number or distribution of mitochondria within a cell may alter the ability of the cell to carry out such energy-dependent processes as cell reproduction, DNA synthesis, and protein synthesis.

Ribosomes

Messenger RNA, which transports information from the nucleus, combines with protein synthesis machinery within the cell to convert the RNA message into explicit protein molecules. The sites of synthesis for cellular proteins are clusters of RNA called ribosomes. Again a mechanical process combines with chemical processes to produce the ability to locate amino acids, to form amino acid chains, and, ultimately, to synthesize the macromolecules. Forces exerted by ultrasound may alter the ability of the proteins to attach to a ribosome or may fatigue macromolecules during the process of formation, which could alter cell processes.

Lysosomes

Within many cells are structures called lysosomes, which contain digestive enzymes surrounded by a special membrane that is immune to the effects of these enzymes [6]. If the lysosome ruptures, the enzymes that are normally protected from the cell interior break loose and cause cell damage or death by digesting the internal cell components. Lysosomes are common in cells specialized for the immune response—cells often used for *in vitro* experiments on the bioeffects of ultrasound.

   These, then, are some of the cell sites that could be affected by pressure waves and forces exerted by a traveling ultrasonic wave or even by an ultrasonic standing wave. To better understand the various effects of ultrasound as a function of the applied ultrasonic intensity, we will look next at the ranges of intensities commonly described in the literature.

Ranges in Ultrasound Intensities

Diagnostic ultrasound generally ranges from 0.002 W/cm^2 to 0.5 W/cm^2 SPTA. Therapeutic ultrasound, on the other hand, usually ranges from 0.5 W/cm^2 to 2.0 W/cm^2. And ablative applications of ultrasound extend above 50 W/cm^2 to 100 W/cm^2.

   At the high intensities used for ablative applications, high compressional and shear stresses appear that rupture and disorganize the carrying medium. The result is a high level of tissue damage and local breakdown of tissue at these intensities.

   An added effect often seen with high intensites and low frequency is cavitation, in which a mechanical resonance is set up between bubbles formed in the tissue and the traveling ultrasonic waves. Cavitation causes gross mechanical damage to tissue and total disruption at both the macro and micro levels [3].

   Accompanying the dramatic effects produced by the mechanical stresses of ultrasound at high intensities is a local heat production that may exceed the mechanical effects of ultrasound in tissue damage. In fact, it appears that much of the local effects of medium- and high-frequency ultrasound are due to heat production.

   Medium-intensity effects appear to follow a dose-response relationship, much like a tissue interaction with a drug or ionizing radiation (this is not to suggest that ultrasound is ionizing). Medium-intensity effects again involve local heating, in which thermal energy appears at a rate faster than conduction and vascularity can carry it away. As the wave intensity increases, the interaction between the tissue and the ultrasound begins to alter the shape of the wave front, making the pressure change of the advancing wave front more steep [3].

Under these conditions, interfaces experience radiation forces along the decreasing energy gradient. Stokes forces appear and are expended on the particles suspended in the propagating medium. Oseen forces exert stress on interfaces and particles because of wavefront distortion. Microstreaming results from the radiation force, and from the microstreaming issue Bernoulli effects that exert lateral forces on the tissue particles and cells.

Bioeffects at Various Intensity Levels

Medium Intensities

Medium-intensity levels produce changes in laboratory animal fetuses, and some of these effects involve intensities as low as 0.2 W/cm^2 to 0.6 W/cm^2. The results of these radiation experiments show that a 1-MHz, CW ultrasonic beam applied for 2 min to 3 min on the 6th and 9th days of gestation produces growth retardation, hemorrhage, and neurocanal damage [7]. These effects were observed both in hamster embryos and pregnant mice. Reference [8] provides a good summary of lesion production from medium and high levels of ultrasound in lab animals.

Diagnostic Intensities

A number of observations in intact laboratory animals and *in vitro* experiments indicate that diagnostic levels of ultrasound can carry a biological response. The effects have not been observed in the intact human.

Some of these observations at various diagnostic ultrasound intensities include the following:

1. Siegal, et al., using a total RMS power of 1.76 mW and exposure times ranging from 0.25 min to 60 min, observed a reduction in cell attachment in cultured human cells [9]. The authors used a 2.25-MHz, 19-mm diameter, unfocused transducer with a PRF of 1,000 Hz.
2. Prasad, et al., observed that DNA synthesis in a standard HeLa cell line was inhibited with an ultrasonic exposure of 4.0 mW/cm^2 for 10 min at 1 MHz [10].
3. Liebeskind, et al., using an intensity of 11 mW/cm^2, observed alterations in DNA and cell synthesis in HeLa and other cell lines after a 20-min exposure at 2.25 MHz [11].
4. Kremkau and Witkofski exposed rat livers to 1.9-MHz ultrasound at an intensity of 60 mW/cm^2, continuous wave, for 5 min and found reduced rates of cell division [12].

Other researchers have found similar results when irradiating lab animals such as *Drosophila* flies and rotifers [13, 14]. The effects seem to fall into two major categories: first, a change in cell activity, and second, a change in the ability of cells to attach to one another.

At the clinical level, the major concern is the exposure of the fetus to ultrasound and what effects that exposure might produce in the offspring. Hellman, reported in *Lancet* a compilation of data of abnormalities in offspring from 1,114 normal pregnant women who had undergone sonography (cited in [3]). In total, 3,297 women were examined, and they found an overall rate of abnormality of 2.7%. These data were compared to 63,238 single births in 26 hospitals, where the observed abnormality was 4.8%. This study, however, has received a great deal of criticism, not only because of the way in which the experimental subjects were selected but because of the methods used to compare one group of women against another. Although it does not show that ultrasound improves the rate of abnormalities in pregnant women, it does not suggest that diagnostic ultrasound has an adverse effect on the fetus.

Another study, by Lyons, is an ongoing program of examining fetuses from 10,000 women who have experienced single or multiple exposure to ultrasound (cited in [15]). Preliminary data show that neoplasm formation in 3,000 children up to 9 years of age is currently zero. A complete preliminary report is expected soon.

Conclusions

It is clear that we can no longer be unconcerned about the bioeffects of ultrasound at diagnostic levels. Interactions between the cell and ultrasound occur and appear not to be related to regional heating. On the other hand, the effects so far observed *in vitro* have not been observed *in vivo* for the same typical diagnostic ultrasound intensities. These data suggest that we should take a more cautious view of ultrasound in nonmedical situations. Diagnostic ultrasound may turn out to be as harmless as a cold stethoscope, but until the evidence is clear, a conservative approach is prudent.

The eagerness to know the bioeffects of ultrasound has generated various laboratory experiments. But some "natural" experiments are also in progress. One such experiment, although it has not as yet included any clinical data collection or measurements, involves individuals who make and test ultrasound devices in industry. Many of these persons have been exposed to ultrasound for prolonged time periods in the course of scanning themselves and one another to test new designs or to manufacture standard devices. And in many manufacturing facilities for real time, this sort of scanning is also conducted. We have no information on what the effects of prolonged exposure to low levels of ultrasound might be. This group of individuals, however, could provide some indications of the potential effects of chronic exposure to ultrasound; they have only to be tapped by the medical community.

References

1. Kossoff, G. 1978. On the measurement and specification of acoustic output generated by pulsed ultrasonic diagnostic equipment. JCU 6:295–382.
2. AIUM Committee on Bioeffects. 1976. Biological effects of ultrasonic energy on living mannals. Ultrasound Med Biol 2.
3. Hussey, M. 1975. Diagnostic ultrasound: An introduction to the interactions between ultrasound and biological tissues. London: Blackie & Sons.
4. Lehninger, Albert L. 1970. Biochemistry. The molecular basis of cell structure and function. New York: Worth Publishers.
5. Kessel, R.G., and R.H. Kardon. 1979. Tissues and organs: A text-atlas of scanning electron microscopy. San Francisco: W.H. Freeman & Co.
6. Bloom, W., and D.W. Fawcett. 1968. A textbook of histology. Philadelphia: W.B. Saunders Co.
7. Fry, F.J., et al. 1978. Ultrasonic toxicity study. Ultrasound Med Biol 3:351–366.
8. Fry, F.J. April 1979. Biological effects of ultrasound—A review. Proc IEEE 67:604–619.
9. Siegal, E., et al. October 1979. Cell attachment as a sensitive indicator of the effects of diagnostic ultrasound exposure on cultured human cells. Radiology 133:175–179.
10. Prasad, N., et al. 29 May 1976. Ultrasound and mammalian DNA. Letter to the Editor. Lancet 1:1181.
11. Liebeskind, D., et al. April 1979. Diagnostic ultrasound: Effects on DNA and growth patterns of animal cells. Radiology 131:177–184.
12. Kremkau, F.W., and R.L. Witkofski. June 1974. Mitotic reduction in rat liver exposed to ultrasound. JCU 2:123–126.
13. Fritz-Niggli, H., and A. Boni. 28 July 1950. Biological experiments on Drosophila melanogaster with supersonic vibrations. Science 112:120–122.
14. Dunn, F., and S.A. Hawley. 1965. Ultrahigh-frequency waves in liquids and their interaction with biological structures. In Ultrasonic energy, ed. E. Kelly. Urbana, IL: University of Illinois Press.
15. Arehart-Treichel, J. 12 June 1982. Fetal ultrasound: How safe? Science News 121:396–397.

Chapter 11

Testing B-Scanner Function: Quality Assurance at Home

At a time when all medical procedures are coming under increasing public and private scrutiny for their effectiveness and advisability, diagnostic ultrasound is no exception. The fundamental question with ultrasound extends beyond when to use ultrasound to whether or not it is being used to its maximum efficiency. To answer the second part of this question, sonograph users must first determine whether their machine is working properly. By measuring the machine's performance in a variety of circumstances we can determine whether or not it still performs to the original specifications. This chapter describes the measurements that an ultrasound laboratory can make to evaluate a sonograph's functioning.

The task of determining machine function is called *quality assurance* (QA). Maintaining peak performance in a sonograph requires that machine parts be checked regularly, that records be kept of machine performance and of necessary repairs, and that preventative maintenance be provided. Although such measures have yet to be introduced in most ultrasound departments, once initiated, the rewards are quickly realized and are ongoing. This chapter focuses primarily on performance evaluation activities recommended for the B-scanner. Although real-time systems have nearly the same imaging requirements as the B-scanner, they also incorporate some major differences, and therefore are covered separately in Chapter 12.

Early sonographs were prone to drift and to misalignment, which prompted the development of digital sonographs. But even ''going digital'' did not fully solve the quality assurance problem. Computers and digital scan converters—like any other such devices—have component failures too. Often, the failures are catastrophic, preventing further machine operation. At other times, small failures in program logic can cause subtle changes in the execution of a program, altering not only how a sonograph operates but the results of analysis by an adjunct computer. Digital systems must be examined as frequently and carefully as analog systems, with an eye to these subtle failures that can alter system operation.

Essential Operations

Most digitally based sonographs still have a large part that is analog-based. While digital functions appear in key segments of the organization in such machines, digital electronics has not taken over completely. Whether digital or analog, the static B-scanner still has pivotal functions in the imaging process. When these functions are changed by drift, component failure, or maladjustment, the image and its information content suffer. The goal in any quality assurance program is to detect these changes and apply corrective measures to restore the sonograph to original specifications.

Sonograph function begins with the transducer producing and receiving ultrasound. The transducer must convert the transmitter voltage into ultrasonic energy. On the other hand, the returning echoes must stress the transducer to produce the echo signal. Machine performance can quickly deteriorate if the transducer fails either to make ultrasound or to convert properly the returning echoes into electrical signals.

The electrical signals representing echoes are first processed through the transmit/receive switch located between the transducer and the receiver. If the signals are distorted or modified at this juncture, they cannot be processed later into effective signals in the machine.

Once past the transmit/receive switch, the echo signals enter the radio frequency amplifier, where they are amplified and modified by time-gain compensation (TGC). The rf amplifier should increase the echo-signal level without distortion. Further, the amplifiers should respond to the time-gain compensation (TGC) curve instructions in a linear, predictable manner. Nonlinear TGC responses can introduce surprises and errors in the final image.

After passing the rf amplifiers, the detector operates on the signal, removing the rf and leaving only the signal envelope. A nonlinear detector can increase the range of signals and the shape of each. In addition, such detectors can respond poorly to higher-frequency components, changing the signals that finally reach the display.

At the analog-to-digital converter, or ADC, the analog signal is digitally sampled at a high rate and converted into a set of binary numbers. In systems with fewer than 32 gray levels, nonlinear preprocessing handles the assignment of numerical values to signal amplitudes. The image is acutely sensitive to changes in this signal assignment process at the ADC.

Following the ADC, the system controller stores the digital signals in the scan converter memory. The controller needs to know the assignment sequence for each memory location for later reconstruction of the image. Poor assignment algorithms can be too lengthy for rapid scanning, and access to all or part of the memory can be lost through component failures. The random access memory (RAM) may be digital, but it is still part of the physical universe we live in.

To bring the image stored as numbers onto a cathode ray tube (CRT) display, the numbers in the RAM must be brought from memory in a sequence that looks as though the image were being scanned with an electron beam in a standard television format. Once out of the memory, the digital numbers are turned into analog television signals by the digital-to-analog converter, or DAC. At the DAC, the numbers are assigned to a television intensity. As in the case of preprocessing, the image is sensitive to the assignment rules used for the post processing function.

The display monitor takes the signals from the DAC and converts them into intensity information. The operating qualities of the monitor, its response to fast-changing video signals, its range of intensity, and contrast response all help to develop the final display image. No amount of proper signal handling along a well-designed signal path, however, can survive a defective display.

To function properly, both the static B-scanner and the real-time sonograph need to know the ultrasound beam position in space. The scanning arm performs this function for the static B-scanner. Correction of location errors is especially critical for the accurate operation of static B-scanner. Compound scanning places a heavy requirement for positional accuracy on the scanning arm. Manufacturers offer a variety of systems, both analog and digital, to improve arm accuracy. But even digital encoders in an arm can produce positional error. The scanning arm registration should be carefully evaluated in any quality assurance program.

With the above pivotal points in image-making as background, the section following looks at some means of evaluating sonograph function.

Transducer Performance

The first place to look for information on transducer performance is the beam profile provided by the manufacturer. This profile is arrived at by directly testing the beam characteristics with a set of known, identical targets. The beam profiler scans the beam over a set of evenly spaced steel rods, all with the same diameter, and plots or graphs the signal levels as a function of position. The result is a graph such as that shown in Figure 11-1.

The most obvious piece of information contained in a profile is the location of the transducer focal point. The focal point represents the narrowest and most intense portion of the ultrasound beam. Extending in either direction, the signals decrease in amplitude.

The rate of focus and defocus is evidenced by the way amplitudes increase into the focal point and decrease on the way out of the focal point. Rapid focusing with fast and large increases in beam intensities can be hard to remove from the image with a simple TGC system. Badly positioned or poorly formed focal zones are all evident in a beam profile.

Along with considerations of focusing, the ultrasound beam needs to be perpendicular to the face of the transducer housing. A beam profile will show any lack of symmetry in the beam geometry. The example in Figure 11-2 shows such a misaligned transducer beam.

In addition to analyzing the beam geometry information, an evaluation is often made of the transducer passband or band width. The quantity is usually expressed as a percentage of the center operating frequency. For example, a 3.5-MHz transducer with a 45% band width has 6-dB frequency components at 1.89 MHz and

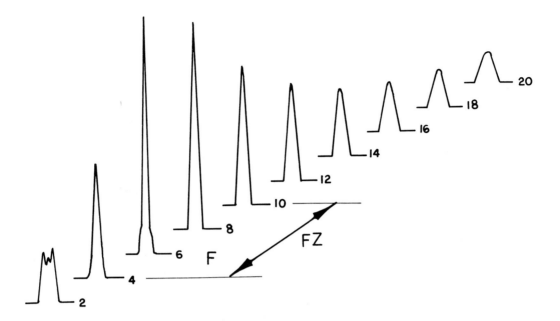

11-1   Typical beam profile for transducer. A beam profile gives information on the characteristics of the transducer focusing. It yields information on the rate of focus and defocus, focal-point position, range of focal zone, and effective lateral resolution throughout the beam length.

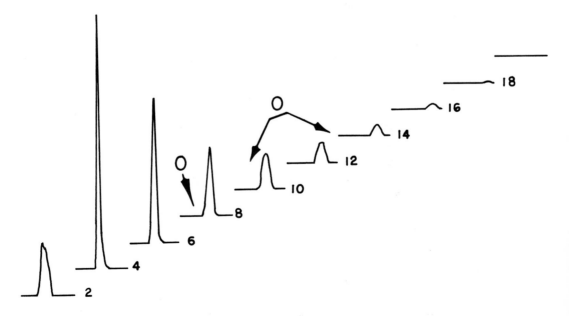

11-2   Beam profile for a poorly aligned transducer. This beam profile shows a transducer poorly aligned within the casing. The first evidence of offset, *O,* appears at 8 cm and becomes progressively worse with distance.

5.11 MHz. The higher-frequency components will affect the image texture close to the transducer, and the low-frequency components will influence effective tissue penetration.

One early indication that a transducer is not operating properly is the appearance of large dots in the image. These larger dots (often called "blobby dots") can come from extended ring-down time, loss of effective beam formation, or an alteration in signal processing within the sonograph. In general, transducers are rather well behaved and do not offer too many problems, and relative to the sonograph, are stable and unchanging.

Passive Devices for Measuring Performance

Passive devices for measuring the sonograph performance can be divided into two classes. The first class is the *test object,* and the second is the *tissue-equivalent phantom.* A test object uses no materials that attempt to imitate tissue characteristics. The tissue-equivalent phantom, on the other hand, may have many of the measurement elements of the test object, but the elements sit inside a material that provides attenuation and scattering, much like soft tissue [1]. Some measurements are common to both the phantom and the test object. Others are unique to only one or the other. Each testing device is examined in more detail later in the chapter.

One of the first truly controlled devices used to measure the B-scanner performance was the AIUM 100-mm Test Object. It is generally a plastic container with small metal rods distributed in patterns shown in Figure 11-3. The container holds a fluid mix with a propagation velocity close to 1540 m/s, but with very little attenuation to the ultrasound. As a result, attenuation-dependent processes within the sonograph cannot be adequately tested with a test object. Using the distributed pins, however, a large number of other performance aspects of the sonograph can be tested. As few as four scans of the test object can measure the more important parameters of the operating B-scanner [2].

Within the test object are pin arrangements to measure axial resolution, lateral resolution, range accuracy, minimum sensitivity, and the dead zone. Scanning from different sides of the object evaluates the scanning arm registration. The protocol for each of these measurements is examined in more detail below.

In contrast to the test object, the tissue-equivalent phantom carries a different set of internal structures. To begin with, the ultrasound propagates through a material with a rather steady attenuation rate that can be set by the manufacturer. In addition, the material carries small carbon particles that scatter ultrasound much like small scattering bodies of soft tissue [1]. Aside from an array of pins to measure the spatial elements in image formation, the phantom often contains "cystic" and "solid" structures to test the portrayal of circular structures in various parts of the display. The amounts of enhancement behind the cyst and of shadowing behind the solid structures provide an additional assessment of gray-scale resolution in the sonograph. The pins offer a means of measuring axial and lateral resolution, focal-point position, scan uniformity, and overall machine sen-

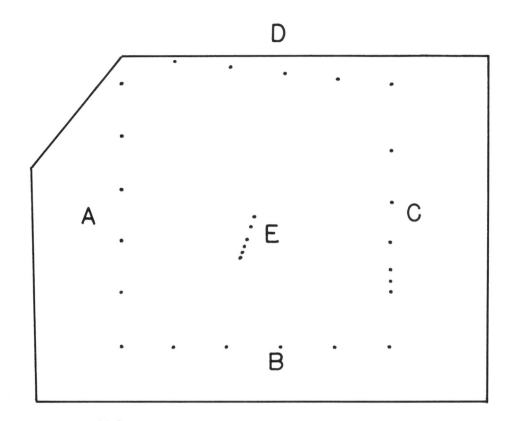

11-3   Schematic pin Arrangement for AIUM Test Object. *A* is a set of pins, each separated 20 mm apart. *B* is a set of horizontal pins separated at 20-mm intervals. *C* is a set of pins with separations decreasing with depth, in the sequence: 25 mm, 20 mm, 15 mm, 10 mm, 5 mm, and 3 mm. *D* is a set of pins separated at an increasing distance from the top, increasing from left to right: 2 mm, 4 mm, 6 mm, 8 mm, and 10 mm.

sitivity. In some models, the phantom can be scanned from different sides to show scan-arm registration. A schematic tissue-equivalent phantom is shown in Figure 11-4.

Common to all the devices that test the sonograph signal path from the transducer to the display is a need to hold certain parameters within the device to a set of specific values. For example, the velocity of propagation must be 1540 m/s or must match the machine velocity assumptions, and furthermore, must not change rapidly with changing temperature. If the device does change rapidly with the temperature, then a thermometer should be included as part of the device's construction and a chart kept of changing propagation velocity with temperature. In addition, the attenuation rate should be a steady, known value, also slow to change with temperature. Whether the attenuation rate is higher or lower than normal tissue is not as important as knowing what the rate actually is. The spatial separation of pins and special reflectors must be known and accurately placed within the testing device. And any internal structures with an attenuation higher or lower than the surrounding material should be well defined. These reflectors, too, should not

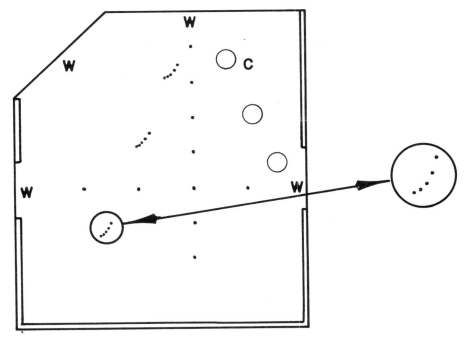

11-4 B-scanning tissue-equivalent phantom model. Unlike a test object, a phantom contains attenuating material with evenly distributed scattering bodies. Within the phantom are simulations of typical scanning situations. To scan from several different directions, the phantom has several windows, W. Included are a set of vertical pins, separated by 20 mm; a horizontal set of pins at a 10-cm depth, separated by 20 mm; three sets of axial resolution pins separated by, 3 mm, 2 mm, 1 mm, 0.5 mm; and three vertically positioned cysts, approximately 0.75 cm in diameter. Courtesy of Radiation Measurements, Inc., Middleton, WI.

change with temperature, but should remain as steady as the surrounding material. The scattering bodies should be uniformly distributed within the material, creating no visual "hot spots" or "dead zones." Such anomalies alter the ability to correctly check the scan uniformity of the sonograph. The scattering bodies should mimic as closely as possible the normal scattering and dot size of typical soft tissue.

With these facts in mind, we can now look at specific protocols for testing the B-scanner with an AIUM Test Object and a tissue-equivalent phantom.

Measurements with the AIUM Test Object

General Test Conditions

All of the measurements following use coupling gel between the transducer and the test object. The test object is, in turn, placed on a *stable* surface for scanning. The internal temperature of the test object should be recorded for final determination of the propagation velocity.

Normal Sensitivity Measurement

The object of this test is to obtain a reproducible scan of the test object that will permit a determination of both the minimum sensitivity and the normal sensitivity of the sonograph. The protocol is:

Set the TGC flat at the minimum gain settings.

Set the power output from the transducer to the range normally used for tissue scanning.

Set the reject control to its minimum setting, allowing the largest range of signals to reach the display.

Scan the test object along its top.

Reduce gain until one of the bottom rods is just visible. The same rod must be used for each test.

Record the gain setting under the label, *Minimum Sensitivity.*

If the gain setting varies more than 3 dB over a period of time, then the sonograph needs internal adjustment, and a service representative should be called.
To obtain the *normal sensitivity* measurement:

Increase the system gain just until all the rods are clearly seen in the image.

Record this new gain setting under the label, *Normal Sensitivity.* All the remaining measurements are made at this gain setting.

An example of a minimum sensitivity image is shown in Figure 11-5.

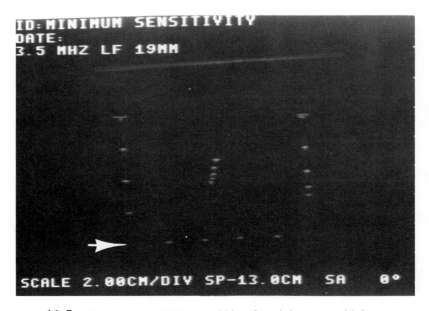

11-5 Scanning an AIUM Test Object for minimum sensitivity. Minimum sensitivity occurs when the system gain and output power are set so the lower left pin is just visible in the image (arrow).

Axial Resolution Measurement

Axial resolution is the ability to distinguish two axially placed echo sources as two. The ability to carry out the discrimination is a function of the spatial pulse length and signal processing within the sonograph. This is quite different from the problem of resolving distances on the display. Despite the AIUM practice of lumping axial resolution with range resolution, we will separate the two here. In this text, range resolution expresses the ability to measure the range between two objects along the beam axis. With digital calipers on most of the newer digital sonographs, range resolution can be quite small, often less than a millimeter.

The primary objective here is to measure the axial resolution and the smallest echo-source separation that can be seen as two. The procedure is:

Set the machine into the normal sensitivity settings.

Scan the center portion of the test object where the pins are separated at decreasing intervals from 5 mm to 1 mm.

Examine the image for the smallest, clearly seen separation. This separation is recorded under the label, *Measured Axial Resolution.*

An example of the axial resolution image is in Figure 11-6.

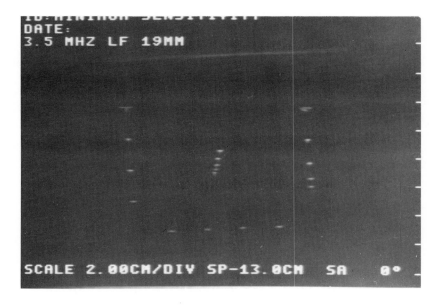

11-6 Scanning the AIUM Test Object for axial resolution. The center pins of the test object are separated to provide a measure of axial resolution. In this image, the 2-mm pins are well separated; the 1-mm pins are not.

Lateral Resolution Measurement

The AIUM Test Object has a set of pins spaced at intervals of 25 mm, 20 mm, 15 mm, 10 mm, 5 mm, and 3 mm. Scanning across this array of pins offers a direct measurement of lateral resolution. Each pin in the array appears as a line on the display. Pins farther apart than the beam width will appear as two lines, whereas pins less than the beam width apart will become continuous on the display. Although this measurement does not represent the best lateral resolution, it is the lateral resolution at a fixed distance from each measured transducer. The protocol is:

With the sonograph at normal sensitivity settings, scan the array of pins from the largest to the smallest separation.

Examine the image for the smallest distance between the lines. Record this separation interval as the *Measured Lateral Resolution.*

Repeat the measurement for each of the transducers in use.

The lateral resolution of a given transducer should not change significantly over time. If the measurement shows a major change in lateral resolution, it usually indicates problems either within the sonograph (most often) or the transducer, and deserves a visit from a factory service representative. An example image for lateral resolution is shown in Figure 11-7.

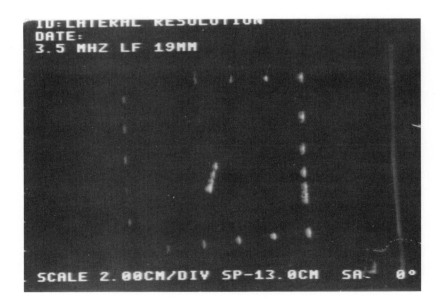

11-7   Scanning the AIUM Test Object for lateral resolution. The vertical pins on the right of the image are separated at intervals starting at 25 mm and decreasing at 5-mm steps. The transducer is on the right side of the image. Lateral resolution for this 3.5-MHz transducer is 10 mm at the measuring range.

Dead-Zone Measurement

After the transmitter voltage excites the transducer, the ring down in the transducer and transmit/receive switch form a refractory period for the sonograph, often called the "main bang." During this period, the sonograph is unable to detect the presence of external echo sources. Problems in the sonograph front end can significantly extend this dead zone. Measuring the dead zone, then, provides an evaluation of the receiver front end.

Within the test object are pins that extend down from the top of the test object at 10 mm, 8 mm, 6 mm, 4 mm, and 2 mm, evenly spaced across the test object. The measurement protocol is:

Scan the top of the test object above the variable range pins with the sonograph at normal sensitivity settings.

Examine the image for the first visible line below the main bang. Record the range of this pin as the *Dead-Zone Measurement*.

A dead zone of 2 mm to 4 mm is most common, but a few systems extend to 6 mm. Dead zones beyond 8 mm indicate problems. Regardless of the starting values, a shift in dead-zone values is more important here than an absolute value.

A scan for dead zone appears in Figure 11-8.

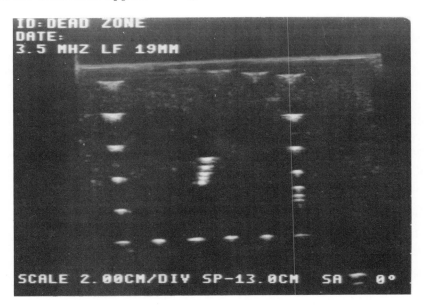

11-8 Scanning the AIUM Test Object for the dead zone. The top pins are separated from the top of the test object at increasing 2-mm intervals, starting at 2 mm and ending at 10 mm. The dead zone for this system is less than 4 mm but greater than 2 mm, an acceptable value for this sonograph.

Arm-Registration Measurement

Measuring arm registration determines whether or not the test-object pins appear in the image at the same place when scanned from three different directions. Each rod in the test object produces a line, and all the lines should intersect for the registration to be close to ideal.

The measurement protocol is:

Be sure to place the test object on a stable surface for the scanning. Scan the test object from at least three sides without erasing the image between scans.

Examine the image for the intersection of lines from each scan. The lines should intersect within a circle 7 mm in diameter, or less if the sonograph specifications so state. Record whether or not the sonograph is within specification under the heading *Arm Registration*.

Determine the intersection by using the centers of each scan line to represent the pin. For most scanners, a registration larger than 7 mm means major distortions in the image, and will require a readjustment by a service representative.

An arm-registration scan appears in Figure 11-9.

Depth-Calibration Measurement

The AIUM-Test Object has a known pattern of pin separations and locations. These patterns and separations should appear on the display just as they appear in the test object. Depth markers can be placed in the image to test the depth or range calibration. This is a measure of the machine time base, representing 1540 m/s, and of how linear this time base remains over the whole image. Placing the depth markers beside the pins separated 20 mm apart offers a chance to examine the accuracy of the markers, as well as any digital calipers on the sonograph. Unless otherwise stated, a 2% error is acceptable, that is, the measurement is permitted to be 2 mm off in either direction for a measurement over 100 mm. The protocol is:

Scan the test object with normal sensitivity settings.

Position the depth markers in the image alongside the regularly spaced, 20-mm separated pins.

Examine the image for alignment of the pins and the 20-mm intervals in the depth markers. The distances in the image and the depth markers should be the same for the top, middle, and bottom of the image.

Bring up the digital calipers and measure the pin separations at the top, middle, and bottom of the image. A measurement from top to bottom should show a range of 100 mm, plus or minus 2 mm.

A failure to fall within the specifications means the time base in the sonograph may be off and thus needs to be repaired.

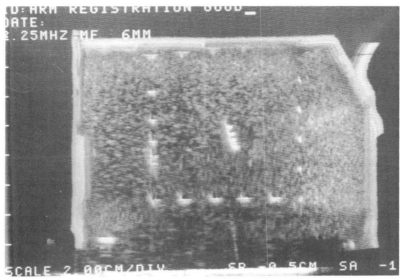

11.9 Part A

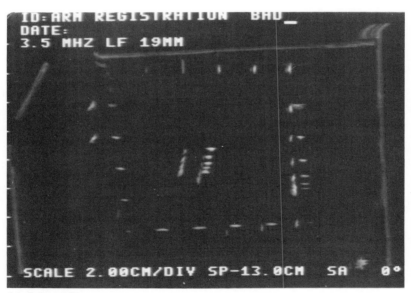

11.9 Part B

11-9 Scanning the AIUM Test Object for arm registration. Part A: This B-scanner shows good arm registration, as indicated by the close intersection of the scan lines for each pin. The texture in the image comes from small scattering bodies within this test object. Part B: This B-scanner is out of alignment enough to compromise compound scanning. The error is about 1 cm.

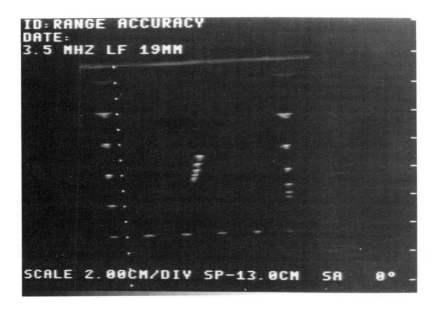

11-10 Scanning the AIUM Test Object for range accuracy. Placing a depth marker next to the left-hand pins shows any timing errors within the sonograph. Here the depth markers are slightly off close to the transducer, but become correct for deeper portions. The range error is less than 2 mm in 100 mm, and therefore is acceptable.

This measurement relies on the fluid in the phantom propagating at 1540 m/s. If the test object has a thermometer, the test object can either be heated to an operating temperature or the error can be calculated from a known velocity-temperature relationship.

A depth-calibration image appears in Figure 11-10.

Measurements with the Tissue-Equivalent Phantom

The outstanding feature of a tissue-equivalent phantom is its ability to present the B-scanner a set of attenuation, reflection, and scattering situations that test overall function. Importantly, the testing occurs at normal power, gain, and TGC settings found in typical soft tissues. Some of the parameters measured with the AIUM Test Object are also measured by the tissue-equivalent phantom. Others, like the dead-zone measurement, are unique to the test object.

All the measurements following assume use of a coupling gel or oil between the transducer and the phantom windows.

The scanning requirements of a static B-scanner differ from those of real time, and these differences are reflected in the shape of the phantom used for each. A B-scanner phantom needs at least three windows to the interior to test scanning-arm registration.

Depth-Calibration and Range-Resolution Measurements

Placing depth markers next to the evenly separated pins reveals any alteration in depth calibration over the whole image formation. Most phantoms change velocity slowly with changing temperature; thus, normal room variations in temperature will introduce little error in the phantom propagation velocity. The protocol is:

Scan the top of the phantom over the region of the pins.

Place the depth markers from the sonograph next to the regularly separated pins in the phantom image.

Examine the image for depth-marker variations away from the pin separations in the phantom. Record any observed variations.

Position the top cursor of the electronic calipers over the top pin. Place the second cursor at the 8-cm or 10-cm range. Record the displayed range as the *Caliper Calibration*.

Variations greater than 2% or greater than the manufacturer specifications indicate a need for a service call.

An image showing a determination of range accuracy appears in Figure 11-11.

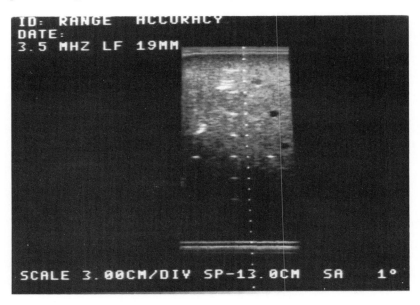

11-11   Scanning a tissue-equivalent phantom for range accuracy. The depth markers passing through this image of a tissue-equivalent phantom are well placed for measuring. The timing in the sonograph is within the 2% tolerance (2 mm in 100 mm) range.

Determining Spatial Accuracy

The sonograph should produce an accurate portrayal of structures anywhere in the image format. One of the best tests of this ability is to examine a circular cyst structure within various parts of the image. B-scanning phantoms usually have such structures placed at different depths within the phantom. A circular structure is a good test of spatial accuracy, and most people can quickly detect distortions in a circular pattern. The protocol is:

Scan the top of the phantom over the region of the cysts.

Repeat the scanning with the cysts in different portions of the image format.

Examine the image for distortions in the circular pattern of the structures as a function of lateral or axial position.

Measure the diameter of the cysts using the electronic calipers in each of the image locations. Record the variations under the heading *Spatial Accuracy*.

The ability to show the shape of a lesion depends upon the image-production techniques within the sonograph. Subtle changes can cause image distortion either over the whole screen or in small segments. By scanning circular structures the image production may be tested in all directions. Large deviations in the circular patterns indicate the need for a service call.

A second method uses the horizontally placed pins that appear at the 10-cm depth. These pins can be measured horizontally with the calipers or depth markers. Spatial accuracy requires that the sonograph depict the correct separation to within 2%.

An example of a horizontal measurement and cyst depiction appears in Figure 11-12.

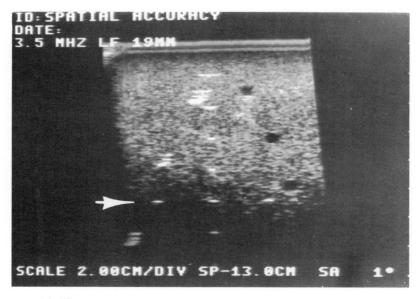

11-12   Scanning a tissue-equivalent phantom for spatial accuracy. This scan is seeking to determine if axial and lateral portrayal of echo-source locations is accurate. The horizontal pins at the 10-cm depth (arrow) are separated 20 mm in the image. In addition, the cysts are circular. This sonograph has good spatial accuracy.

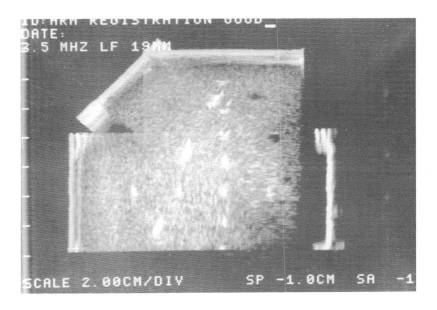

11-13 Scanning a tissue-equivalent phantom for arm registration. Scanning a phantom from at least three directions will show the intersection of pins in the image. This sonograph has good arm registration.

Arm-Registration Measurement

Just as in measuring the scanning arm registration with the AIUM Test Object, the pins within the phantom are scanned from different directions. The degree of registration shows up in how well the signals from the pins overlap in the final image. The protocol is:

Scan the pins within the phantom from three sides.

Examine the image for the intersection of the signals from the pins. The center of each scan line should fall within a 7-mm diameter circle or a circle specified by the manufacturer. Record whether or not the arm registration is within or outside acceptable limits.

The criteria developed for arm-registration measurements using the AIUM Test Object still apply to arm-registration measurements in the phantom. An arm-registration error exceeding 7 mm indicates need for adjustment or repair.

Figure 11-13 shows the image typical for determining arm registration.

Maximum Penetration and Sensitivity Measurement

Most tissue-equivalent phantoms attenuate ultrasound at a rate close to normal tissue, at about 1 dB/cm/MHz. This can be a one-way or a two-way attenuation rate. Whatever the selected value, the attenuation should prevent the scattering bodies from being seen all the way to the bottom of the phantom when the lowest frequency is used. "Bottoming out" on the phantom means the sonograph cannot be used at its maximum sensitivity and maximum power out.

The object of this test is to measure the maximum penetration into the phantom using the maximum gain and power for the sonograph. The protocol is:

Set the TGC flat at maximum values. Increase the system gain and the system power to maximum.

Scan the phantom along its top.

Examine the image and measure the maximum penetration, using either the internal depth markers or the electronic calipers on the sonograph.

Record this depth as the *Maximum Phantom Penetration*. This number represents the best that the sonograph can do.

A variation in this depth greater than 0.5 cm is significant, but does not merit a service call unless it also represents a change in gain greater than 3 dB. For example, a 3-MHz transducer used on a phantom with a 1-dB/cm/MHz attenuation rate attenuates 3 dB for each centimeter traveled, or 6 dB for a centimeter round trip. Thus, a shift of 0.5 cm represents a shift of 3 dB in system sensitivity.

The image from a scan for maximum sensitivity appears in Figure 11-14.

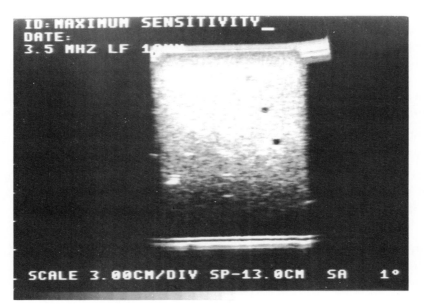

11-14 Scanning a tissue-equivalent phantom for maximum sensitivity. This test requires scanning for maximum penetration into the phantom. The system gain and output power are maximum. The range of the last scattering echo signal is recorded as the maximum sensitivity range. The last scattering signals vanish at 15 cm for this sonograph.

Dot-Size Measurement

Distributed within the phantom gel are small particles of carbon that produce scattering. The pattern produced by these carbon particules should be uniform over a major portion of the penetration, and then should rapidly fall off to zero. The size of the dots that make the pattern is a function of the transducer frequency, transducer size, degree of focusing, and band width. Superimposed on the transducer characteristics are the distortions introduced by the sonograph signal processing. The protocol is:

Scan the phantom with typical machine settings, using the same settings for each scan.

Photograph the resulting image as a record of dot size and texture formation.

Examine the image for evidence of poor dot formation or gray-scale contouring around the dots.

Major changes in the dot size and texture of the image will require a service call. An example of textural information from a phantom scan appears in Figure 11-15.

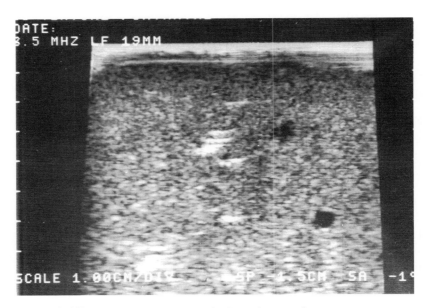

11-15 Scanning a tissue-equivalent phantom for texture portrayal. The texture of the phantom image should change from top to bottom, becoming increasingly coarse with increasing range. The texture should consist of large and small echo signals in a regular mix that is repeatable in additional scans.

Axial Resolution Measurement

Within many phantoms are axial resolution pins set at different depths. These pins provide measurement of the axial resolution as the ultrasound pulse shape is

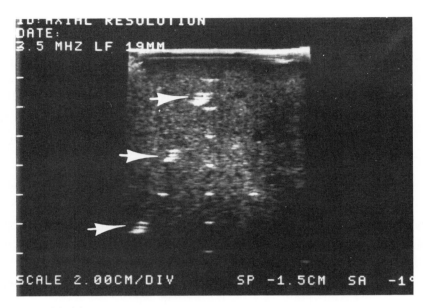

11-16   Scanning a tissue-equivalent phantom for axial resolution. Axial resolution can change as a function of range from
the transducer. The three sets of separated pins (arrows) permit
a measurement of axial resolution with increasing range. This
sonograph has an axial resolution of less thn 2 mm but greater
than 1 mm.

changed by frequency-dependent attenuation. The separations are usually smaller
in a phantom than in the AIUM Test Object. The protocol is:

Scan the top of the phantom with maximum power and with the TGC set to
produce a uniform texture.

Examine the image for the smallest separation between successive signals.
Record this value as *Axial Resolution*.

If the phantom has more than one set of axial resolution pins, use the value
derived from the center set as representative of axial resolution. Typical values
approach but do not exceed three wavelengths for the center frequency in use.
Axial resolution exceeding three wave lengths warrants a service call.

The image of a scan for axial resolution appears in Figure 11-16.

Lateral Resolution Measurement

Within the B-scanning phantom should be a set of equally spaced pins, separated
by 1 cm or 2 cm. These pins offer a rapid-beam profile when the transducer is
scanned over this region of the phantom. The equally spaced pins will appear as
lines, with the line length showing the width of the ultrasound beam at that point.
The narrowest line shows the position of the focal point and the extension of the
transducer focal zone. The protocol is:

Scan the top of the phantom over the region of the pins.

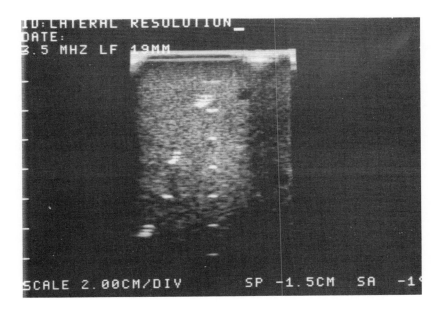

11-17 Scanning a tissue-equivalent phantom for lateral resolution. Scanning the center pins of the phantom shows the effective beam width at 2-cm intervals down the beam. This 3.5-
MHz, long-focus transducer has a focal point close to 6 cm and
a focal zone that extends from less than 6 cm to about the 10-
cm range. The beam is nearly 1 cm wide at the 12-cm range.

Locate the smallest line in the image and record this number as the *Focal-Point
Range*.

Measure the length of the smallest line and record it as the transducer *Lateral
Resolution*.

Significant alterations in lateral resolution can signify a change in either the
transducer or the signal processing within the sonograph, and indicate a need for
a service call.

An example of a scan for lateral resolution appears in Figure 11-17.

Testing B-scanner Transducers

Although we would like to believe that all transducers with identical markings
behave identically, they can, in fact, vary widely in performance. The tissue-
equivalent phantom offers a clear opportunity to test one transducer against another,
comparing any of the standard transducer parameters such as frequency, focal
point range, focal zone range, and degree of focus. The protocol is:

Scan one-half of the phantom with the first transducer.

Change transducers and scan the second half of the phantom with the second
transducer. This produces a split image, containing data from both the first and
the second transducer.

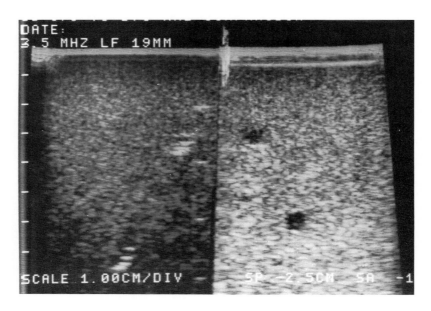

11-18 Scanning a tissue-equivalent phantom to compare two transducers. Transducers can be easily compared by scanning a phantom with both transducers in sequence. On the left is a 5-MHz transducer; on the right is a 3.5-MHz transducer. Notice the marked difference in texture and amplitudes for these two transducers.

Examine the image for differences in dot size, penetration, textural qualities, and variations in intensity over the image.

Record the observations or make a photograph of the display.

Variations among transducers can be subtle and hard to describe in words. The most effective way to compare supposedly similar transducers is to photograph the image for long-term comparisons.

An example of a two-transducer scan appears in Figure 11-18.

Active Electronic Phantoms

The transducer does not have to be the only source of signals for the sonograph. The electronic processing and the signal path can also be examined with an rf signal source. This signal source is called an *electronic phantom,* or an *electronic gray-scale generator,* and is shown in Figure 11-19. The device emits a burst of rf signals that change amplitude at a fixed rate. The cue for the burst is the transmitter pulse from the sonograph. With signals falling at a fixed rate, the maximum sensitivity, TGC response, and malassignments in preprocessing or postprocessing are easy to detect. The electronic phantoms, unlike the passive phantoms, need maintenance and calibration at regular intervals. An A mode display and image produced by a gray-scale generator is shown in Figure 11-20.

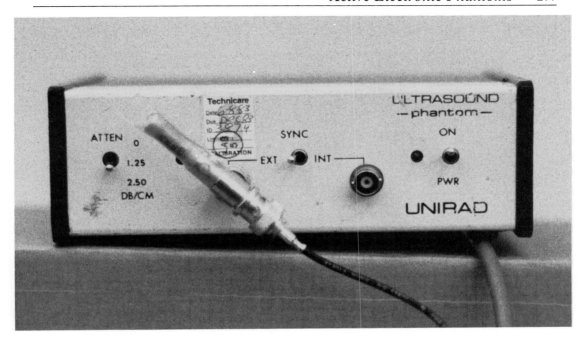

11-19   An active electronic gray scale phantom. An electronic gray scale phantom replaces the transducer and generates electronic radio frequency (rf) signals synchronized by the transmit voltage from the sonograph. The signals are used to set TGC response and gray scale characteristics of the sonograph. Courtesy of Technicare Ultrasound Division, Englewood, Colorado.

In order to test particular portions of the sonograph, often a special signal source is needed. This is the case for the digital scan converter. The adjustment and functional tests for the digital scan converter are best examined with a signal source that highlights the important steps in the scan-conversion process. Like the electronic phantom, the gray-scale generator places a set of signals into the analog-to-digital converter to examine sampling rate, preprocessing assignments, and proper storage of the signals into the RAM. With the input signal-stream characterized, the postprocessing functions can be checked for correct operation.

The electronic phantoms permit a detailed examination of the TGC system. Time-gain compensation relies on two elements in the sonograph: first, the correct production of the TGC curves by the TGC curve generator; and second, the correct response by the rf amplifiers or video amplifiers to the applied TGC voltage. Variations in the TGC system greater than 3 dB will appear in the image, and can create unexplained intensity variations within an image.

In general, most ultrasound departments do not have electronic phantoms or special signal generators. These devices are usually installed by the service representative as part of a regular check of the sonograph. In some of the newer machines, these rf sources are located within the sonograph already. The repair person simply connects the rf sources into the signal stream and performs an established protocol for testing the major steps in the signal path. In addition, many of the newer sonographs that use large amounts of software to control the device employ "self-test" electronics to verify that the software is operating in the proper sequence and amplitudes.

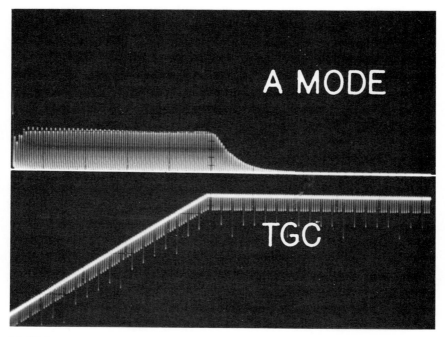

11-20A

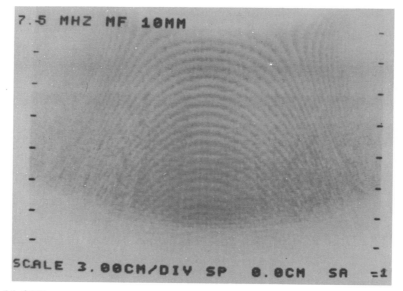

11-20B

11-20 The output of an electronic gray scale phantom on display. A) The most frequent use of an electronic phantom is to calibrate the TGC response in the sonograph. B) The gray scale B-mode image can also be tested with the phantom. Courtesy of Technicare Ultrasound Corporation, Englewood, Colorado.

A QA Program at Home

Perhaps the most difficult aspect of any quality assurance program is getting started. In answer to the question, Where do I begin? any quality assurance program must be composed of three components:

1. Making regular measurements of essential machine capabilities;
2. Maintaining an equipment history of all the QA measurements and a service history on each sonograph; and
3. Assuring that regular service calls are made by the factory service representative to perform the "deeper" equipment checks.

All three components contribute to an ability to follow the normal trends and changes in the sonograph.

To initiate a QA program, a department first needs something to measure, either an AIUM Test Object or a tissue-equivalent phantom with the necessary internal structures. These devices are now available from a number of commercial sources.

Although the AIUM Test Object is not an overly complex device, a tissue-equivalent phantom requires a more sophisticated manufacturing ability. Thus, it is best to buy phantoms from experienced companies or newer companies that demonstrate a firm grasp of the principles of ultrasound science, including the ability to distinguish between acoustic impedance and attenuation.

Once the department has a phantom or test object, the next step is to develop an equipment history form for recording measurements and findings. This form should follow the measurement protocol as closely as possible, thus making recordkeeping simple. The record can, in turn, prompt the measurement protocol. A well-designed program of measurements will take no more than 20 min on the morning of the test day. Although the measurements can be taken daily, weekly, or monthly, measurements at weekly intervals are recommended, interspersed with spot measurements when a malfunction is suspected. The simpler the routine, the less chance that the program will be abandoned out of frustration or boredom.

Along with the use of phantoms and test objects, equipment can often be tested by applying postprocessing to the images or by using testing circuits designed into the sonograph. For example, contouring can be examined with postprocessing. Internal signal sources can inject signals that can be read at the A-mode display or on the B-mode display. Whatever the procedure, the goal is to gain enough information to know whether or not the sonograph is working to specifications, and if not, the degree to which the machine diverges from the specifications.

One of the more difficult decisions in a quality assurance program is knowing when to call the service representative based on QA measurements, even though the sonograph may still seem to be working. The decision is often based on an intuition or "guess." A much-more-reliable method is to ask the question: Does the equipment malfunction produce sufficient error in the sonograph to permit a diagnostic mistake? If the malfunction is not serious, the repair can probably wait until a routine service call. More serious mistakes, however, require an immediate service call. The service engineer's respect will hardly be gained, however, if the "emergency" service call is solved by simply plugging in the sonograph or turning a single control. A careful inspection of the problem before telephoning the service engineer can quickly sort out equipment problems from operator problems.

A general rule for responding to equipment failure is: Panic first, but do nothing; then check the machine; and, finally, call the service representative.

Conclusion

Because of the internal complexity of the contemporary static B-scanner, a quality assurance program is necessary to determine whether or not the sonograph is operating within manufacturer's specifications. Day-to-day variations in function are not necessarily visible even to the experienced sonographer, but these variations can affect the performance of the sonograph as a diagnostic tool.

Effective testing requires giving the B-scanner a known set of targets and conditions that can test machine function. The AIUM Test Object and tissue-equivalent phantom are such targets. In conjunction with an understood testing procedure, the static sonograph can be tested for key point functions. Because of its design, the B-scanner carries a number of "soft spots" that require regular attention. These critical points include:

1. The scanning arm;
2. The TGC signal generator;
3. The rf amplifier response to the TGC signals;
4. The rf amplifier gain and noise figure;
5. The system gain and output power control;
6. Preprocessing functions;
7. Postprocessing functions; and
8. Display monitor linearity.

A carefully organized and maintained quality assurance program can regularly monitor these soft spots.

References

1. Burlew, M.M., et al. February 1980. A new ultrasound tissue-equivalent material. Radiology 134: 517–520.

2. Goldstein, A. August 1980, Quality assurance in diagnostic ultrasound. AIUM.

Chapter 12

Reliable Real Time:
Testing Real-Time Sonographs

Although considerable literature is available for sonographers who wish to test static B-scanners, this is not the case for any of the real-time systems now in use. In an effort to begin to correct this inadequacy, this chapter discusses a method of testing real-time sonographs. The techniques described here are not the last word in testing, but they have served us well over years of evaluating real-time sonographs for customers and manufacturers.

At the outset, testing a real-time sonograph appears complex. The transducer is not connected to an arm, the AIUM Test Object has a surface too hard and inflexible for many of the sector scanners, and even those systems testable with the AIUM Test Object can be examined in only a limited manner. Still, a real-time sonograph has the same imaging end points as the B-scanner—namely, size, shape, position, texture, and dynamics. We thus need to test the real-time sonograph in terms of each of these components.

The testing tool is the tissue-equivalent phantom, which offers a mixed set of targets in a stable environment. In all, 14 tests and comparisons are available in an appropriately designed phantom to evaluate the imaging characteristics of a real-time system. But not every phantom can be used successfully to test a real-time sonograph. Our first requirement, then, is to define the phantom characteristics needed to test a real-time system.

General Phantom Characteristics

The tissue-equivalent phantom requirements for real time are slightly different from those needed for the static B-scanner. For example, the scanning surface on the phantom must be able to handle both small and large real-time scan heads. The B-scanner can scan a very hard surface, such as found on the AIUM Test Object. A real-time sonograph with a small mechanical scan head, however, cannot adequately scan through such an inflexible surface because of the limited contact area. As a result, the typical real-time tissue-equivalent phantom uses a soft scanning surface. Often this surface is flooded with coupling material to project the whole scanning field into the phantom.

The physical size of the phantom depends upon the types of real-time devices and the frequencies involved in the testing process. If the scanhead is large, such as a linear array or a sizable rotating transducer, then a physically large phantom is required to visualize the whole scanning field at one time. High attenuation rates can make a phantom shorter, but a high attenuation rate is not a typical scanning situation. A better choice is an attenuation rate close to normal tissue values. In general, a good phantom for real time should be 18 cm to 20 cm deep, about 16 cm wide, and 4 cm to 5 cm thick. In addition, a small lip around the top of the phantom can hold a reservoir of oil, water, or gel to help test the mechanical sector scanners.

Part of the testing will be a depiction of circular structures. The phantom, then, needs circular cysts at least ¾ cm in diameter to help test the spatial accuracy of the real-time system and its contrast sensitivity. The cysts should have a low attenuation rate, at perhaps one-tenth of the surrounding material, to permit an easy portrayal of acoustic enhancement. With a 10:1 ratio in attenuation rates, the enhancement will be obvious in an operating real-time sonograph.

A pattern of pins is used to represent separated structures within the tissue equivalent phantom. The pins should be separated in a manner that tests axial resolution and the range accuracy of the machine. The range-accuracy pins are usually located down the center of the phantom, equally spaced at 20-mm intervals. Axial resolution pins are separated by intervals of 3 mm, 2 mm, 1 mm, and 0.5 mm, and are placed at several different depths. These internal structures, in conjuction with the normal tissue-like characteristics of the phantom, permit a wide range of tests and comparisons to be carried out on the real-time sonograph.

The protocols discussed in this chapter can be used for the linear array or sector scanner with frequencies ranging from 2.25 MHz to 7.5 MHz. Within this range of frequencies, the scattering body size and characteristics are well defined for most phantoms currently available. The remainder of the chapter examines in detail some testing protocols.

Testing Protocols

General Conditions

The starting conditions for the test assume that the tissue-equivalent phantom has a propagating velocity of 1540 m/s, an attenuation rate of 1 dB/cm/MHz to 1.5 dB/cm/MHz round trip, and contains cysts, pins, and windows to permit viewing of all of the interior structures. Gel, oil, or water couples the ultrasonic energy into the phantom. The phantom should not "bottom out," that is, when operating the sonograph at its maximum sensitivity and maximum transmitting power, the scattering signals should not reach the bottom of the phantom for the lowest frequency in use. This insures that as the test proceeds, any variations in the total performance of the sonograph can be readily observed and measured.

The phantom should rest on a stable surface for scanning, and should be positioned on the surface within easy reach for the sonographer to do the testing. Most phantoms respond slowly to major temperature changes, but operate best at a stable room temperature. When not in use, the phantom should be stored in a secure area at room temperature.

Information such as the above—and much more—can be found in the manufacturer's instructions on the phantom. For example, the temperature coefficients for propagation velocity and attenuation are measures of phantom stability, and these should be known for any phantom in use.

The protocols described below depend upon a phantom containing the following specific characteristics: an attenuation rate of 1 dB/cm/MHz to 1.5 dB/cm/MHz round trip; a propagation velocity of 1540 m/s; axial resolution pins positioned 4 cm, 6 cm, and 8 cm from the transducer, with a separation starting at 3.0 mm and progressing down to 0.5 mm; the pins are made of monofilament line with a reflectivity at least 10 dB above the surrounding scattering bodies; the phantom should have cysts positioned in the near field, focal point, and far-field portions of the phantom; the cysts should be 0.75 cm or larger; and the phantom should have a set of axially positioned pins separated either 20 mm or 10 mm apart, extending over a range of at least 14 cm; the phantom should also have a set of horizontal pins, separated 30 mm apart, spanning the phantom at the 10-cm depth. A diagram of such a phantom appears in Figure 12-1.

With these conditions in mind, let us examine the 14 tests available for the real-time sonograph.

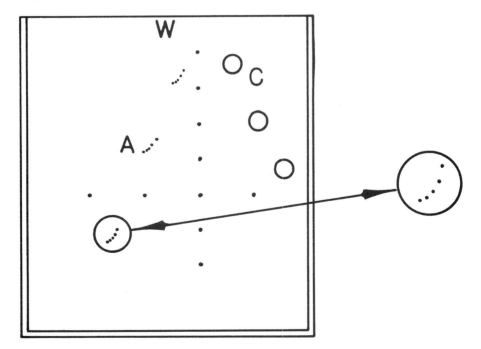

12-1   Tissue-equivalent phantom for testing real-time sonographs. The phantom contains a regularly attenuating material with a known attenuation rate and propagation velocity. In addition there are scattering bodies, evenly distributed, to mimic the signal mix from soft tissues. Inside is a vertical pin-set, each pin 20 mm apart; a horizontal pin-set at 100 mm deep, each pin spaced 20 mm apart; three pin-sets at different depths with separations of 3 mm, 2 mm, 1 mm and 0.5 mm; and three cysts, *C*, at different depths, each about 0.75 cm in diameter. The top is one large window, W. Courtesy of Radiation Measurements, Inc., Middleton, WI.

Ray and Scanning Field Formation

The first machine test is to examine ray formation and formation of the scanning field. This is a particularly critical portion of the real-time evaluation. If the sonograph fails these early tests, the remaining evaluations will not be as meaningful. The test is as follows:

Scan the phantom from the center of the top. Look for any problems in forming the imaging field. We need to show that the scanning field is properly formed, either as a sector or a rectangle. If it is a sector, we need to determine if the sector is, for example, 90° or 60°. A 90° sector can be measured by using the corner of an 8 ½-by-11-inch sheet of paper. Sector angles less than 90° can be drawn on tracing paper and fitted over the image to test for the correct sector formation. A linear array should form a rectangular field, and this field should be linear across the bottom, top, and both sides. The straight edge on a piece of paper or plastic ruler can quickly show any nonlinearities.

We next examine the formation of the rays, or lines of sight, that create the image. They should be evenly distributed across the scanning field, with no "drop outs" in rays, no variations in ray intensity from one to another, and no missed pixels. Malformation of the rays will prevent depiction of structures and the proper making of later determinations in the testing procedure. It is essential that the sonograph pass this test before relying on any of the subsequent tests.

Position the vertical pins down the center of the image. The centers of these pins should form a straight line down the image, with no lateral displacements. The horizontal pins should form a pattern at 90° to the vertical pins, with their centers along a straight line. Placing a straight edge along the centers of the horizontal pins will quickly show whether or not they are displaced in the image.

Slowly scan the pins in the center of the phantom, moving the pins on either side of the image center. Look for sudden decreases in lateral line widths as they approach the center of the scanning field. Disappearing lines or abruptly short lines indicate a scan converter that is not showing all the scan lines in the center of the image.

Position the vertical pins in different portions of the image to demonstrate linearity in the center of the image and the edges of the scanning field.

With the transducer positioned over the center pins and held steady, examine the image for any flickering in intensity or wavering in the image. These variations indicate problems in positioning the ultrasonic beams or in handling position information within the sonograph.

It should be reemphasized here that unlike the static B-scanner, which permits the sonographer to "scan out" problems that appear in the sonograph, the early conditions described above need to be met in the real-time system for the system to function properly for both the remainder of the tests and diagnostic imaging. A good sector image appears in Figure 12-2.

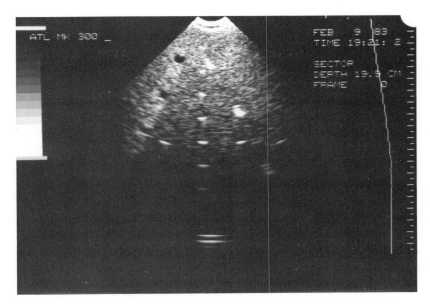

12-2   Good real-time image of tissue-equivalent phantom. During this scan, the formation of the scanning field should permit visualization of the phantom components: vertical pins, cysts, axial resolution pins, and lateral pins.

Range Accuracy

Scan the center pins of the phantom, placing the pins along one of the rays near the center of the image. Move the system depth markers close to or onto the image of the pins and freeze the image if the sonograph has a scan converter. Measure any differences in the anterior, middle, and posterior pin positions. The depth markers and the phantom pins should align with an error not greater than 2%. That means the sonograph should not vary anymore than 2 mm out of a total distance of 100 mm.

Some sonographs have depth markers displaced from the start of the image. In this instance, the *distances between* phantom pins and depth markers should be the same, even if they are not exactly aligned.

After testing the accuracy of the depth markers, place the electronic calipers on the image of the pins and measure the distances between pins. As in the case of the depth markers, an error of 2% or less is considered adequate. The manufacturer's specifications may be larger or smaller than 2%, in which case, the published specifications for the particular sonograph should be used. Errors in either the depth markers or the electronic calipers that are greater than either 2% or the manufacturer's specifications indicate potential problems in the imaging time base. This sort of error requires a visit from the field service engineer. Record the results under the heading *Range Accuracy*.

Scan the phantom with the vertical pins down a center ray and position the scanning field to display the horizontal pins. Measure the distances between the

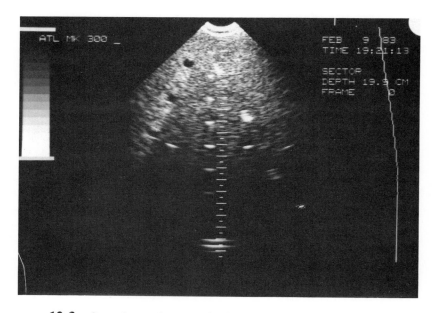

12-3 Scanning a tissue-equivalent phantom for range accuracy. A frozen image of the phantom permits easy placement of depth markers on the image. A comparison shows these markers slightly out of alignment with the pins because of pressure on the phantom top. Depth accuracy, however, is within 2%, that is, a 2-mm variation out of a total distance of 100 mm.

horizontal pins. They should be within 2% of the phantom dimensions. An example of a range-accuracy test appears in Figure 12-3.

A mechanical sector scanner can run into problems here if the scan head scanning surface is curved and the coupling material is gel. In this instance, the gel will form a wedge between the scan head surface and the phantom surface. The wedge will look like a lens to the ultrasound, causing the ultrasound beam to bend, giving an error of up to 10% in lateral measurements. If the coupling material is oil or water, however, this lens effect is reduced, and the measurements will be restored. The same effect does *not* happen on the body because the skin conforms to the curve of the scan head; thus, gel works well on the body. The problem appears only with the flat surface of a phantom.

If these measurements prove to be outside accepted limits, then the remainder of the test protocol can be carried out to see what else is happening, while keeping the early limitations in mind.

Spatial Accuracy

We have already been given a grasp of spatial accuracy by measuring the pin separations both horizontally and vertically. The cysts located within a tissue-equivalent phantom represent a circular and therefore continuously changing line within the image. The circular body of a cyst tests the spatial accuracy of the sonograph, and this portrayal can be tested by looking at the cyst in various parts

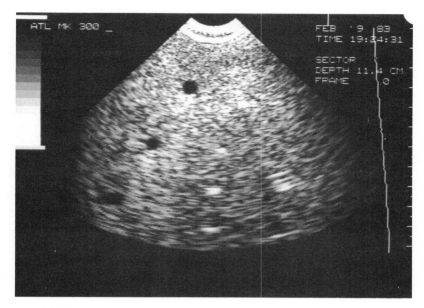

12-4 Scanning a tissue-equivalent phantom to show cyst portrayal. The best cystic portrayal will occur in the focal zone of the transducer. This transducer has a 4-cm focal point, and the cyst closest to the transducer has a well-defined border. Border definition becomes poorer with increasing beam width.

of the scanning field. The tissue-equivalent phantom should carry at least three separate cysts, located at three different distances from the transducer.

Scan the cysts within the tissue-equivalent phantom and move the cysts slowly to the anterior, middle, and posterior portions of the field. Be sure the scanning plane is perpendicular to the cylinders that form the cysts within the phantom. Scanning the cysts away from normal can change their shape in the image. Look for variations in the circular characteristics of the cysts and for poor boundary definition. In many phantoms, the cyst boundaries that are perpendicular to the beam will take on specular reflection characteristics. The lateral walls, which depend on scattering signals for portrayal, will provide information on the spatial accuracy of the sonograph. An image showing phantom cysts appears in Figure 12-4.

While scanning the cysts, look for any changes in the circular characteristics of the cyst image that are not a result of the scan plane position. Record any variations from normal under the general heading *Spatial Accuracy*.

Maximum Sensitivity

Set the sonograph output power, TGC, and system gain to maximum. Scan the center portion of the tissue-equivalent phantom, and examine the image for the maximum penetration into the phantom. Look for the last echo signals from the scattering bodies. If the sonograph has an A-mode display, confirm on the A-mode

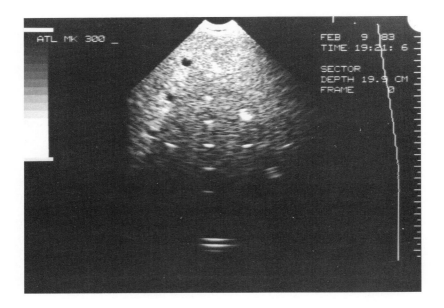

12-5   Scanning a tissue-equivalent phantom for maximum sensitivity. This test requires the output power and system gain to be maximum. The range of the last scattering echo-signal marks the best penetration. This sonograph shows a penetration to 14 cm with a 3-MHz transducer.

display that the last scattering signal in the image is disappearing at the same range as the two-dimensional image. The two should differ by not more than a distance equal to 3 dB.

If this is a first-time measurement of the sonograph, record the results as "expected" or "initial" penetration characteristics of the sonograph. Record this number under the heading *Maximum Sensitivity*.

If this is a secondary measurement of maximum penetration, then the penetration distance can be compared with the first-time evaluation. If the penetration changes by an amount representing more than 3 dB at the center operating frequency, the system's gain and signal-processing systems should be checked by the field service engineer. Record the results under the heading *Maximum Sensitivity*. A measurement for maximum sensitivity is shown in Figure 12-5.

Variations in sensitivity are determined by multiplying the center operating frequency by the attenuation rate of the phantom. For example, at 2.25 MHz and an attenuation rate of 1 dB/cm/MHz, a distance variation exceeding 1.3 cm represents a variation greater than 3 dB. As the frequency increases, the amount of variation permitted decreases. For example, a 3.5-MHz sonograph should be serviced if the scattering signal depth varies more than 1 cm.

Axial Resolution

Move the scan head to the portion of the phantom containing the axial resolution pins. Set the time-gain compensation for an even image in which the axial resolution

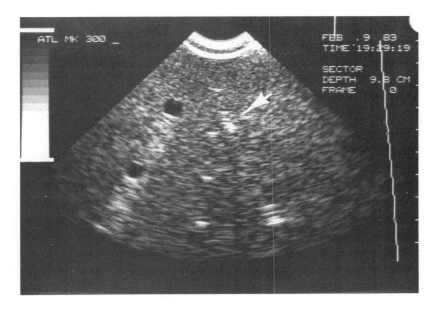

12-6 Scanning a tissue-equivalent phantom for axial resolution. The axial resolution of a sonograph is a function of distance, and the various pin sets in the phantom permit measurements at different depths. This 3-MHz transducer has an axial resolution of 1 mm, which can be easily separated in the image (arrow).

pins can be clearly seen against the background echo signals. Set the output power to a typical scanning level and use the same power setting for all future tests. Slowly move the scan head until the smallest pin separation appears on the screen. Record this value under the heading *Axial Resolution*. Record also the results from the pins close to and more distant from the scan head. The most representative axial resolution will be that found in the pins closest to either the focal point or the focal zone of the transducer. An axial resolution image is shown in Figure 12-6.

The expected value for axial resolution is less than or equal to three wavelengths. Sonographs that change axial resolution markedly or that have axial resolution greater than three wavelengths, provide an unacceptable resolution for clinical applications. Axial resolution greater than three wavelengths merits a service call.

Lateral Resolution

Some tissue-equivalent phantoms now have a "plane" of bubbles inside the phantom to provide a complete picture of the beam profile. Other phantoms have an equidistant set of pins extending 14 cm to 16 cm from the surface of the phantom, evenly spaced either 20 mm or 10 mm apart.

Scan the tissue-equivalent phantom along the pins or bubble interface. Obtain the clearest and best picture of the phantom pins and locate the narrowest portion of the transducer beam. Measure the width of the beam at this point using either

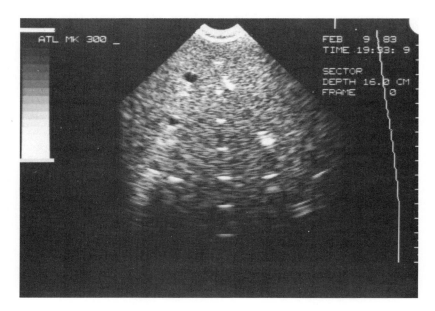

12-7 Scanning a tissue-equivalent phantom for lateral resolution. The vertical pins separated at 20-mm intervals give a
good look at the beam formation for a real-time transducer. This
sonograph has a focal point close to 4 cm, and a beam width of
approximately 1 cm at a range of 10 cm.

an external set of calipers or the electronic calipers inside the sonograph. Record
this width as the *Sonograph Lateral Resolution.*

If the earlier test on the scan-field completeness showed a sudden ''shrink'' in
line width, that is not a good place to test lateral resolution. Move off center, then,
to make the measurement. An example of a lateral resolution image is shown in
Figure 12-7.

The half maximum beam width (HMBW) calculation can provide a measure of
the expected beam width that can be compared with the measured value. This
equation appears as:

$$HMBW = 1.22 \lambda \ F/D \qquad (12.1)$$

Where λ is the wavelength in millimeters, F is the focal point range in millimeters,
and D is the transducer diameter in millimeters.

Focal-Point Position

While scanning for lateral resolution, identify the range of the narrowest beam
width. A continuous source of echoes in the beam shows the exact position of the
focal point. If the pins, on the other hand, are 2 cm apart, the focal-point position
is approximate, but is still valuable.

Record the range of the narrowest pin, or the range of the narrowest portion of
the beam, under the heading *Focal Point Position.* The narrowest line is quite
evident in Figure 12-7.

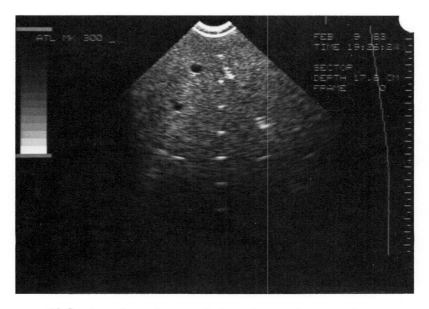

12-8 Scanning a tissue-equivalent phantom for textural portrayal. The texture of the phantom should change with increasing range from the transducer. The texture close to the transducer should include small echo signals that vanish with increasing depth. The major transition for this sonograph is about 3 cm into the phantom.

Solid-Texture Portrayal

Set the TGC for a uniform intensity portrayal of the phantom scattering signals. Echo sources that produce the textural information are small carbon particles distributed in a random but uniform manner. These scattering bodies should yield a combination of echo signals originating from both the primary scattering process and a secondary, phased-dependent speckle. The resulting texture should consist of a set of large and small echo signals that span a narrow range of gray levels but that are still distinguishable from one another. If the sonograph has difficulty portraying speckle and scattering information, the image dots from the phantom will run together and contour, forming large regions of continuous echo signals that have the same gray intensity. A good textural image is illustrated in Figure 12-8.

Set the TGC controls to a setting typical for a smooth-appearing image and examine the image texture for a uniform portrayal of gray levels. This interrogation of the image can employ either the system-reject control or, if possible, manual postprocessing in the sonograph (see Chapter 14 for a postprocessing protocol).

Look for a uniform texture portrayal over the region of compensation, extending from the TGC initial point to the TGC knee. If possible, make a photograph of the image. This photograph will be used as a reference to compare existing machine conditions with past photographs or for future evaluations. Store the image and write any observations under the heading *Gray-Scale Texture*.

Motion Portrayal

With the TGC set for a normal image, slide the scan head slowly over the phantom window. Examine the image at the edges of the scanning field. Look both for evidence of "paradoxical motion" (inappropriate motion) within the scan field as the scattering echo-signals move within the image, as well as for missing or rapidly changing texture within the field. If the scan converter and the scanning field are functioning properly, the movement of scattering bodies into, out of, and through the image should be uniform and clearly shown as lateral movement only.

Contrast Sensitivity

Along with providing the ability to test spatial accuracy, the cysts offer an opportunity to test the contrast sensitivity of the sonograph in two areas. The first area deals with the ability to portray echo-free structures as echo free; the second area is the ability to show small differences in echo-signal levels as different gray-scale intensities. These characteristics are shown in Figure 12-4.

Continue to scan the tissue-equivalent phantom with the same normal TGC settings. Slowly scan the cysts and examine the anterior, middle, and posterior cysts for an echo-free portrayal of the cyst interior. Cysts that appear echogenic in the phantom indicate that the sonograph will have trouble portraying simple cysts in real scanning situations. Note which cysts are filled or appear complex in the image.

The cysts should have a low attenuation rate—a difference in attenuation that produces enhancement behind the cysts. This enhancement should be evident in the anterior, middle, and posterior segments of the image. Record under *Contrast Sensitivity,* any failure to portray the enhancement behind any of the cysts.

Some phantoms have "solids" that carry higher-than-normal attenuation rates. These structures will produce shadowing within the image. Any shadowing should be easily seen behind these structures. Shadowing, however, is more dramatic with small changes in attenuation. Examine the image for both shadowing enhancement; each should be visible if the system is functioning properly.

Dot Formation

The dots that form the image texture are created by an interaction among the ultrasound beam, signal processing in the sonograph, and the phased-dependent processes of small scattering bodies. The dots, on the other hand, collectively contribute to the image texture. Here, however, we are interested in how the dots are formed. The dots produced by the phantom-machine interaction should create a wide range of dot sizes, some large, others small, but no free-standing dot should exceed three wavelengths in axial distance. Dots that exceed three wavelengths usually indicate difficulties in internal sonograph signal processing. Failure to portray the dot formation and texture of the tissue-equivalent phantom indicates

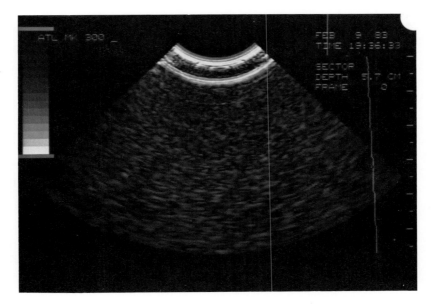

12-9   Scanning a tissue-equivalent phantom for dot formation. Poor dot formation from this 3-MHz transducer can lead to large, blobby dots that hide textural information; it can come from poor signal processing in the sonograph or from gray-scale contouring in the display. These dots show some contouring from a limited gray scale (16 gray levels), but present a good signal mix and variations in size and intensity.

an inability to portray textural differences between normal and abnormal tissue. An image showing dot signal mix appears in Figure 12-9.

Scan the phantom slowly and interrogate the image for evidence of dot formation that would prevent normal dot portrayal. This evidence includes such things as dots that are pulled axially on large amplitudes and contouring that places all the dots on the same intensity step, forcing them to run together in the image. Contouring within the phantom image will almost guarantee the same process in imaging tissues.

If the real-time scanhead has more than one frequency, or if scanheads with different frequencies are available, then an increase in frequency should change the character of the dot formation and overall texture. An example of a high-frequency transducer image is featured in Figure 12-10. A higher frequency usually means a greater scattering interaction and larger amounts of scattering energy returned to the transducer. This produces a change in the phantom echogenicity, increasing as the frequency cubed. Groups of scattering bodies that were previously medium-level signals may now become higher-level signals, and the normal smooth distribution of dots may be highlighted with more specular-appearing dots. This is a normal and expected change in the portrayal of the phantom as the result of an increase in frequency.

Record under the heading *Dot Formation* all observations of the dots as a function of frequency, and provide a photograph for future reference and comparison.

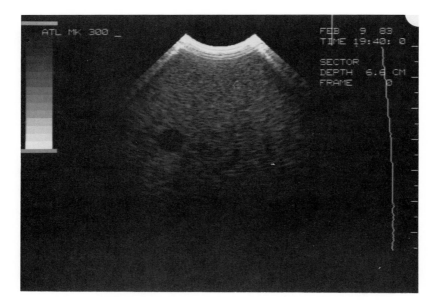

12-10   Changing the image texture of a phantom with a high-frequency transducer. This 7.5-MHz transducer forms a much-more-uniform and finer texture than the 3-MHz transducer in Figure 12-9. Examining texture can show if a high-frequency transducer is making a texture like a lower-frequency transducer, defeating any benefits from moving to a higher frequency.

TGC Response

Many current real-time sonographs do not utilize a calibrated TGC system. Moreover, TGC circuits are often not examined during routine service calls. A tissue-equivalent phantom provides an opportunity to test the ability to handle a uniform attenuation rate with a uniform scattering process, using the sonograph TGC curve.

Set the time-gain compensation for a uniform image. Examine the A-mode display and the image for any regions with lower or higher intensities than the surrounding material. This interrogation applies only over the ramp portion of the TGC. Variations in intensity greater than 3 dB are visible in the phantom image. We can make these variations more visible by using either the system reject or any resident postprocessing controls to enhance or visually separate the regions of nonlinearity (see Chapter 14 for a postprocessing protocol). Large variations in TGC response that cause either high- or low-intensity areas will affect the image under normal scanning conditions. This problem will require repair, calibration, and resetup by the field representative. A uniform sector image is shown in Figure 12-8.

When making this test, users should be aware of transducer focusing, which can increase signals within the region of compensation. Unless the sonograph has beam-profile compensation, this is an acceptable intensity change.

Record any variations in intensity, the range of the intensity variations, and the direction of the intensity changes (that is, too high or too low) under the heading *TGC Response*.

Preprocessing Response

Preprocessing establishes the relationship between the analog signals and the numbers stored in the scan converter memory. This assignment can change significantly the qualities of an image and affect such parameters as dot size, penetration, and the ability to perceive enhancement or shadowing in the phantom. The goal in this test is to determine whether or not the preprocessing curves have changed, and whether or not they are still carrying out each primary function.

Scan the phantom with the TGC and preprocessing set in normal positions. These are the same settings used for most of the previous measurements and comparisons on the phantom. Note the character of the texture formation. Note also dot size and apparent penetration into the phantom. An example of image changes with preprocessing appears in Figure 12-11.

Now change the preprocessing switch to a new curve and examine the image again for changes such as: 1) dissapearing enhancement or a more contrasting portrayal of enhancement; 2) larger or smaller dots, or an increase or decrease in the number of dots in the texture; and 3) changes in penetration. For a permanent record, make a photograph of the result, with a separate photograph for each preprocessing curve.

If this is a starting set of tests, then the photographs will represent a reference for comparing future photographs. If this is a routine test, compare the photographs from this test with the originals for any overt changes in the preprocessing response.

Changes in the image due to preprocessing assignments can be predicted based on the characteristics of the preprocessing curve. For example, a curve with a sigmoid shape will provide a wider range of response in the center signals than at the upper or lower end of the signal range (see Chapter 15). Knowing the shape and characteristics of the preprocessing curves can help determine what to expect for small-and medium-signal portrayal, as well as any recasting of small and medium signals onto new gray-scale steps.

Report any changes in the preprocessing curves under the heading *Preprocessing Response*.

Postprocessing Response

Not all real-time sonographs have variable or alternative postprocessing curves. If the sonograph does have variable postprocessing, the postprocessing responses can be tested by using the tissue-equivalent phantom.

Set the TGC preprocessing and the postprocessing into normal or typical settings for examinations. Examine the image for the character of the texture, texture formation, dot size, and dot distribution.

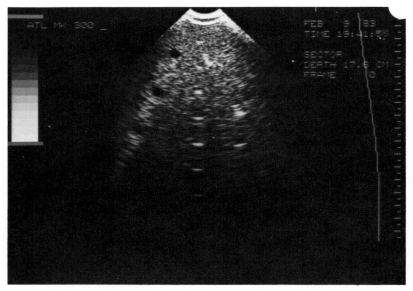

12-11A

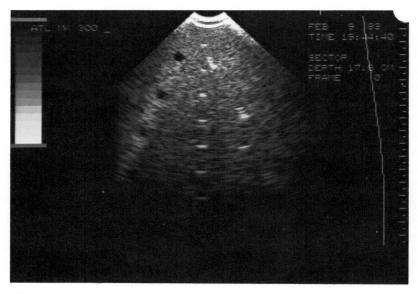

12-11B

12-11   Changing phantom gray-scale image with preprocessing. Preprocessing changes the assignment of the video signal to scan-converter values. Part A: This processing curve widens the visual separation between large and small signals. Part B: This processing curve compresses most of the smaller signals onto similar gray-scale steps, forming contours in this image.

Change to a new postprocessing curve and examine the image for the following: 1) disappearing enhancement or increased contrast in the portrayal of enhancement; 2) changes in the dots that form the texture, in which the dots either increase or decrease in size or increase or decrease in number (the dots may alter intensity considerably); and 3) changes in apparent penetration.

Proceed through each of the postprocessing curves and note or photograph the result of each curve. The goal is to determine whether or not the postprocessing curves are functioning properly. Often this can be carried out with some understanding of what the postprocessing curves are doing to the signal-to-gray-scale assignments. Because the characteristics of the postprocessing curves subtly modify the image, the best record of these tests is to photograph the image and retain the photograph for future comparisons. Record any observations and photographs under the heading *Postprocessing Response*.

Conclusions

The tissue-equivalent phantom is an effective means of looking at the real-time sonograph, owing to the common visual end points for the static B-scanner and the real-time sonograph. Still in need of further exploration, however, is the ability of the real-time sonograph to portray motion accurately. Although we can partially test motion depiction with this protocol, high velocities and high frame rates have not been tested.

The 14 tests outlined in this chapter involve measurements, observations, and comparisons that together provide a broad evaluation of the real-time machine function. Many ultrasound departments still have not initiated such tests. However, given the importance of regularly monitoring real-time systems in the interval between routine service visits, these tests offer an easy, quick means of implementing a weekly quality assurance program. With these tests, a user need not wait for the service representative to appear. The phantom and its protocols can be employed at any time to assure real-time function.

As sonographs improve in design, they will have better-defined end points for imaging. Such improvements will require more sophisticated tests, using a phantom or an active electronic phantom that may be part of the machine.

Along with the phantom, a valuable tool to the service representative is an equipment history record generated by consistent testing and recording the responses of the sonograph. To help assure the reliability of information, the preparation of an equipment history should be closely allied with the test protocal design, and the tests should be as easy and natural as possible. The order of testing should also be logical. For example, measurement processes should not be last in a protocol, but should appear early in order to establish measurement accuracy for later images.

A phantom and a protocol can go far toward helping insure that an ultrasound department's real-time sonograph is working properly, thus permitting a diagnostic confidence not otherwise possible. Nevertheless, a call to a service engineer is sometimes deemed necessary. Before requesting a service visit, however, the user should endeavor to be certain of any test results. In this connection, at least two questions should be asked: Can the test results be attributed to a practice that is peculiar to the sonographer testing the machine or to a particular control being set improperly? If these questions can be answered in the negative, then the next question is: Could the problem cause a diagnostic error? If so, then the service call is right and proper. It is the sonographer's responsibility to carry out the protocols carefully and consistently in order to answer the above questions as accurately as possible.

Another trap we can fall into is that of asking more of the sonograph than it can deliver. This presents another reason why it is important to know the sonograph's design specifications and how they translate into phantom images. By answering the above questions accurately and living within machine specifications, we can limit service calls to only those that are essential, thus lowering maintenance costs while still assuring proper machine operation.

Chapter 13

TGC and the Sonographer: Building Informative Images

Through the years, sonographers have been offered all sorts of protocols for setting time-gain compensation, or TGC. Some have used calculations based on the attenuation rate; others have used the displayed anatomy as an indicator. As might be expected, the results have also been highly variable, and the literature abounds with images showing equivocal information because of a TGC setting that does not match the tissue. Too often, this maladjustment seems to be the result of users not knowing the events in ultrasound well enough to formulate a successful TGC set up protocol.

This chapter, then, seeks to build a rational model for time-gain compensation that predicts events and explains observations. It does more, however, than simply outline a TGC protocol. It describes the principles that show how and why a good TGC protocol works, in the hope that readers will gain an understanding not only of the imaging needs for TGC setup but of the design needs for any sonograph. Let us begin at the heart of the problem.

Tissue Attenuation and TGC

As ultrasound travels through the tissues, the tissues remove energy at a fairly steady rate. This attenuation is applied to both the transmitted wave and the reflected wave. The identified mechanisms of this energy loss appear to be largely energy absorption, which converts the ultrasonic energy into heat, and wave scattering, which spreads wave energy away from the main path of travel through the tissues. (These two processes and effects were discussed in detail in Chapter 9.)

The method of expressing this attenuation in relative signal strength is the decibel unit, or dB per unit distance. For example, a reduction in signal strength of 30 dB over a distance of 10 cm produces an attenuation rate of 3 dB/cm. The attenuation rate is also a function of the ultrasound frequency, with attenuation rate increasing directly with frequency. By expressing attenuation in units of dB/cm, the attenuation rate becomes almost a linear function of frequency, expressed as dB/cm/MHz. For most soft tissues in the body, the frequency-dependent attenuation rate is about 1 dB/cm/MHz, measured *one way* through the tissue. Taking this frequency dependence into account means an attenuation rate of 3 dB/cm for a 3-MHz ultrasound wave.

An examination of the compiled information on mammalian soft tissue shows just how much an approximation 1 dB/cm/MHz turns out to be. In addition, many tissues change attenuation rate at a frequency greater than the power of one [1, 2]. Still, a simple attenuation rate tells a great deal about how to set the TGC.

Despite its link with tissue attenuation, the application of time-gain compensation is an electronic function within the sonograph and affects nothing physically in the tissues. For example, adjusting TGC will not change the output of the transducer or the reflectivity of the interfaces within the tissue. It will, on the other hand, change the way the echo signals are portrayed within the sonograph, which in turn changes image content and quality dramatically.

Limits on the overall signal range available for any TGC circuit are set by the amount of power coming out of the transducer and the dynamic range of the transmit-receive (TR) switch (see Chapter 2.) As the power generated by the transducer increases, the largest echo signals close to the transducer soon reach the highest amplitude that can go through the TR switch unclipped. This power setting fixes the upper limit on echo signals presented to the receiver for processing at any tissue depth. From the largest, the signals fall off in a manner shown in Figure 13-1. Decreasing the transmitter power moves this signal line downward, simultaneously reducing the largest anterior signal and the effective penetration. This relationship between effective penetration and transducer power is used later in setting the sonograph output power for specific imaging goals.

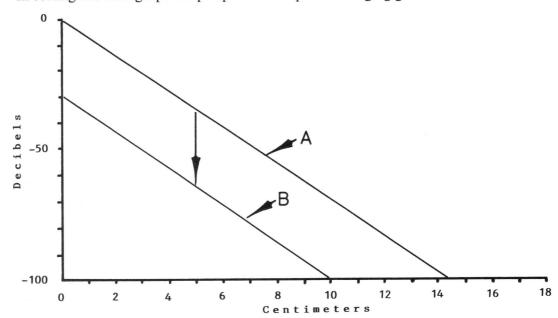

13-1   Echo-signal amplitude as a function of distance. Because the attenuation rate in tissue is not a function of echo strength, a reflector 30 dB below a maximum reflector *B* will lose signal strength at the same rate as the maximum echo *A*. Echo signals below the − 100-dB line will not pass the transmit-receive switch. Y-axis is echo-signal amplitude in decibels; X-axis is distance in centimeters.

Below the maximum signal line are all the smaller biological and interference signals, extending nearly 50 dB below the maximum echo signals from specular reflectors [1]. As the output power decreases, so do the signals from these smaller reflectors, limiting both effective penetration and the range of useful signals available for display. Thus, we are dealing with two dynamic ranges: first, the range of signals from all sources that can pass through the sonograph TR switch, which we will call the *input dynamic range;* and, second, the range of signals produced by the different reflectivities and interference processes within the tissues, which we will call *tissue signal dynamic range*. The input dynamic range extends over the largest to the smallest echo signal at the input to the rf amplifier (see Chapter 2). This range of signals is defined by the level of transmitting power to the transducer and the acceptance range of the transmit-receive switch. The tissue signal dynamic range is a component of the input dynamic range, and can vary by as much as 50 dB (Chapter 9).

The goals in setting TGC are two-fold: first, to make all of the like echo sources within the image look alike, so that the differences among echo-sources may be appreciated; and second, to portray this information over the largest amount of tissue possible. In other words, we would like to obtain the greatest possible *effective* penetration. The method of reaching these goals seems clear—we simply set the gain of the sonograph to follow the rate of attenuation over depth (Figure 13-2). However, the concept is deceptively simple.

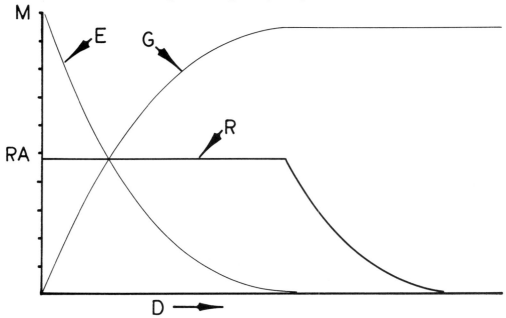

13-2   Classic model for time-gain compensation. In the classic model for TGC, echo signals from like reflectors *E* fall off with distance exponentially. The sonograph should portray like reflectors alike. The solution is to apply a gain that changes similarly to the attenuation rate *G,* producing the resulting curve *R*. Beyond the region of changing gain, the signals again fall off exponentially. *RA* is relative amplitude; *M* is maximum signal level; *D* is distance into the tissue.

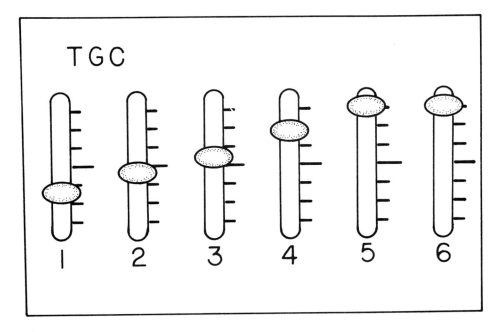

A

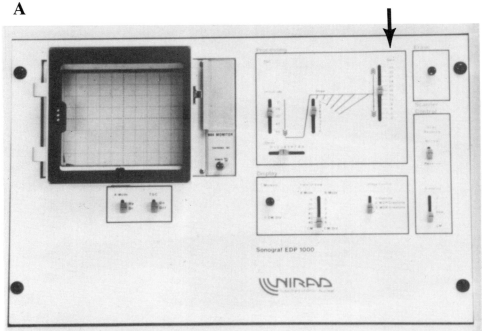

B

13-3   Two basic methods of setting up time gain compensation controls. A) The segmented TGC control breaks the field of view into segments with a single control setting the gain for each segment. B) The TGC parameter controls (in the box marked processing) set components of the TGC curve such as initial gain, delay, and slope. Courtesy of Technicare Ultrasound Corporation, Englewood, Colorado.

Depending on machine design, TGC is known by several other names, including swept gain and depth-gain compensation (DGC), as well as TCG, or time compensated gain. Although any of these names is appropriate, the controls among different machine designs tend to vary and can be classified according to the type of manipulation used to set the TGC curve. The first type of controls is a set of rotating or linear controls that specify TGC initial, slope, and delay in a smooth manner, controlling each variable of the TGC curve. The second type is a segmented control that divides the displayed depth into segments, each with its own gain control. The various TGC curve parameters are formed by changing the gain in each segment. Examples of both controls are shown in Figure 13-3.

Whether segmented or nonsegmented, the TGC controls are used to manipulate the same things, namely: the initial gain; the ramp; the knee; and the delay. Each of these components is explained below.

The initial gain sets the starting point for the TGC ramp, and also the start of the compensating region of the TGC curve. The ramp shows the rate of gain change from the initial gain to the final gain. The initial gain represents the start of compensation and the knee represents the end of compensation at the maximum gain in the sonograph. In some sonographs, the TGC curve is further modified with posterior TGC controls to handle the problem of depicting the posterior left ventricular wall in echocardiography. This wall has a wide range of signals extending from small endocardial signals to large pericardial-lung interface signals, all of which are close together and need visual separation and separate gains.

The TGC delay permits the ramp to begin later, placing the start of compensation deeper into the tissue. In the delay portion of the TGC curve, the gain is constant, set to a value by the initial gain control.

To this point, the problem and its apparent solution seem clear. But appearances are deceiving. To understand the gap between the model as so far described and the real events, we will first examine a simple, single-frequency model of the TGC adjustment and then expand that model to include a more complete transducer response and an expanded description of events.

A Single-Frequency Model

Our single-frequency model is a 5-MHz transducer. And in accordance with general sonograph design, we will consider the output of the transducer set so that the largest anterior signals just reach the upper edge of the TR switch dynamic range. In addition, the smallest biological signals are 40 dB below these larger signals. These basic conditions are shown in Figure 13-4. The attenuation rate is 1 dB/cm/MHz × 5 MHz, or 5 dB/cm. Because the attenuation is a one way value, the ultrasound loses 5 dB/cm on the way out and 5 dB/cm on the return trip. The total attenuation is the sum of the two, or 10 dB/cm for the round trip. This pattern of attenuation was detailed in Chapter 9.

The TR switch dynamic range is 100 dB, which means that the largest of the 5-MHz signals go to zero at 10 cm (see Figure 13-4). On the other hand, the smaller

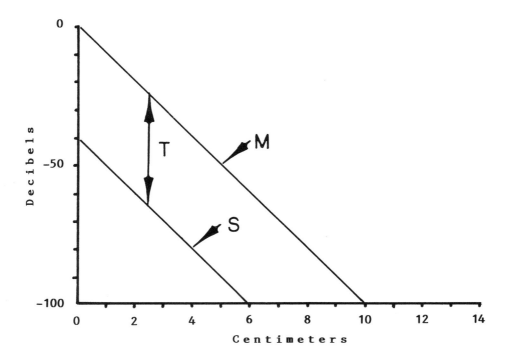

13-4   The dynamic range of tissue reflectors. The range of tissue reflectances is over 40 dB, which means that tissue echo signals will vary at least 40 dB *(T)* among themselves, regardless of tissue attenuation. The maximum echo signals in a 5-MHz ultrasound field will decrease with distance following *M,* while the smallest will follow *S.* Between 6 cm and 10 cm, the echo-signal dynamic range shrinks to zero, and will form a region of changing texture on a gray-scale display. Y-axis is signal strength in decibels; X-axis is distance in centimeters.

signals begin to vanish much sooner. For example, the smallest biological signals (40 dB below the largest) vanish at 6 cm. Thus, an increasing portion of the smaller signals will not be seen beyond 6 cm, and such signals cannot be recovered by increasing the system gain. They simply never made it past the TR switch into the machine.

The imaging task is to recover from the input signals the 40-dB variation among signals that represents tissue variations, and recover these signals as deeply as possible in the tissues. Moreover, the compensated region of tissue should show like echo signals with like intensities on the display. The smallest biological signals just above the signal floor will receive the highest gain; the medium signals will receive a medium gain. This means that the large anterior signals will receive the lowest gain. The result is that all the unlike echo-signals from like echo-sources will look alike at the display. The first requirement, then, is to reduce the anterior signals so that the largest is 40 dB above the signal floor, thus showing the 40-dB differences among echo signals as deeply as possible. By matching the rate of gain in the TGC curve to the rate of echo-signal amplitude decrease, like echo signals will turn out to have the same amplitude. This relationship is shown in Figure 13-5.

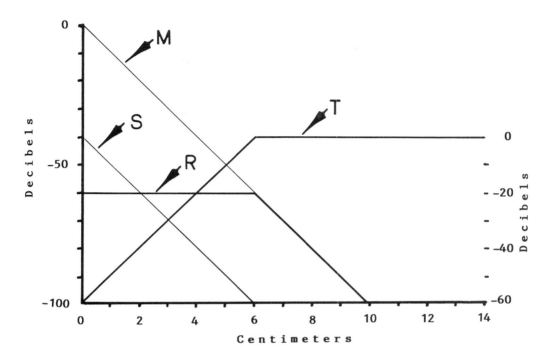

13-5 An ideal application of TGC. The goal in applying TGC is to include the largest amount of tissue-signal variation over the greatest depth. In this example of 5-MHz ultrasound, the smallest reflectance *S* is 40 dB below the greatest *M*. By setting the TGC initial gain 60 dB below the maximum gain, the maximum signals are portrayed with like amplitude *R*, until compensation ends at 6 cm. The resultant *(R)* is 40 dB above the zero signal level, including the whole tissue reflectance dynamic range. Relative signal strength is on the left Y-axis; receiver gain in dB is on the right Y-axis; X-axis is distance in centimeters.

A closer look at Figure 13-5 yields some interesting facts. First, the location of the knee (6.0 cm) and initial-gain setting (−60 dB) hardly look like those of a typical, real TGC setting for a 5-MHz transducer. (For example, a 5-MHz, medium-focus transducer will have a 40-dB initial gain and a knee close to 10 cm on a Technicare EDP 1000.) Second, despite the single-frequency concept, the falloff of signal amplitudes within this model looks like the events we considered earlier in the classic TGC problem (Figure 13-2). Thus, signals of like amplitude appear alike in the ramp portion of the TGC, and then decrease at a standard rate beyond the knee.

Clearly, the knee represents more than just the end of the compensation region; it represents the largest gain applied to the arriving echo signals. Echo-signals, then, can appear below but never above the top echo-signal line. Thus, setting the TGC to reach a maximum gain where the *weakest* reflector's signals vanish ensures meeting our two imaging objectives: first, to have like echo signals look alike over the region of compensation; and second, to have the region of compensation include the 40 dB of biological signals over the largest range possible. The initial gain is 60 dB below the maximum gain in order to match positioning the weakest

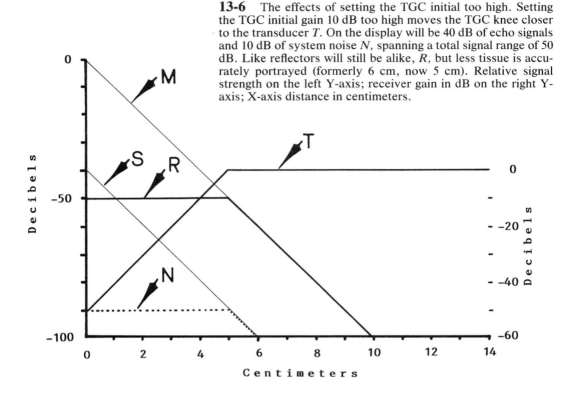

13-6   The effects of setting the TGC initial too high. Setting the TGC initial gain 10 dB too high moves the TGC knee closer to the transducer T. On the display will be 40 dB of echo signals and 10 dB of system noise N, spanning a total signal range of 50 dB. Like reflectors will still be alike, R, but less tissue is accurately portrayed (formerly 6 cm, now 5 cm). Relative signal strength on the left Y-axis; receiver gain in dB on the right Y-axis; X-axis distance in centimeters.

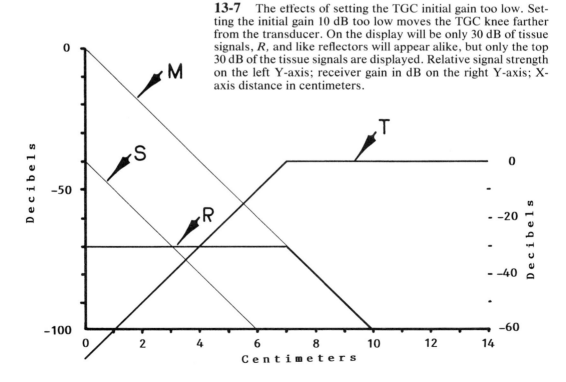

13-7   The effects of setting the TGC initial gain too low. Setting the initial gain 10 dB too low moves the TGC knee farther from the transducer. On the display will be only 30 dB of tissue signals, R, and like reflectors will appear alike, but only the top 30 dB of the tissue signals are displayed. Relative signal strength on the left Y-axis; receiver gain in dB on the right Y-axis; X-axis distance in centimeters.

reflector echo signals just above the signal floor. The initial value is the difference between the input dynamic range (DR) and the biological signals dynamic range (dr), or: DR − dr. To test whether or not this is the best TGC setting, let us see what happens when the TGC curve is changed.

First, set the initial gain at 50 dB below maximum rather than 60 dB below maximum, and keep the same TGC slope (Figure 13-6). The 40 dB of biological echo signals are well above the smallest displayable signals (10 dB above, in fact) and over the region of compensation, they have the same amplitude. But the compensation extends over a depth less than the first setting (Figure 13-5). Therefore, we have met only one of the two TGC criteria because the region of compensation is less than the best possible.

If the initial gain is now set to 70 dB below maximum gain, keeping the same slope, the region of compensation now extends over a much greater depth (Figure 13-7). At the same time, however, the displayed dynamic range among biological signals is now 30 dB rather than 40 dB. In this case, the region of compensation is greater than the original setting, but we have failed to keep the first criterion of depicting the 40 dB of biological signals.

Clearly, to obtain the best compensation curve, TGC must be set for the smallest signals we hope to depict. With these principles established, we next examine a more complex model that begins to include more of the machine and transducer qualities.

The Multiple-Frequency Model

Chapter 3 stated that highly damped transducers produce a wide range of ultrasound frequencies extending above and below the center operating frequency. For example, a 5-MHz transducer with a 50% passband at 6 dB below the center operating frequency amplitude will have a significant amount of energy at both 3.75 MHz and 6.25 MHz. Figure 13-8 shows how these frequency components fall off as a function of distance. The 6.25-MHz energy will contribute to the textural information close to the transducer. The 3.75-MHz energy, however, penetrates deeply into the tissue, providing significant energy beyond the vanishing depth for the 5-MHz energy. It is this low-frequency energy that extends the effective penetration of a highly damped transducer.

If we also begin to consider that the dynamic range of the biological signals extends some 40 dB below the maximum, then the character of the TGC setting begins to change. These additional signals are shown in Figure 13-9. With a 100-dB input dynamic range and a 50% band width on the transducer, the smallest biological signals from the 3.75-MHz energy vanish at the same range as the largest 5-MHz signals. Thus, if we hope to set the TGC for a uniform intensity of signals over the region of compensation, it cannot follow the 5-MHz rate; it must follow the 3.75-MHz attenuation rate.

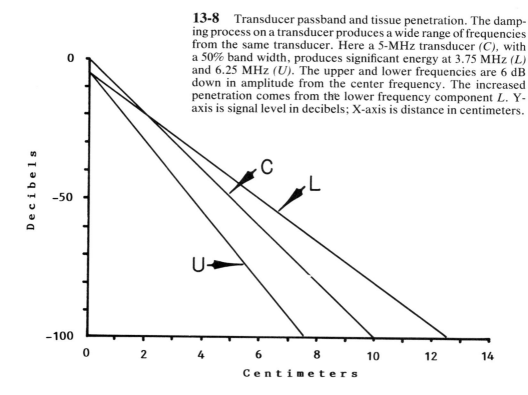

13-8   Transducer passband and tissue penetration. The damping process on a transducer produces a wide range of frequencies from the same transducer. Here a 5-MHz transducer *(C)*, with a 50% band width, produces significant energy at 3.75 MHz *(L)* and 6.25 MHz *(U)*. The upper and lower frequencies are 6 dB down in amplitude from the center frequency. The increased penetration comes from the lower frequency component *L*. Y-axis is signal level in decibels; X-axis is distance in centimeters.

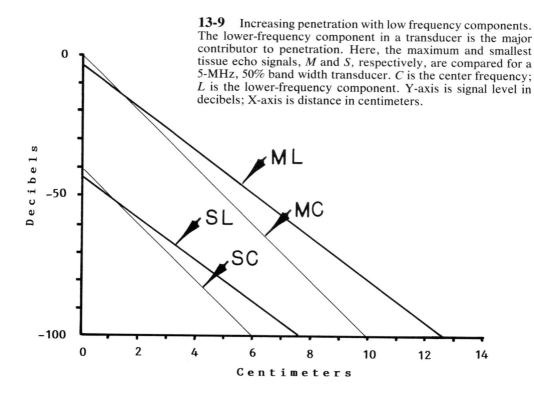

13-9   Increasing penetration with low frequency components. The lower-frequency component in a transducer is the major contributor to penetration. Here, the maximum and smallest tissue echo signals, *M* and *S*, respectively, are compared for a 5-MHz, 50% band width transducer. *C* is the center frequency; *L* is the lower-frequency component. Y-axis is signal level in decibels; X-axis is distance in centimeters.

It is the wide passband of the highly damped transducer that helps explain why a one-way tissue attenuation rate of 1 dB/cm/MHz nearly works in two-way calculations. In fact, as the TGC is adjusted for a uniform image intensity, all of the frequency components below the center operating frequency are included in the compensation. These lower-frequency components make the final attenuation rate represented by the TGC ramp look different from a slope calculated on the center operating frequency alone. It is, in fact, the failure to include these low-frequency components that makes TGC calculated settings using a simple attenuation model and the real TGC settings so different from one another.

Other factors also affect the beam intensity profile and, thereby, the TGC setting. One of these is transducer focusing.

Transducer Focusing and TGC

As pointed out in Chapter 3, transducer focusing produces an uneven beam intensity as the ultrasound beam narrows to the focal point and expands beyond it. Because of this geometry, the intensity of the beam increases into the focal zone and decreases at distances beyond the focal zone. Although this process can disrupt the uniformity of the beam intensity, it usually does not significantly increase the effective penetration at any given frequency, as shown in Figure 13-10. In large diameter, short-focus transducers, focusing may even decrease the effective penetration and the TGC settings.

The gain produced by any transducer focusing is a function of each frequency component. For example, an expected gain of about 17 dB results from focusing a 13-mm diameter, 5-MHz transducer at 6 cm. At the same time, a 3.75-MHz wave component in the transducer beam would have a gain of only 11 dB. This reduced gain is a consequence of the poorer focusing at lower frequencies, as predicted by the HMBW equation (equation 3.3).

In the image, the question of a proper TGC setting is answered by examining the gray-scale intensity of like reflectors in the image. Thus, the TGC will be set to include not only variations due to the transducer frequency mix, but also the variations in intensity due to the inability of the transducer to focus all the frequencies the same amount at the same range.

Having outlined the major variables in the TGC problem, we will next integrate them into a coherent picture of events surrounding TGC setup.

A Coherent TGC Model

The Initial Gain Value

The first task in setting the TGC on the sonograph is to determine the initial gain value. The goal is to place the full dynamic range of the tissue signals on the display, starting right at the skin line. As we learned earlier, an initial gain set too

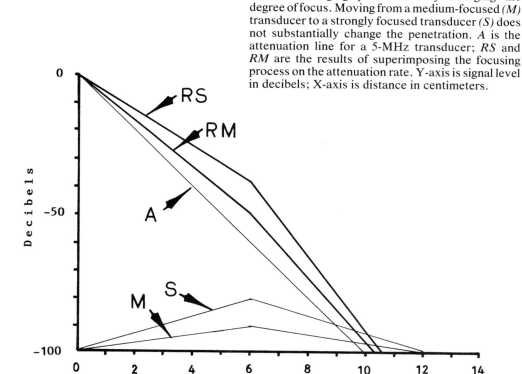

13-10   Changing penetration by changing the degree of focus. Moving from a medium-focused *(M)* transducer to a strongly focused transducer *(S)* does not substantially change the penetration. *A* is the attenuation line for a 5-MHz transducer; *RS* and *RM* are the results of superimposing the focusing process on the attenuation rate. Y-axis is signal level in decibels; X-axis is distance in centimeters.

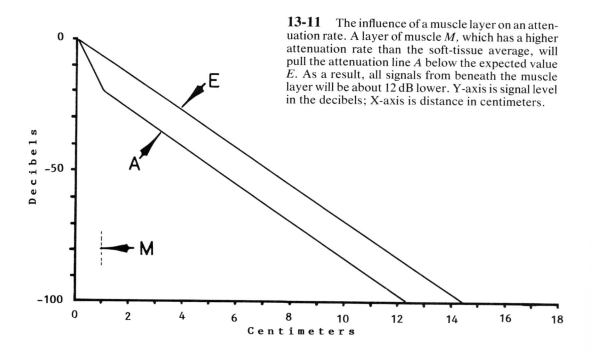

13-11   The influence of a muscle layer on an attenuation rate. A layer of muscle *M,* which has a higher attenuation rate than the soft-tissue average, will pull the attenuation line *A* below the expected value *E.* As a result, all signals from beneath the muscle layer will be about 12 dB lower. Y-axis is signal level in the decibels; X-axis is distance in centimeters.

high will have a limited range of compensation, and an initial gain set too low will remove the smaller signals from the image.

In the conditions shown in Figure 13-5, the initial gain value for the 5-MHz transducer was -60 dB. This value was arrived at by working backward from the TGC knee to the initial gain value, following the attenuation of the signals. The result was an initial gain value representing the difference between the input dynamic range, DR, and the tissue signal dynamic range, dr. Thus, as we might expect, if the input signal dynamic range is decreased because of a low transmitting power, the initial gain value is not as far below the final gain value. But the input signal dynamic range can be modified dramatically by the architecture of the tissue. For example, placing a highly attenuating tissue up front greatly modifies the echo-signal levels from deeper tissues. In the abdomen, this attenuating tissue is the abdominal muscle, with an attenuation rate close to 3 dB/cm/MHz across the fibers. The change in the attenuation profile is shown in Figure 13-11.

Setting the initial gain value, then, becomes a problem of identifying events at the beginning of the image, in the first centimeter or so of tissue. We would like to get the highest echo signals possible for the deeper tissues. Often this means saturating some of the skin signals in order to start the internal tissue signals at a higher value. And the saturation occurs at the TR switch, controlled by the transmitter power. If we have a system with a fixed power and variable system gain, then setting the initial is rather routine, as in -38 dB for the EDP 1000. But changing the system response with a transmitting power change requires determining the proper power setting.

An ideal transmitter power setting would place the largest early echo signals just under saturation at the TR switch. We might produce this setting by viewing the echo signals on an A-mode display, with an initial gain setting of -60 dB. The early tissue signals will be much-less-than maximum in the sonograph and will not saturate at the video level. Increasing the transmitter power will bring up the anterior echo signals until they saturate on the TR switch. On an A-mode display, they would flatten on the top. On a B-mode display, they would not increase in intensity any further with increasing power, but would become axially wider with increasing power. Once saturation is found, we back off the power to just *under* saturation. Now the initial gain value can be set to write the largest tissue echo signals to the most intense gray level. In practice, this will provide initial gain values in the -30 dB to -50 dB range, depending upon anterior tissue reflectivities. Higher values such as -60 dB seldom happen because of the layer of attenuating muscle on the abdomen.

With an initial gain value set, we can now look at knee position.

Locating the TGC Knee

To get the full dynamic range of the tissue signals to the display, TGC is set for the smallest echo signals, giving them the highest system gain. Once an initial setting is achieved, the next task is to determine a starting position for the TGC knee, based on the combined parameters within the transducer and the sonograph. The events are examined easiest through an equation.

The knee position will be a function of the input signal dynamic range at the TR switch, the dynamic range of the biological signals we wish to image, the center operating frequency of the transducer, and the frequency response band width of the transducer at 6 dB (amplitude) below maximum. If these parameters are known, they can be entered into a single equation that will indicate the TGC knee position. The equation appears as:

$$KP = DR - (6 + dr)/AFc(2 - BW), \tag{13.1}$$

where KP is the knee position in cm, *DR* is the input signal dynamic range in dB, *dr* is the sonograph signal-processing dynamic range for display (for example, 30 dB or 40 dB), the 6 comes from the 6 dB-down amplitude, Fc is the transducer center operating frequency in MHz, *BW* is the transducer 6-dB band width expressed as a decimal fraction (i.e. a 50% band width is 0.5) of the center operating frequency, and *A* is the attenuation rate in dB/cm/MHz.

Equation 13.1 is derived from a simple geometric consideration of the signal decrease due to a regular attenuation rate, but at the lowest significant frequency from the transducer. By inserting in different values for the parameters, we can see how the TGC curve changes with different conditions.

An examination of equation 13.1 shows some of the observed relationships among machine parameters. For example, if the transmitting power decreases, the signal dynamic range (DR) decreases, and the TGC knee position comes closer to the transducer. The same thing happens if the transducer frequency increases. The transducer 6-dB band width will influence the TGC knee position as well. For example, should the band width decrease, less energy appears in the lower frequencies and the knee moves closer to the transducer. Although this equation does not include all of the factors that can influence TGC setup, it does include enough of the major elements to permit an excellent estimate of the knee position.

The attenuation rate is included in the equation. Thus, tissue attenuation can be varied to look for changes in knee position and, thereby, changes in the TGC slope. On the other hand, we could work backward through equation 13.1 from the TGC slope to the tissue attenuation rate.

If we have some idea of the initial gain value, equation 13.1 can be modified to include this value, thus enabling a prediction of the knee position from that value. Earlier we noted that the initial gain value was DR − dr. Replacing that difference with Ip to indicate the initial point, equation 13.1 becomes:

$$KP = Ip - 6/AFc(2 - BW) \tag{13.2}$$

In equation 13.1, knee position changes with the transducer band width. The degree of change is shown in Figure 13-12, where the knee point and band width are compared. In addition, the knee point changes with the input signal dynamic range, as shown in Figure 13-13. Changes in knee position with varying attenuation rate are illustrated in Figure 13-14.

The resulting TGC now represents not the final TGC curve, but the *starting TGC curve*. If the patient is close to the expected normal values, then little if any additional adjustment is needed to finish the TGC setup. If the patient's reflectivity deviates from normal, then the initial value may have to be changed up or down to place the biological signals' dynamic range within the display dynamic range.

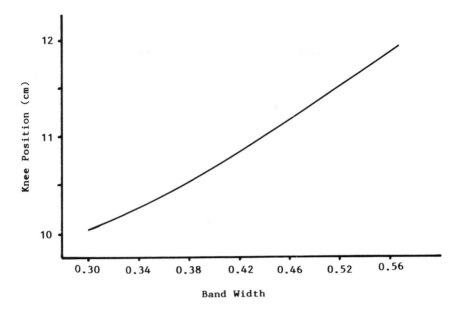

13-12   The change in TGC knee position as a function of transducer band width. As a transducer band width increases, the lower-frequency component gets progressively lower in frequency, increasing effective penetration and increasing the TGC knee position. Calculations are for a 5-MHz transducer and an attenuation rate of 1 dB/cm/MHz.

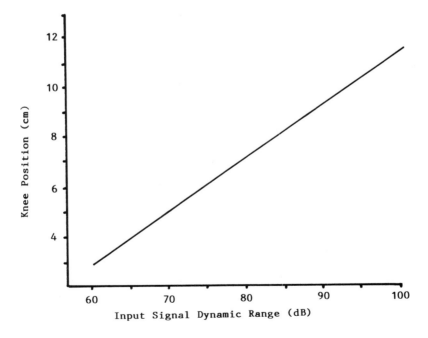

13-13   The change in TGC knee position as a function of input signal dynamic range. The input signal dynamic range is strongly controlled by the transducer output power. Decreasing output power will decrease the input signal dynamic range, moving the knee position closer to the transducer. Calculations are for a 5-MHz, 50% band width transducer and an attenuation of 1 dB/cm/MHz.

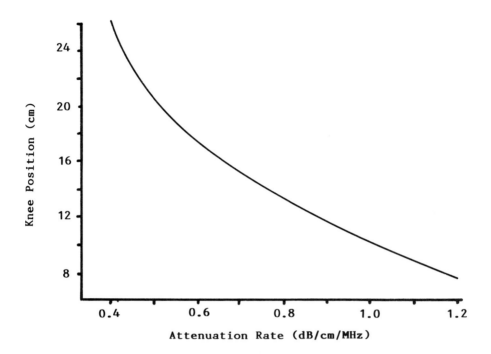

13-14   The change in TGC knee position as a function of tissue attenuation rate. Tissue attenuation rate has a strong influence on TGC adjustment and the position of the TGC knee. Calculations are for a 5-MHz, 50% band-width transducer and an input dynamic range of 100 dB.

If the patient's attenuation rate is greater than normal, the knee will have to come toward the transducer. If the patient's attenuation rate is less than normal, the knee will have to move away from the transducer.

The end point for determining the TGC slope is to have like reflectors appear alike in the image. The likeness of signals at the display can be tested by using either the system reject function or by using variable postprocessing.

In the first case, the reject control is advanced while watching either the A-mode display (if the sonograph is a standard B-scanner) or the image (if the sonograph is a real-time system with no A-mode display). As the reject function is increased, the echo-signals *over the region of compensation* will all vanish at the same rate.

This test is more easily performed with a postprocessing system. First, the postprocessing display signal-window is decreased to make the display bistable, and then the window is slowly moved from the lowest to the highest signal levels. As the window moves up to higher signal amplitudes, all the echo signals in the region of compensation should vanish at the same rate on a correct TGC curve, and all should finally vanish when the window reaches the highest signal level. This postprocessing protocol is detailed in Chapter 14.

Examples of different TGC settings and evaluation of TGC settings with postprocessing are shown in Figures 13-15, 13-16, 13-17, and 13-18.

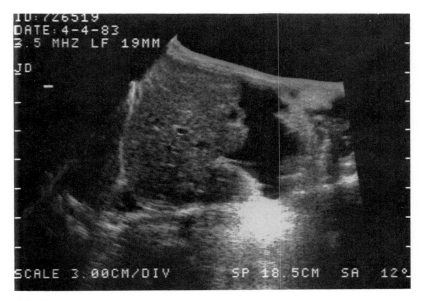

13.15A   Part A

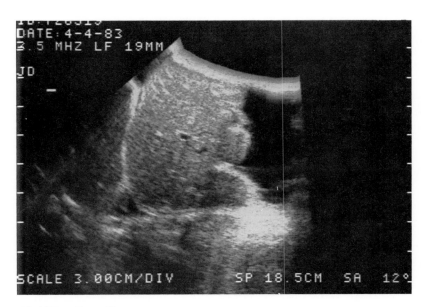

13.15B   Part B

13-15   Changing image content by changing the TGC initial setting. Part A: A correctly set TGC for the patient and conditions. Part B: The TGC initial gain is set too shallow (-30 dB) below the final gain setting. The anterior portion of the image contains noise that adds to the echo-signal mix.

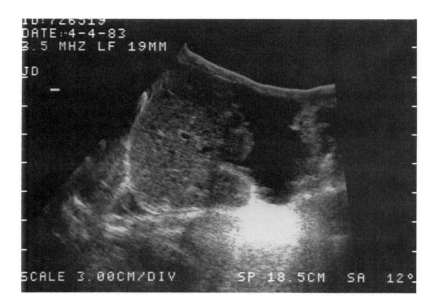

13-16 TGC initial gain set too far below the final gain. The TGC initial setting is set too far (−60 dB) from the final gain values. The anterior portion of the image contains too few tissue echo signals.

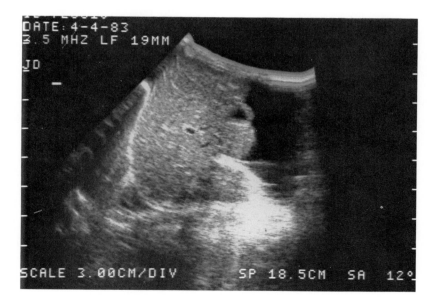

13-17 TGC knee set too close to the transducer. The TGC knee is set too far forward for the tissue, creating a bright band at the position of the TGC knee and transducer focal point. The posterior tissue patterns shown in Figure 13-15, Part A, are gone.

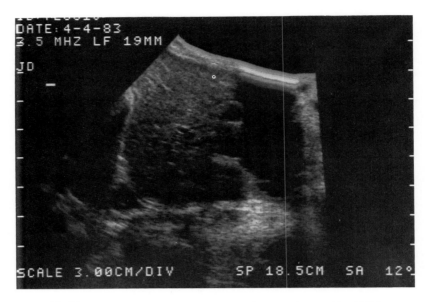

13-18   TGC knee set too far from the transducer. The TGC knee is set too far back in this image, not giving the smaller echo signals sufficient gain for portrayal. The posterior texture is inadequate to show the more-distant tissue patterns.

Normally, TGC delay is not used in abdominal scanning. It is utilized, however, to delay the start of the TGC curve and is helpful when some sort of material layer with an unusual attentuation rate exists between the transducer and the organs being imaged. A thick layer of subcutaneous fat, for example, would be handled with a delay through the fat layer, after which the TGC ramp would be started into the organs.

Another layer often seen in imaging is a water path that has a low attenuation rate compared to the organs being imaged. Delaying through the water path permits a proper use of TGC on the underlying tissues. A delayed TGC setting is shown in Figure 13-19 for a water path used in a small-organ scan. This specialized TGC setting is not necessary in sonographs with water paths included as part of machine design. Any necessary water path delays are already integrated into the machine's operation.

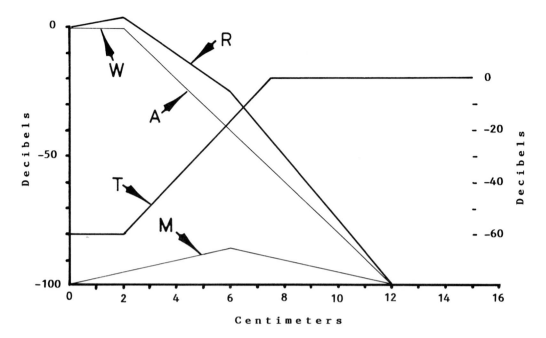

13-19   Setting TGC for a water-path delay. Because of the focusing process of a transducer, *M,* a water layer (or any low attenuator) *(W),* will combine to form an attenuation result that follows *R.* Setting TGC requires a delay through the water path and then a compensating slope *T.*

Conclusion

Setting TGC can be carried out by rote learning, without analyzing why it works the way it does. As this chapter has shown, though, setting TGC is just the tip of the iceberg. In addition to the simple setup, measurements, equations, and assumptions must be made relating to processes within the tissue that are not generally considered in usual TGC setup protocols. The typically simple TGC setup, in fact, is the reason that many protocols do not conform to the final adjustments needed to correctly image the patient. Others come close but provide no real insight into why they work. For example, the authors originally developed a TGC protocol that used twice the focal-point range of the transducer to set the knee position. It provided an acceptable estimate of the starting knee position, but the reason it worked was unclear. Equation 13-1 shows why this estimate was close. For most transducers, the knee position is almost but not exactly twice the focal-point range. Given an understanding of the events and assumptions inherent to using TGC, the final time-gain compensation curve offers a means of evaluating the patient's tissue-ultrasound interactions.

Even more obvious are the influences of TGC on the image formation and image content. Setting TGC requires both a firm knowledge of events within the tissues and a well-designed sonograph that can give the sonographer the right sort of information. Many current sonographs, real time and static, offer the sonographer an uncalibrated TGC, with no values to rely upon and no A-mode display to help determine true signal levels. A minimum of experimentation will quickly show a wide range of possible TGC and power values that seem acceptable. But are they acceptable? What information is lost? Clearly, this chapter's discussion has demonstrated that the values are not all alike. With uncalibrated, unmarked, and undisplayed TGC, we are left trying to make a "pretty picture," while also being faced with a set of unanswerable questions about the accuracy of the image.

References

1. Wells, P.N., T. 1969. Physical Principles of Ultrasonic Diagnosis. Academic Press, New York.
2. Le Croissette, D.H. et al. April 1979. The attenuation of selected soft tissue as a function of frequency. NBS Special Publication 525. Ultrasonic Tissue Characterization II. Melvin Linzer, Editor. U.S. Government Printing Office, Washington, D.C. 101–108.

Chapter 14

Interrogating Gray-Scale Images with Postprocessing

With the arrival of the digital scan converter for the B-scanner came the first major controversy in B-scanning, with the exception of arguments over the pros and cons of individual machine designs. The debate, which is ongoing, surrounds the question of whether it is better to manipulate information before it gets into memory or after it comes out of memory. The controversy pivots on the issue of four versus five or six bit memories. Although preprocessing can alter the image contents, interrogating the image contents is strictly the domain of postprocessing, which is the subject of this chapter.

B-scanners with 32 or more gray levels usually have a set of controls that vary both the apparent intensity and contrast of the image. In the face of this sort of presentation it is easy to believe that the image is being manipulated only in terms of its intensity and contrast. It is clear, however, that changing the analog contrast and intensity controls on a TV display and changing the window width and window position for a postprocessing function are entirely different functions.

Variable postprocessing was featured first on the analog scan converter, but lacked some of the stability present in current B-scanning equipment using digital scan converters. This stability and reproducibility provide opportunities to use the postprocessing functions as a means not of manipulating the intensity and contrast of the TV image, but, rather, of interrogating the image contents for qualitative and quantitative information.

To perform many of these postprocessing functions, however, the sonograph and the sonographer must work in concert in order to control variables that would normally take the information away from the image. For instance, one of the primary requirements is a separation of the incoming analog signals into even dB signal steps. In this process, signals prepared for display that span a dynamic range of 40 dB are divided into 32 equal steps. This separation produces a signal separation of 1.25 dB per step. With display signals separated into equal steps, counting steps can provide numerical relationships among signals that would not be available if the preprocessing involved nonlinear, unequal separations.

Let us now look at postprocessing signal processing with the aim of developing an understanding of how to apply postprocessing in different ways to extract both qualitative and quantitative information from the image.

The Postprocessing Technique

The first step in a digital scan converter is to convert the analog video signals into digital numbers that are stored in memory. Chapter 5, on digital scan converters, established that this number conversion process is controlled by the preprocessing function in the scan converter. In turn, the range of numbers available to the scan converter is a function of the number of bits available in each storage location. The only real requirement for using the postprocessing to quantify is that the conversion of the signal levels to numbers must occur in a linear dB format. This linear separation of the signal dynamic range permits the comparison of one numerical value to another in dB units, by noting the appropriate gray levels on the display.

After storing the signal levels in memory as binary numbers, the scan converter then pulls the binary numbers out of memory in a sequence that reconstructs the image. As the numbers are retrieved from memory, they are assigned a gray-level intensity on the display screen. In many scan converters this conversion is digitally controlled. The intensity range of the TV display is divided into 128 to 256 steps or discrete values. By digitally dividing the intensity range on the TV into specific steps, the assignment process becomes straightforward. Bringing the number out of the memory and assigning it directly to the gray level is then a numerical relationship.

Under most circumstances, a nonmedical digital image has almost the same population of pixels occupying each display intensity. In other words, all intensities in such images have an equal frequency of occurrence in the image [1]. Ultrasound images, on the other hand, do not seem to adhere to this rule and require a much-different population to provide clinically acceptable images. In a series of evaluation experiments, the most desirable ultrasound image was found to be one that had a constant pixel population over only the lower half of the intensity range (the upper half of the intensity range pixel population drops off at a constant sine function [1]). This assignment of relative intensity levels to the signals stored in memory is, in fact, part of the postprocessing mechanism. By changing this assignment of gray levels in a regular and predictable manner, the appearance of the image can be altered dramatically.

The assignment of the number stored in the random access memory (RAM) to the gray-scale intensities on the screen can be linear or nonlinear. Various nonlinear assignments can be used to provide preferred visual images from an aesthetic point of view, or they can be used to create an interrogation scheme to visually separate the various signal levels into preferred gray-level assignments. By manually moving through the curves, the image can be quickly interrogated for large as well as subtle changes in image content. All this interrogation is possible without rescanning the patient, because the interrogation is carried out on stored information rather than signals acquired during scanning.

Postprocessing Controls

Postprocessing controls come in two varieties: first, a manual selection of preprogrammed, postprocessing curves and, second, manual postprocessing controls that manipulate the gray-scale assignment to form display signal "windows." This section focuses on the second type of control.

The first process needed for manual postprocessing is a signal "window" of variable width (Figure 14-1). This window functions in much the same manner as a signal window on a computed tomography (CT) system. It offers an opportunity to present as few as two signal levels or as large as the full dynamic range of the signals presented to the scan converter, but always with the signals spread over the full display intensity range. It is, in fact, a window on the range of numbers possible within the scan converter, offering a gray-scale view ranging from bistable to the full gray-scale compliment of the display. Along with the control, we need to show exactly which of the signal levels or numbers stored in the memory are available to the postprocessing window. This window-width indication can appear as either digital numbers on the screen or as the number of gray-scale steps appearing on a gray bar permanently located at the bottom of the display. Coupling the gray-scale, gray-bar display with the gray-scale image and a window-width control produces an effective means of interrogating the image.

The second control we need is a window-position control that permits the window to be moved over the full range of the stored numbers (Figure 14-2). Added to the variable window-width control, this control lets us position a window over any of the stored numbers and select out of the numbers only those we wish to

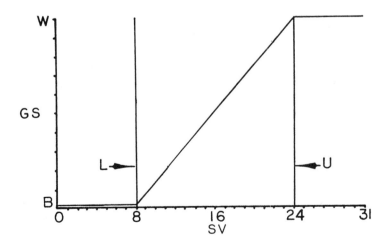

14-1 The variable postprocessing window. Variable postprocessing systems often permit the creation of a display window with adjustable width and position. *L* is the lower window edge; *U* is the upper window edge; *SV* represents the scan converter stored values; *GS* is the gray scale on the display, extending from black *(B)* to white *(W)*. Within the window, the stored values are spread over the full gray-scale range.

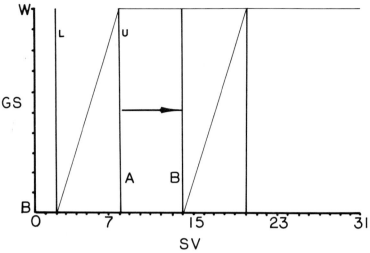

14-2 Moving the postprocessing window over the stored values. In this example, the window is adjusted to span six values and to display these values over the full gray-scale range. Moving from *A* to *B* places the same window over a middle range of values. *L* is the lower window edge; *U* is the upper window edge; *SV* represents stored values; *GS* is display gray scale from black *(B)* to white *(W)*.

display. These two controls will be used in concert to interrogate the image for qualitative and quantitative information.

With the machine organization and postprocessing controls in mind, we can now examine a few protocols for testing and evaluating images and image content.

Testing Time-Gain Compensation

The visual goal in setting TGC is to have like signals have the same intensity within the image, over a distance defined by the TGC ramp. Because of the adjacency principle in our visual processes (see also Chapter 16), a uniform image is not always self-evident. Using the postprocessing controls, TGC settings can be objectively evaluated, and users who are learning correct TGC settings can be provided with a verification of a correct setup.

The first step in this protocol is to set the image format as either white-on-black or black-on-white, depending on your preference for viewing the image (see Chapter 16 for reasons for the choices). In this example, we will use a white-on-black display. Second, decrease the window width until the image is bistable. The lower edge of the window should be on the lowest signal present on the display. This will produce an image that is white anywhere in which signals exist and black where signals are absent. Third, move the window along increasing values of the stored signals. As the window moves along larger numerical values, the image will change as the lower signals appear to drop out of the image (Figure 14-3). When the full range of the stored signals is spanned by the window movement, the image will turn completely black. We are most concerned with the region of the image spanned by the TGC ramp.

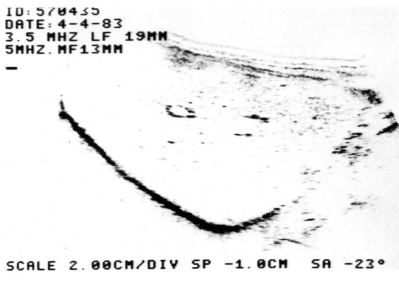

14-3   Part A

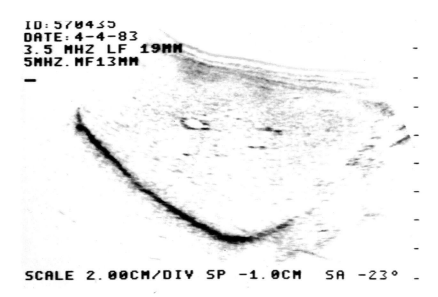

14-3   Part B

14-3   Changing the Image with variable postprocessing. Part A: Gray-scale image with the postprocessing window expanded over the full 40-dB video signal range. Part B: The postprocessign window is set over the center 12 dB of the 40-dB echo-signal range. All the echo signals below the midrange level are set to the same gray level, making the image look incomplete. The gray-bar pattern on the image bottom shows the gray-scale assignment.

If the TGC slope is set too high, the anterior portion of the image will vanish *before* the posterior portion. On the other hand, if the TGC is set too low, the posterior portion of the image will vanish *first*. When the TGC is set properly, the anterior and posterior portions of the image will vanish together, as in Figure 14-4. And again, we apply these visual properties only to the portion of the image spanned by the TGC ramp.

Measuring the Range of Organ Echo Signals

The following protocol is used to examine the range of signals found in any particular organ, or it can be used to examine the total range of signals presented to the digital scan converter. In the first instance, we are interested in the range of signals characteristic of an organ; in the second, we are concerned with assuring that the total dynamic range of the digital scan converter is used.

The first step is to move the zoom box over the portion of the image being tested. Later the display will become bistable. At that point, locating the signals we want to measure will become difficult, and the zoom box will hold the image position for us. For example, if we wish to look at a kidney, then the zoom box is expanded and positioned over the kidney.

Next, decrease the postprocessing window to form a bistable display. Position the postprocessing window with the lower edge on the first signal step on the gray-scale display.

Slowly move the window upward until the first indication of signals leaving the organ appears (Figure 14-4). These signals represent the lowest signals for the organ. Note the position of the window on the gray bar in order to fix the starting point for the next step.

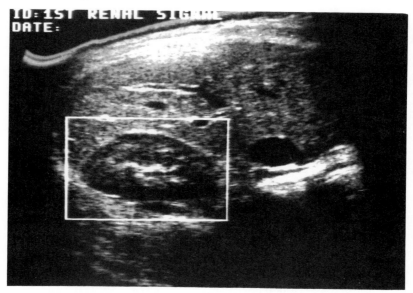

14-4   Part A

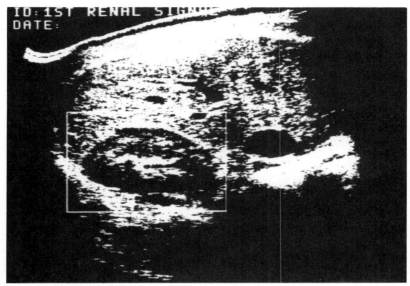

14-4   Part B

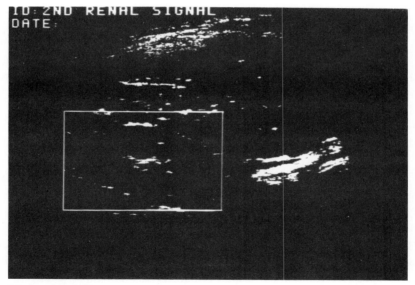

14-4   Part C

14-4   Measuring the range of echo signals using variable post-processing. Part A: Normal gray-scale assignment, with the zoom box over the kidney. Part B: The image is bistable, with postprocessing window set to a single step width. The window has been advanced until the smallest echo signal from the renal tissue just disappears. Part C: The window is now advanced until the largest signal in the organ just vanishes, marking the upper range of the echo signals. The echo signals span 7 steps in this image, which represents nearly 9 dB in echo-signal range.

Continue moving the window upward along the increasing signal levels and count the steps on the gray-bar display until the last organ signal just vanishes. This represents the highest signal in the total range of signals within the organ. The actual range of signals presented by the organ can be calculated by multiplying the digital step size by the number of steps spanned by the moving window. The result is the organ signal range expressed in decibels. The imaging results appear in Figure 14-4.

Measuring Shadowing and Enhancement

A layer of material that has an attenuation different from surrounding tissue can form a region of higher-than-normal or lower-than-normal signals posterior to it. Measuring the amount of attenuation or enhancement behind such a tissue can provide clues to tissue characteristics causing the change and is a valuable tool in sonography.

Making measurements of enhancement and attenuation requires that we follow some basic rules to prevent poor judgements about the results. These basic rules for making measurements include the following: 1) The TGC must be properly adjusted (we now have a protocol to determine this); 2) The comparison with normal tissue must include similar tissue types and similar signals; 3) The measurements must be made at the same tissue depth or range from the transducer. Violating any one of these three rules can prevent the making of useful comparisons. And, in turn, the accuracy of any judgements made from the results will depend entirely on how well these rules are followed in the protocol.

Measuring Acoustic Enhancement

Move the zoom box over the region of interest and change the zoom box size to just fit over the signals being measured. This will help identify the signals picked for the measurement process when the display becomes bistable.

Decrease the window width to produce a bistable display. Slowly move the window upward until a medium-level signal just disappears on the display. Pick the same sort of signal to be used behind the enhancing structure. The difference between the levels of these two signals will represent the amount of acoustic enhancement present because of the low attenuating medium in front. For the sake of comparison, be sure to choose signals at the same range from the transducer.

Slowly move the postprocessing window upward in level until the same kind of signal chosen for comparison just vanishes behind the enhancing structure. Count the number of steps between the point of the first signal vanishing and the second signal vanishing. An example of the imaging results appears in Figure 14-5.

The number of steps multiplied by the step size in decibels gives the range or difference in signal levels in decibels between the normal signal and the signal enhanced by the low attenuating material. A method of expressing the difference

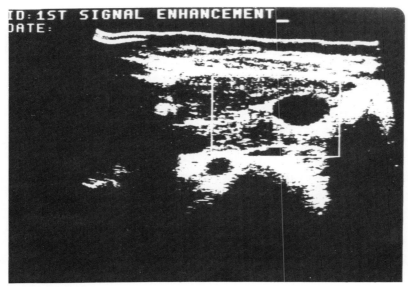

14-5   Part A

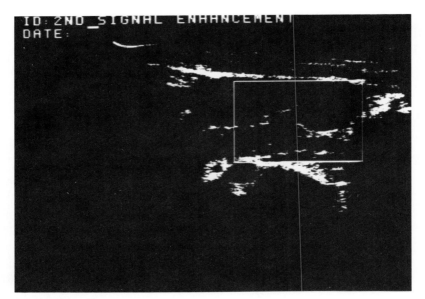

14-5   Part B

14-5   Measuring acoustic enhancement with variable postprocessing. Part A: The postprocessing window has been closed to a single step and moved until the first tissue echo signal outside the enhancement just disappears. The zoom box surrounds the area of interest. Part B: The postprocessing window has been advanced to the point at which a like reflector just disappears within the enhancement. The two reflectors for comparison are at the same depth. The enhancement in this image increased the echo signals by nearly 9 dB.

is an *enhancement index* that can be calculated by dividing the enhancement in dB (the difference between the two signals) by the thickness of the enhancing structure. This process provides a rough evaluation of the attenuation rate within the low attenuating medium.

Measuring Acoustic Shadowing

Applying the same technique to shadowing offers an insight into the attenuation rate of a higher-than-normal attenuating material.

Move the zoom box over the region of interest. This again will provide a means of keeping track of the signals we are trying to measure.

Decrease the window width to produce a bistable display. Move the window upward along the stored signal values until one of the medium-level signals behind the shadowing structure first disappears on the image. This disappearance will mark the starting point for evaluating the difference between signals. An example of the imaging results is shown in Figure 14-6.

Continue to move the window upward while counting the steps, until the same sort of signal outside of the attenuating shadow just vanishes.

Multiplying the step size by the number of steps between the two signals gives a value of the amount of signal decrease due to the higher attenuating material between the transducer and the echo signals. As before, be sure that the two signals being compared are at the same distance from the transducer, with one signal being within the shadow and the other signal outside of the shadow.

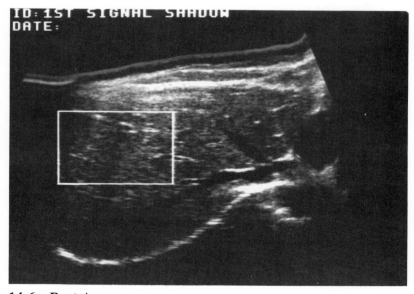

14-6   Part A

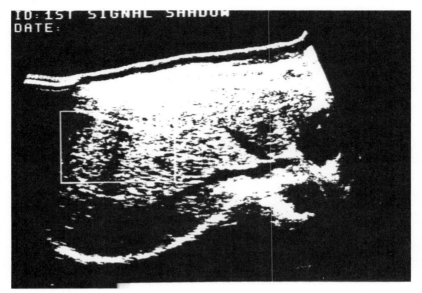

14-6   Part B

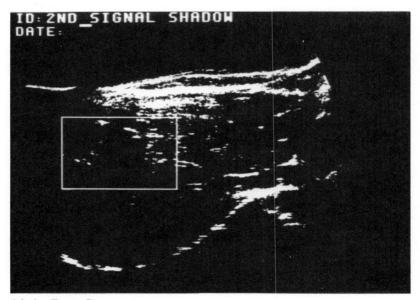

14-6   Part C

14-6 Measuring acoustic shadowing with variable postprocessing. Part A: An image containing shadowing with linear postprocessing. The zoom box is set over the region of measurement. Part B: The postprocessing window was closed to a single step and advanced until the first echo signal within the shadow just vanished. Part C: The postprocessing window was moved along the echo signals until a like signal at the same depth just vanished outside the shadow. The shadow produced echo signals 15 dB below normal.

In the same manner that we calculated the enhancement index, we can calculate a shadowing index by dividing the decrease in signal, or the signal difference between the largest and the smallest echo signals, by the thickness of the attenuating structure. This provides an approximation of the attenuation characteristics within the attenuating material.

Using Preselected Curves

With a set of properly chosen postprocessing curves, the operator can rapidly interrogate an image for its contents, simply by switching from one curve to another. The secret in using this technique is to know what each of the processing curves does to the signals, what signal levels are being expanded, and what signal levels are being compressed together. For example, a curve can be shaped to enhance or separate the smaller signals within the total signal mix. Alternatively, the signals in the medium range can be preferentially separated. Another form of processing could involve rejecting signals below a certain level, while presenting the remainder in a linear format. Some examples of postprocessing curves are shown in Figure 14-7.

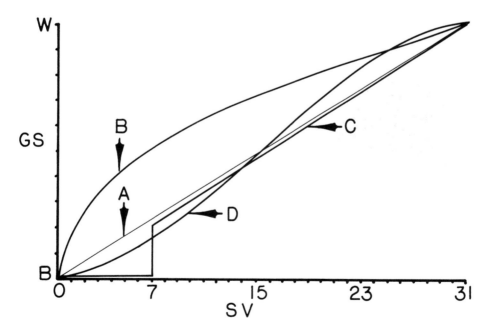

14-7 Switchable postprocessing curves. Switchable postprocessing curves are often available to quickly interrogate some of the subtle qualities of an image. *A* is a linear curve; *B* enhances separation of the lower signal range; *C* drops out the lower signals by assigning them the same intensity; *D* enhances the separation of the middle-range signals. *SV* represents stored values; *GS* is display gray scale from black *(B)* to white *(W)*.

The purpose of a postprocessing mechanism is to provide preferential separations of signals. Often this kind of separation does not lead to an aesthetically pleasing image. Instead, the images appear contoured and contrasty (Figure 14-8). In this instance, however, we are more interested in obtaining diagnostic information than in achieving balance or beauty within the image.

With the curves as knowns, the different curves can be selected while the image is visually examined with each new curve. The important thing to remember is that each curve has a region or range of signals that it prefers to present; thus, knowing not only the curves but what you are looking for in the image can make postprocessing a valuable tool.

Off-line Postprocessing

Postprocessing analysis need not be just part of the machine interior. In fact, dedicated analysis carts and dedicated software are available to help the sonographer and the sonologist analyze ultrasonic images. Although dedicated analysis carts have been available for some time, dedicated software is only now becoming available. Below is a description of some of the general characteristics of analysis carts and analysis software.

In general, analysis carts use some type of microprocessor and memory in combination to handle the analysis. Frequently, information input is through such objects as video images from a video camera, bit pads, or key-entry techniques from a keyboard. Most analysis carts tend to be very dedicated to a specific use, a dedication that often makes the machine appear more constricted than it actually is. The dedication, however, can make the cart valuable in high-volume analysis situations.

Analysis software, on the other hand, uses a much-different approach. Instead of using a dedicated microprocessor and memory, it employs a general microcomputer often available through local business stores or through dedicated computer sales shops. As with the analysis cart, the general microcomputer inputs information through objects such as bit pads, key entry, or sometimes other special entry devices such as magnetic tapes. The analysis software is usually able to run on only one make of microcomputer. Although the analysis software can be quite dedicated, the analysis machine, which is the microcomputer, is not. In this sense, the microcomputer continues to be able to carry out the normal and specialized functions of the microcomputer, and is not dedicated only to a particular task.

Both analysis carts and analytical software have strong points and weak points. At the same time, it is clear that the increased volume of information in ultrasonic images needs to be processed in faster and more efficient ways. Off-line postprocessing is one means of handling this problem.

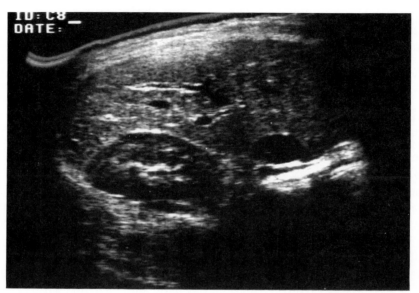

14-8   Part A

14-8   Changing the image with preset postprocessing assignment curves. Part A: A linear postprocessing assignment of stored values in the scan converter to the display gray-scale intensities. Part B: A nonlinear postprocessing curve that places the lowest 12 dB signals on the same intensity. Part C: A nonlinear postprocessing curve that places the highest 12-dB signals on the same intensity contouring the larger echo signals together.

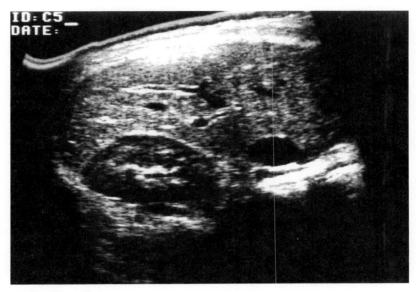

14-8 Part B

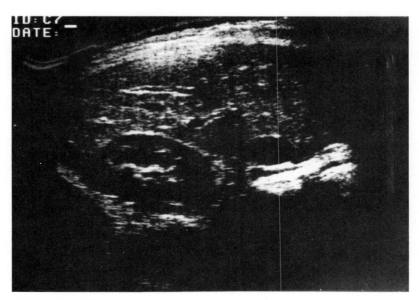

14-8 Part C

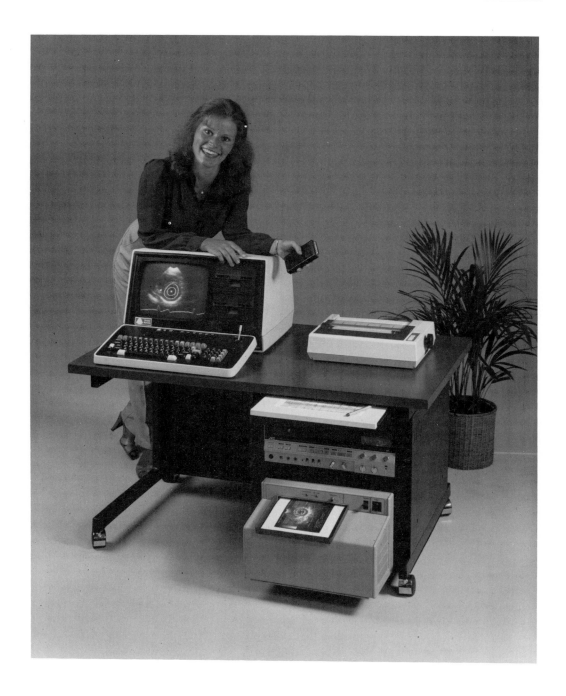

14-9   A dedicated, off-line image analysis system. Combining a computer with video image information permits a variety of postprocessing techniques. This system provides a number of computer-controlled analyses of real time images and hard copies of selected images. Courtesy of MicroSonics, Inc., Indianapolis, Indiana.

Conclusion

Postprocessing is not a means of necessarily obtaining a "pretty" image. Rather, postprocessing provides an opportunity to interrogate the stored image contents either on a programmed or a personal basis for specific pieces of information. The ability to perform quantitative tasks in postprocessing depends upon specific characteristics contained in the imaging process itself.

Applying quantitative techniques imposes major limitations on how the data are originally collected. The TGC must be set properly to portray like echo sources similarly within the image. One of the first requirements in applying quantitative techniques, then, is to test the image for proper TGC setup.

With a good image in memory, we can proceed to interrogate the amount of acoustical enhancement or shadowing in an image. Postprocessing means more, however, than simply varying the intensity and contrast on the display. It involves the opportunity to test the image for its numerical content. As we gain experience in applying these techniques, we can expect the characteristics of ultrasound to change, thus making new postprocessing designs available for the knowledgeable user.

References

1. Robinson, D.E., and P.C. Knight. July 1981. Computer reconstruction techniques in compound scan pulse-echo imaging. Ultrasonic Imaging 3:217–234.

Chapter 15

Making Use of Preprocessing

In earlier chapters, we explored the basic issues of variable preprocessing versus variable postprocessing for both the B-scanner and the real-time sonograph. The use of variable preprocessing is fairly direct in the applications of real-time sonography. This does not extend to the B-scanner, however, which requires rescanning to effectively utilize any available preprocessing curves.

It is this requirement for rescanning that has created problems in using preprocessing effectively in the B-scanner. Equipment manufacturers have provided a wide range of preprocessing that goes unused in most ultrasound departments, and understandably so. With the pressures of a large patient load and the time required to determine an appropriate curve, most sonographers simply pick one curve and always scan with it. As a consequence, however, important information can be missed, and the sonograph is not used to its full potential.

This chapter, then, outlines a protocol for selecting and using the preprocessing that is available on many B-scanners.

Preprocessing and Signal Separation

The problem of choosing an appropriate preprocessing curve is inherent to the design of small digital scan converters with a storage word of 4 or fewer bits. A 4-bit scan converter, for example, generates 16 values that can be used to represent variations in signal amplitude. In general, a linear separation of 40 dB or more into 16 parts provides too much separation between signals to show adequately the textural differences among tissues. To solve this problem, most manufacturers have offered several ''selectable'' preprocessing curves for the sonographer. In general, as the number of grays available to the B-scanner decreases, the shape of the preprocessing curve becomes more critical and the number of curves as options decreases.

The first step in digital image processing is to convert the analog signals into a set of binary numbers that are stored in the random access memory (RAM). The number of values available to the RAM is a function of the word size in the analog-to-digital converter. After the numbers are stored in memory, they are recovered in a programmed sequence to produce the image. At this point, the numbers are assigned a gray level for final display.

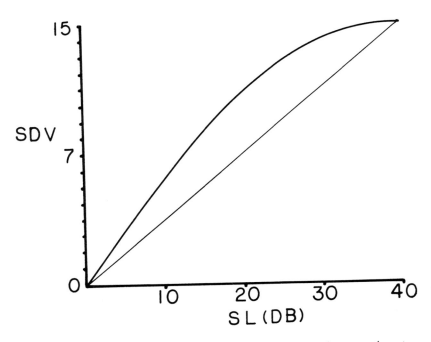

15-1   Preprocessing curve to enhance gray-scale separation at low signal levels. Preprocessing assigns the analog signal level *(SL)* to the stored digital values *(SDV)*. The curve enhances the gray-scale separation of echo signals below 25 dB.

Preprocessing governs the events before the data are stored in memory. Once the image is stored, it cannot be changed without erasing the memory contents and rescanning the patient, using a new preprocessing curve. Thus, it is incumbent upon the operator to choose the appropriate preprocessing curve for the job at hand.

The connection between the shape of the preprocessing curve and the ultimate visual emphasis of echo signals is an essential point to understand. The catch, if one exists, is to know the design purpose for each available preprocessing curve. The shape of the curve determines which segment of the total range of signals arriving into the memory will be assigned the numbers finally stored in memory.

For example, the preprocessing curve can emphasize small signals as a result of spreading the lower-range signals over a larger portion of the available digital numbers. This sort of signal separation is shown in Figure 15-1. Such a curve can differentiate the more subtle characteristics of the small echo signals that aid in tumor and cyst definition. This curve, then, would be a poor selection for a survey in which overall signal characteristics are under examination during the scan, but would be appropriate for scanning the details of a mass.

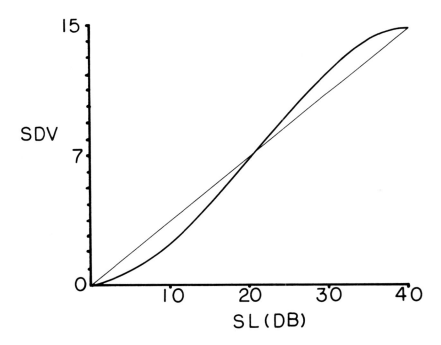

15-2 Preprocessing curve to enhance gray scale separation at medium signal levels. This curve assigns the center 20 dB of the signal levels *(SL)* to most of the available stored digital values *(SDV)*.

Preprocessing can also shift the signal emphasis into medium-level signals, as shown in Figure 15-2. This type of sigmoidal curve spreads the medium-range signals into more of the available digital numbers. It is a good curve for survey work, where small signals and large signals are compressed together, but in which the medium-range signals that produce much of the textural information and the larger signals that are associated with structures and boundaries are seen easily.

Preprocessing can, moreover, shift the emphasis into the higher signal levels. The curve appears exponential, sweeping upward over the larger signals, as shown in Figure 15-3. A separation such as this is useful when trying to delineate a number of closely spaced specular reflectors, such as the boundaries between an organ and a highly reflective tumor. Another application is in separating the anatomy of a mid- and late-term fetus. Biparietal diameters, however, are more difficult to make with this curve, because the intracranial anatomy needed to determine position would be poorly portrayed.

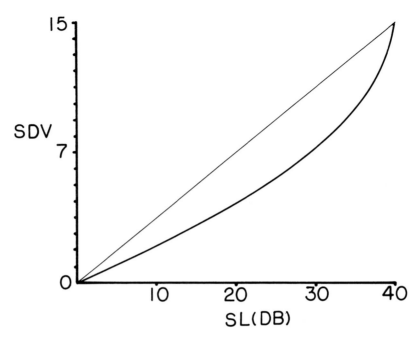

15-3   Preprocessing curve to enhance gray-scale separation at higher signal levels. This curve assigns a large number of the stored digital values *(SDV)* to the upper 15 dB of signal levels *(SL)*.

Preprocessing and Image Content

The position of the preprocessing function in the signal stream means it influences all incoming signals. Because it governs the assignment of available values in memory, preprocessing can have a major influence on such things as axial resolution. Changing preprocessing curves while making measurements on an AIUM Test Object or tissue-equivalent phantom shows how each curve can affect the apparent resolution of the sonograph. We should expect, then, to see changes in axial resolution in scans of the same part of the body while using different curves. Examples of image changes with different preprocessing curves were illustrated in Chapter 12.

Preprocessing can also influence the apparent lateral resolution of a sonograph. Moving small signals into brighter intensities can make the ultrasound beam appear wider. Being able to select the preprocessing curve for the task at hand involves understanding the changes and influences made by altering the assignment of analog signals to digital numbers.

Along with axial and lateral resolution changes, preprocessing also affects the apparent penetration of the sonograph. The assignment of the first gray-scale step will change the apparent penetration of a sonograph by influencing which analog signal level is assigned the first visible gray-scale step. Such changes are included in Chapter 12.

Along with these readily apparent influences on the image, preprocessing can modify our imaging in subtle ways, such as influencing our choice of transducer frequency for a given task. As we increase the transducer frequency used for imaging, the amount of energy scattered back to the transducer increases according to the square or cube of the frequency (see Chapter 9). This has the effect of changing the position of low- and medium-level signals on the preprocessing curve, and thus, their portrayal. Further, if the sonograph has reject control that changes the amplitude of the signals presented to the analog-to-digital converter, then using a reject function not only removes structural echo signals but also changes the gray-scale assignment and texture within the image.

With an awareness now of how preprocessing can influence the image, let us look at a preprocessing selection protocol.

Preprocessing Selection Protocol

The use of preprocessing with the B-scanner is not as easy as it might appear. For one thing, the B-scanner requires rescanning to change any preprocessing effects. In addition, no amount of postprocessing can recover information lost in the preprocessing. Whenever rescanning is required, it decreases the number of patients a sonographer can examine in the course of a day. When facts such as the above are combined with the problem of selecting a preprocessing curve without a protocol, a sonograph's signal-processing capabilities often wind up either being underutilized or abandoned.

We need a means, therefore, of rapidly seeing the effects of a preprocessing selection, just as we do in real time. The means to do this is available in most B-scanner digital scan converters in the form of the survey mode.

The survey or last-value mode in a B-scanner replaces the scan converter contents with the results of the most current values, not the peak values (see Chapter 5). Thus, scanning the transducer over the abdomen, for example, in a series of single-pass scans will produce a new image with each pass of the transducer. By slewing the arm position and scanning at the same time, a whole series of rapid scans can be used to survey a portion of the abdomen. By not slewing the arm position and holding the transducer to a single plane, a series of repeated scans can be used to look for a desired preprocessing curve.

As noted in Chapter 2, the survey mode reduces the signal-to-noise ratio and requires an increase in the output of the sonograph or an increase in system gain in order to restore the ratio to the same levels as peak detection. Using the survey mode, a new preprocessing curve can be selected for each pass of the transducer and the curve measured for the imaging task. And the time required for the selection is not much more than would be required for a real-time sonograph. Once the curve is selected, we can return the system to a peak-value mode and the system output or gain can be reduced to normal compound scanning values.

Of course, using this technique requires an understanding of the curves and what segments of the signal spectrum each curve works on. Again, a good place to start is by looking at the shape of the curves in material provided by the manufacturer. Knowing the appearance of the curves from the beginning permits a more systematic match of the preprocessing curve to the problem. The alternative is to execute a blind trial in order to find the curve that will work, and that takes far too much time.

The preprocessing curves that are available are often not selected for the best information transfer. Companies choose curves not so much on the clinical information available in the final image, but for the aesthetic qualities of the image; in other words, the curves are selected for "beauty," not utility. Choosing the appropriate preprocessing curve requires looking beyond beauty, however, to the information that is presented in the image. Pretty images are not necessarily clinically useful, although the reverse can be true.

Conclusion

While all digital scan converter systems use preprocessing, machines differ according to whether the preprocessing curves are linear or nonlinear, and the number of curves that are available to the sonographer. Nonlinear preprocessing curves are found on all sonographs with 16 or fewer gray levels. In the B-scanner, the curves seem largely unused because of the inconvenience of rescanning and the lack of a good selection protocol.

As this chapter has underscored, the first step in selecting an appropriate preprocessing curve is to know and understand the relationship between the shape and function of each curve. Once the shape and function are known, the appropriate curve can be chosen in the survey mode for the specific scanning task at hand.

Preprocessing can help extract diagnostic information from an image by visually separating signals that offer diagnostic clues. In the end, choosing the curve will depend upon the signal-to-noise ratio in the sonograph, the range of signals presented by the patient and sonograph in combination, and the overall quality of the displaying system.

Chapter 16

Gray-Scale Vision and the Human Eye

In preceding chapters, we have dealt entirely with the processes that occur within the tissue or within the machine that makes the images. Between the displayed information and the decision-making human brain is the eye. Because all ultrasonic information is funneled through our sense of vision, the eye deserves special attention in this book.

Sonographers should not only understand the physiology of the eye but should be able to answer questions such as: Can we see only 10 shades of gray? Is the video inverse switch on the TV display really useful? Can postprocessing aid visualization? Are more than 10 shades of gray valuable within a sonograph? These are but a sampling of questions related to the transfer of ultrasound information through the eye. Not uncommonly, the answers to such questions have been clouded by myths surrounding the workings of the eye.

This chapter exposes some of these myths about vision and imparts, it is hoped, enough understanding of the information transfer mechanism to enable readers to comprehend the limits of vision and, thereby, the limits of any information transfer.

Mechanical Organization of the Eye

A cursory look at the physical eye as shown in Figure 16-1 is enough to convince the viewer that the eye is a camera made of living parts. Each functional element of the eye as depicted in the figure has an analogue in the camera, including parts that refract, focus, absorb, and detect light.

The cornea of the eye is the first surface that light encounters on its way to the retina. The cornea has a regular organization of proteins that gives the tissue its transparency. When these proteins lose this organization because of pressure or disease, the cornea becomes partially or completely opaque. The radius of curvature at the first surface of the cornea forms a first-surface lens, and light crossing the corneal surface at an acute angle is refracted away from its normal path.

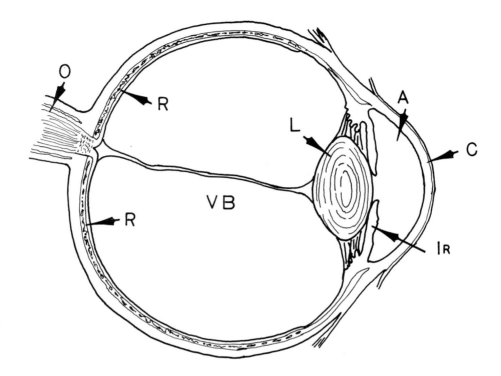

16-1   Anatomy of the mammalian eye. *C* is the cornea; *IR* is the iris; *A* is the anterior chamber; *L* is the lens; *VB* is the vitreous body; *R* is the retina; *O* is the optic nerve.

Behind the cornea are the lens and iris. The lens connects to muscles that change the lens thickness during adaptation. The radius of curvature for the lens changes with muscular contraction and relaxation, causing a change in the focal point for the lens. Adjusting the focal point of the eye brings different portions of the visual field into focus on the retina as an inverted image.

Between the lens and the cornea is the iris. This structure rests on a sphincter muscle that opens and closes the iris aperture under neural control. Because of the geometry of the eye, the iris limits the amount of light reaching the retina, and at the same time, changes the depth of focus. Despite the dynamic qualities of the iris, it provides only a small portion of the light control for the retina. Although the eye can adapt to 10 or more logarithmic units, the iris can manage light over only 3 logarithmic units [1]. The iris seems to play a much greater role in communications than that of a simple regulator of incident light to the retina [2].

Both the space between the iris and the cornea and the space between the lens and the retina are filled with fluid that is constantly circulating and refreshed. The fluid, called aqueous humor, fills the anterior chamber and central portion of the posterior chamber of the eye (Figure 16-1). The remaining portion of the posterior chamber is filled with vitreous humor, which appears to be a transparent gel.

As the light from an outside image passes to the retina, the image is inverted and focused onto the surface of the retina.

Thus, except for the fact that the parts of the eye are made of living cells or the products of living cells, the physical optics of the eye so far described in our discussion do not appear to differ substantially from those of a simple camera. Yet, we know that the range of light over which the eye can function is much larger than that of a camera and, furthermore, that the adaptation of the eye to light is handled largely by something other than the iris. The source of these properties thus must abide somewhere else in the complex neuroanatomy and physiology of the eye. In reality, the eye may be an analogue to the camera, but only as far as the retina. From that point on, the eye far surpasses the camera in sophistication of operation.

Neuro-organization of the Retina

In a camera, light reaches a photosensitive paper to record the image focused by the lens. The retina serves this photosensitive function in the eye, but with a greater range of response and complexity in signal handling than that of a silver halide molecule. The retinal cells convert light energy into electrochemical energy that the neural system can use. And beyond simple detection, the light energy distribution is encoded and enhanced in character before being transferred to the optic nerve, where the information is conveyed to the brain for further encoding and enhancement. Despite all this special signal processing, the "trueness" of the visual perception is retained.

The retinal cells respond in two ways to stimulation. One response is called a graded response, in which the cell responds to its stimulus with a slow change in its transmembrane potential [1]. This response is known also as a slow potential. The second response is called the action potential and represents an all-or-none response by the cell [1]. In this response the transmembrane potential experiences an abrupt change and recovery that represent the action potential cycle. The information is encoded not in the amplitude of the action potential, but in the number of cycles that occur per unit time. In other words, the information is encoded into the frequency of action potentials resulting from stimulation.

Changes in the transmembrane potentials are used normally to handle signals and responses within a single cell. When nerve cells "talk" to other nerve cells, they do so with chemicals called neurotransmitters. This remains true in the retina, with action potentials and slow potentials representing individual cell responses, and with neurotransmitters conveying the visual information from one cell to another.

All vertebrates have retinas that rest on the same five types of cells [1], the organization of which is shown schematically in Figure 16-2 and is described below. The sensory cells convert the light information into a slow potential response. Two types of sensors, called rods and cones, exist in the retina. The rods respond to low light levels, but only to the intensity of the light, forming a simple black and

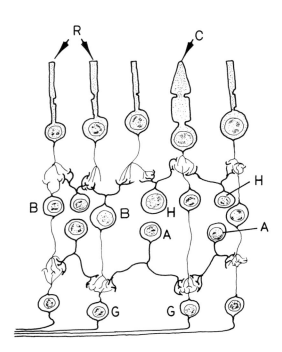

16-2   Simplified organization of the retina. The primary receptive cells are the rods *(R)* and cones *(C)*. They synapse with the
bipolar cells *(B)*, which, in turn, synapse with the ganglion cells
(G). Between the synapse of the bipolar cells and sensory cells
are the horizontal cells *(H)*, providing a set of lateral connections. A second layer of lateral connections occurs between
synapses of bipolar cells and ganglion cells, provided by the
amacrine cells *(A)*. This organization provides contrast enhancement and lateral inhibition at the retinal level.

white visual response [1]. Rods provide low light-level vision at night. The second
group of sensors, the cones, respond to higher light levels and have distinct
responses to different light colors [1]. Experiments clearly show that beginning at
the lowest detectable light levels, the rods provide all the sensory information. At
a fairly low light intensity, the rods saturate, and the remaining response of the
eye is carried by the cones [1]. For normal ultrasonic TV displays, the rods are
saturated, and the cones carry the gray-scale information from the image.

Between the sensory cells and the optic-nerve ganglion cells are the bipolar
cells, conveying the sensory information to the more posterior portions of the
retina (Figure 16-2). In a strict input sense, the light-sensing data are conveyed
from sensory cell to bipolar cell to ganglion cell and finally to the optic nerve.

But the real sophistication of the retina comes from its horizontal organization
and the communications among the different cells. Close to the sensory cells are
the horizontal cells, communicating among both sensory cells and bipolar cells
and linking both rod and cone response together. At a second level of horizontal
interconnections are the amacrine cells that communicate among the ganglion
connections between bipolar cells and ganglion cells [1].

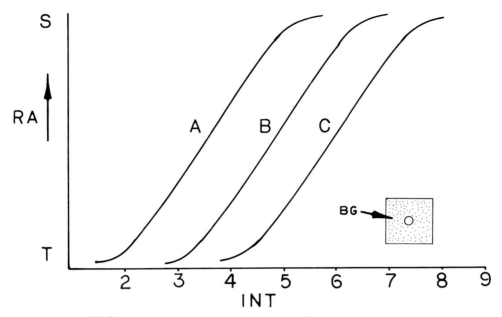

16-3   Adaptive processes of the eye. Measuring the sensing response of the eye shows that it adapts to background intensity levels *(BG)* over a range of about 9 logarithmic units *(INT)*. Within any adapted level, the response of the eye *(RA)* spans about 3 logarithmic units. Movement of the response curves from *A* to *B* to *C* represents an increase in the background field surrounding a small bright dot. *T* is a threshold value, *S* is saturation. By adapting to a wide range of light levels, the eye becomes a relative light sensor, and not an absolute light-intensity sensor.

Curiously, all these structures face toward the posterior of the eye, which means that light reaching the sensors must pass through the optic nerves and retinal cells to finally reach the sensors. This portion of the sclera that is in intimate contact with the sensors is covered on the inside with dark cells to absorb light entering the eye that comes from regions away from the optical pathway to the retina [1].

The nerves within the optic system operate over a functional range of about 100 to 1 [1]. The input range of the eye, on the other hand, is much larger, so the first function of the retina is to compress the incoming light range to 100 to 1. To do this, the retinal cells respond to the general input intensity, adjusting their center of operation to an adapted light level. This response is shown in Figure 16-3, where the range of the individual cells is about 3 or more logarithmic units. The eye simply moves this response curve up or down the overall input light level. Clearly, the adaptation of the eye makes it unable to measure in absolute terms the light intensities reaching the retina.

Because the retinal cells are generally very small, few of them can be examined for electrical activity by placing a microelectrode inside the cell. The ganglion cells, however, are larger cells and do accept microelectrodes for the purpose of investigating the response of individual cells to various patterns of illumination [1]. Because of the interconnection of cells through the horizontal and amacrine

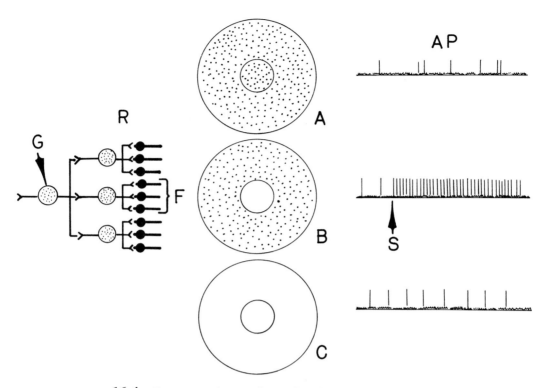

16-4 Response of a ganglion cell to its receptive field stimulation. A ganglion cell *G* receives convergent information from many sensory cells *(R)*, but the cells are organized to respond maximally to an approprite stimulus on the collection of sensory cells, called the ganglion cell receptive field. Part A shows a constantly dark illumination, and the response is a few action potentials *(AP)*. Part B shows an "on" center and an "off" surround that stimulates the ganglion cell to maximum. The stimulus is applied at *S*. Part C shows a low-grade response to a solid illumination.

cells, a single ganglion cell responds to more than a single point of light on the interconnected sensor cell. The pattern of light that causes a maximum response from a ganglion cell is called the receptive field for that cell [3]. The receptive field for the ganglion cell is anything but simple. A great deal of signal organization occurs at the retinal level.

It is interesting to note that the ganglion cell responds well neither to a point of light on one of the sensory cells with which it communicates with, nor to diffuse light over the whole retina [4]. Instead, the cell responds to a specific pattern of light encompassing the sensory cells that are directly or indirectly connected to the ganglion cell. This pattern comprises the visual field for the cell.

The preferred visual field is a circular pattern of light with a small area of "on" in the center of an "off" surround [1, 4]. Some light patterns and specific responses for each pattern are shown in Figure 16-4. As might be expected, along with the "on"-center "off"-surround cells are other cells that respond to "off" centers and "on" surrounds [4].

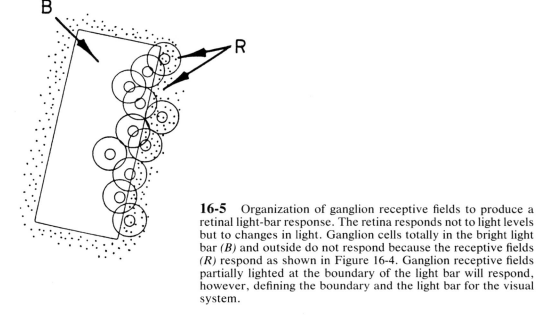

16-5 Organization of ganglion receptive fields to produce a retinal light-bar response. The retina responds not to light levels but to changes in light. Ganglion cells totally in the bright light bar *(B)* and outside do not respond because the receptive fields *(R)* respond as shown in Figure 16-4. Ganglion receptive fields partially lighted at the boundary of the light bar will respond, however, defining the boundary and the light bar for the visual system.

The complexity of the responses grows as other cells in the visual cortex respond specifically to bars of light in various orientations and motion patterns on the retina [5]. The bar-of-light response can be understood by adding together a group of smaller ganglion receptive fields. An example of this summation of smaller fields is shown in Figure 16-5. But the response becomes even more complicated as the orientation of the bar on the retina and its direction of motion begin to determine the cellular response as well [5]. The results of numerous studies support the finding that the eye is most sensitive to motion and boundary information. This fact will be even more evident when we look at whole-organ responses [6].

Of course, the image that falls on the retina is an analogue replication of the outside world, but once inside the retina, this simple relationship of image components is lost in the encoding and enhancement that ensues. The information reaching the optic nerve thus looks nothing like the image, and when it reaches the brain, it is not mapped onto the brain in a one-to-one correspondence. Nevertheless, the brain still does not lose the sense of color, relative intensity, or spatial orientation of the image elements [6, 7]. The eye and brain can be fooled by optical illusions, but this fact offers little justification for holding the data transfer to the brain in suspicion. Rather, optical illusions provide a chance to understand the limits of visual information transfer. Once in the brain, the encoding continues with the segmentation and the channeling of data. The visual information seems to be broken up into separate channels to handle different rates of gray-scale change, motion, and spatial orientation of image elements [4, 8]. Many experiments have been designed to separate one channel's operation from another, with the result that our overall perception of visual events has been expanded.

Whole-Organ Measurements and Reactions

Measurements of the visual system clearly show that although we are looking at gray-scale images with image elements ranging from black to white, the images are bright enough so that the rods are completely saturated. We are using the color portion of the visual system, (the cones) to see ultrasound images. The remainder of our discussion will thus consider gray-scale levels as colors rather than intensities.

One of the first measurements of the visual system was its full range of perceived light. From the faintest just-perceived intensity to just less than the threshold for pain, the eye spans a phenomenal 10 logarithmic units. As noted earlier in the chapter, this represents the adapting range of the retina. The response at any fixed light level is over 3 logarithmic units.

Within any of the adapted light levels, the questions are really: How small a change in contrast can the eye perceive? What are the conditions under which we can expect to see such a transition in color? And how many shades of gray can be perceived in the image gray-color mix?

The methods of measuring contrast sensitivity involve presenting the eye with a fixed level of light and then changing the luminance of a small portion of the visual field by a small amount, ΔL [3]. The fixed light level, L, can come from a circle or a square that occupys a large portion of the retina. Within this field, a smaller rectangle or circle changes a small amount in luminance. The response can be measured subjectively by asking the viewing person to verbally indicate whether or not he or she can see the new intensity [10]. The response can also be assessed by measuring the whole brain-evoked response resulting from any change in the light field [10]. All these measurements place one intensity field in contrast with another, with no intervening lines or other patterns. In more complicated measurements, these other conditions are added to determine special visual characteristics.

Another technique often used employs a set of light and dark lines or bars next to one another [10]. These bars can be changed in contrast and size, and can be stationary or moving. This technique is used to separate contrast-sensing mechanisms from motion-detecting mechanisms in the visual system [8].

One of the earliest reported experiments with whole-eye contrast response was conducted in 1868 [11]. The investigators Konig and Brodhund, graphed their results as a ratio of $\Delta L/L$ against the background luminance, L. The results are shown in Figure 16-6. As the background luminance increased, the absolute change in luminance required to see a contrast change increased at the same time. The fraction, $\Delta L/L$, however, decreased with increasing background luminance. In other words, the relative sensitivity of the eye to contrast improved with increasing light levels. At a medium level of intensity, the contrast sensitivity leveled out, finally becoming independent of the background light level. This fraction yields a discrimination value of about 0.025. In other senses including the eye, this sort of discrimination value turns out to be about 0.1 or less over constant regions of

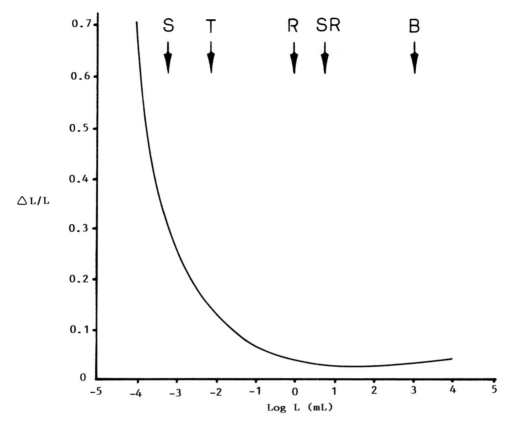

16-6   Earliest Published Data on Whole Eye Contrast Response. Konig and Brodhund published the first measured response of the whole eye to contrast as a function of background brightness in 1889. X-axis is the background brightness in millilumens. Contrast was measured by comparing the change in illumination of the spot in the center of the background field, ΔL to the background illumination, L. The characteristic curve was later called Weber's Law. As the brightness of the background increased, the relative sensitivity of the eye increased. The best value was 0.025. Along the top of the graph are some typical light levels for reference. *S* is starlight; *T* is twilight; *R* is good reading light; *SR* is sunrise; *B* is bright sunlight. From Brown, J.L.; Mueller, C.G.: Brightness Discrimination and Brightness Contrast, in *Vision and Visual Perception,* C.H. Graham, Ed., John Wiley & Sons, New York, 1965, p215.

operation [11]. This ability to discriminate and grade a sensory input was summarized into a sensory law of activity by Ernst Heinrich Weber in 1834 [11]. We now know this to be a general principle of sensory activity, because it is not exact enough to still be called a law.

With improved measurement techniques and experiments that have been better formulated to test specific components of eye function, the threshold for contrast published in 1868 has improved considerably. Values of 0.002 to 0.005 are possible under the right conditions, and values of 0.003 are possible using black-and-white gratings [10, 11]. In addition, the use of gratings to measure and evaluate visual function began to provide new data on visual discrimination processes.

At the heart of understanding what the grating experiments mean is a new concept of frequency called *spatial frequency*. We can form a set of black-and-white bands in which the change in color from white to black changes in a sinusoidal fashion; if we plot the relative intensities of light and dark regions with distance, we would find that the intensities change like a wave. When the image of this grating is projected on the retina, a light and dark pattern forms that can be expressed in terms of the number of light and dark cycles contained in each degree that the image subtends on the retina [10]. This forms the basis of the spatial frequency concept, expressed in units of cycles per degree.

Experiments with stationary gratings show that at the optimum spatial frequency, the contrast threshold for the eye is about 0.003 of the maximum contrast, which has a value of 1.0 [10]. When the grating contrast is further reduced, the differences cannot be perceived. But when the grating is moved, the movement *is* perceived [8]. Thus, two visual contrast thresholds exist, one for a stationary grating and a smaller one for the moving grating [8]. This difference in sensitivity is experienced daily by the echocardiographer who looks at the real-time image of the heart and follows the heart's boundary dynamics, only to lose these same boundaries when the image is frozen. A stationary real-time image needs a much-better signal-to-noise ratio than the same image moving in real time. In terms of visual system physiology, these observations indicate that the mechanisms used to detect motion are different from the mechanisms used to detect contrast, and that motion detection operates at a much lower threshold than does simple contrast detection [8].

The grating experiments also show another unexpected property of the eye, which is that contrast sensing is a function of the spatial frequency of the grating. Above and below a preferred spatial frequency, the ability to detect contrast differences begins to fall off. The spatial frequency best suited for detecting contrast turns out to be about 3 cycles per degree, with the contrast changing over a simple sine function [10]. In this situation, as we learned earlier, the contrast sensitivity reaches a value of 0.003 of the maximum contrast.

The spatial frequencies of an image are often fixed by the physical characteristics of the image. As a result of these fixed characteristics and the preferred spatial frequencies of the visual system, the viewing distance from an image can affect the ability to see contrast. An example of this is shown in Figure 16-7. In Figure 16-7, the spatial frequency changes horizontally and the contrast changes vertically. At spatial frequencies too high and too low, the ability to see the contrast falls off rapidly. When the image is viewed from a greater distance, say 4 feet, the higher spatial frequencies become less visible and the lower spatial frequencies become more visible. These same rules will apply to picking out changes in gray scale representing normal and abnormal tissue differences in an ultrasound image. Just how small the image reduction is with a multiformat camera, as well as our viewing distance from the image, will affect our ability to keep all the spatial frequencies contained in the image within the range of preferred spatial frequencies for the visual system.

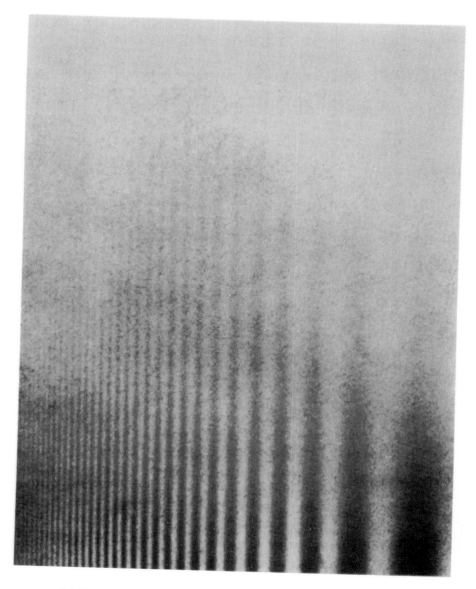

16-7 Sinusoidal grating with varying contrast and spatial frequency. The contrast decreases from the bottom to the top of the image and is constant along any horizontal line across the spatial frequencies, which decrease from left to right. Notice the loss of contrast sensitivity at low and high spatial frequencies with visible contrast reaching higher for the middle frequencies. From Campbell, F.W. and Maffei, L.: Contrast and Spatial Frequency. Scientific American 231 (November, 1974), 106–114.

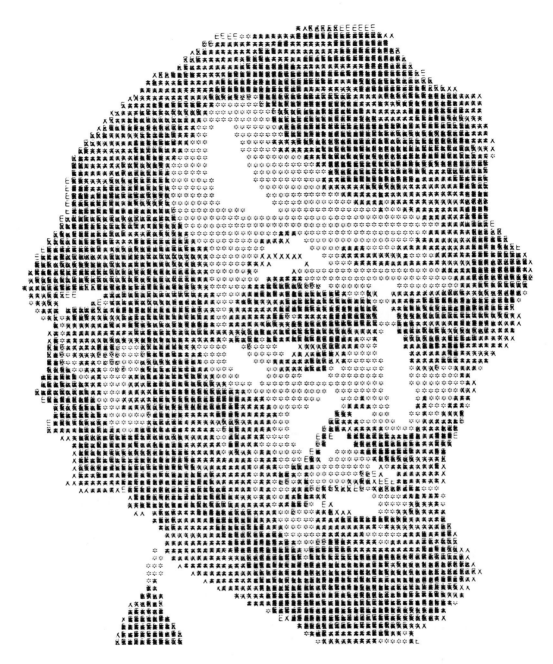

16-8 An example of high spatial frequency aliasing. Viewed close, the characteristics of the figure are hard to see. From a distance, the high spatial frequencies that make up the letters cannot be seen, but the lower spatial frequencies also present in the image are better seen.

Under the right conditions, the clinical information in the image will be carried in the lower spatial frequencies, although the image is made up of components with higher spatial frequencies. The high contrast of the higher spatial frequencies also contributes to an "aliasing" process in which the higher-frequency information dominates the eye in the image, hiding the lower-frequency information. The classic example of this is an image formed by a computer or other printing device using typed letters and other symbols (an example is shown in Figure 16-8). This high-frequency aliasing can be removed by viewing the image from a greater distance or by blurring the image slightly. This was a common problem when the digital scan converter first appeared on the B-scanner. The pixels were large enough to form images with high spatial frequencies. These images were disagreeable, however, to sonographers and sonologists used to the smooth images from the analog scan converter. The solution to this problem was to introduce a means of "blurring" the image, either by limiting the passband of the video to the display monitor or by putting a "smoothing" algorithm in the scan converter controller that would smooth out many of the high spatial frequencies [12].

High spatial frequencies at boundaries produce another phenomenon first observed by Mach in 1865 [3, 13] and known since as Mach bands. These bands appear at the sharp boundaries between one gray color and another. At the boundary, the lighter color appears to become lighter and the darker color appears darker. The greater the contrast at the boundary, the greater are the Mach bands, both in width and intensity [3]. This is a form of contrast enhancement carried out by the eye, beginning at the retinal level, to improve the definition of the boundary. These Mach bands are easily visible in the gray bar patterns displayed by most scan converters. A sample gray bar appears in Figure 16-9.

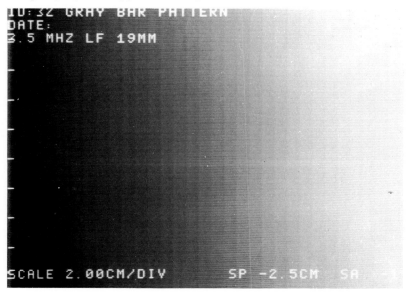

16-9 A 32-step gray bar spanning the display. This gray bar covers the 40-dB video dynamic range evenly, with each intensity representing 1.25-dB signal separations.

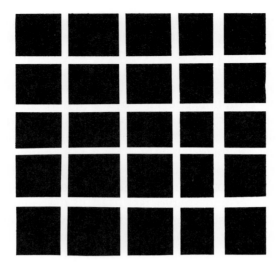

16-10 White-on-black Hermann grid. The Hermann grid is an optical illusion that shows how surrounding intensities influence a center intensity. Looking at the center of the grid will make each of the white-stripe intersections appear gray. Focusing on a single intersection causes the illusion to disappear at that particular intersection. The different white-stripe dimensions and black-square dimensions show independence of size for the illusion.

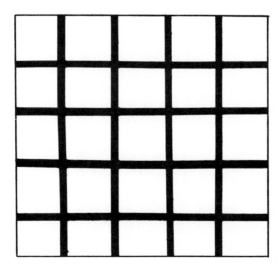

16-11 Black-on-white Hermann grid. In this illusion, the black stripes appear gray at the intersections (lighter), and the illusion disappears when focusing on any particular intersection in the center of the visual field.

The appearance of a particular gray color has been shown time and again to be a function of the surrounding colors [13, 14]. Moreover, the difference in contrast is more than an absolute difference and is enhanced by surrounding cues [6, 7, 14]. This becomes more evident when we discuss the adjacency principle. Let us look first at the "two-dimensional problem."

Often the change in apparent gray-scale color is so subtle that it requires a logical paradox or optical illusion to illustrate the point. One of the best is the Hermann grid, which shows how white can become gray while changing nothing in the image (Figure 16-10). In Figure 16-10, at the intersection of the white lines, the eye casts the white color to an intermediate gray. This occurs in the peripheral portions of the image and not along the center of the visual axis. Thus, the color of an intersection changes depending on its location on the retina and surrounding dark area. Those portions of the white lines surrounded symmetrically with dark areas produce the change in color, whereas the incompletely surrounded portions of the white line do not. The same principles apply for the white-on-black situation shown in Figure 16-11, in which dark strips now become lighter.

But other properties of the image begin to determine just what a perceived color is interpreted to be. For example, a black-and-white photo of a room or hall with variations in intensity will be correctly interpreted according to color despite the rather complex mix of gray colors from changes in illumination. If the change in color is interpreted by the brain as a change in illumination, the shaded and illuminated portions will be integrated to be the same color [6]. If, however, the different colors are seen to be in a common plane, then they are interpreted to result from changes in primary intensity, and contrast enhancement will occur [6]. In other words, the adjacent cues in the image will control how the brain interprets changes in gray color. Two small fields of gray adjacent to one another will appear more contrasting if they are viewed in a more contrasting background [13]. Adjacent grays will not appear substantially different if they are "thought" to be changes in illumination.

The cues for evaluating grays become so important and persuasive that a gray patch can appear white or black, depending entirely on the context in which it is viewed, without changing its own absolute color. The physical arrangement of this experiment is shown in Figure 16-12. When the horizontal tab is seen as part of a three-dimensional corner, the color seems continuous with a lighter color and is interpreted visually to be a shadow and not a primary intensity change [6]. In this context, the tab appears white. When the same tab appears to be in a plane with the same level of intensities, the tab becomes black as part of the contrast-sensing process [6]. It is clear from these results that although we might be able to see a large number of colors within an adaptive range, we are unable to assign an absolute value to any because of the dependence on surrounding cues. This is what is considered a color-dependent *adjacency principle*.

But the adjacency principle extends beyond simple stationary relationships. How things appear to move also is influenced by the movement of surrounding cues [14]. A number of classic optical illusions demonstrate our inability to reference motion in an absolute sense. We are, in fact, *relative* viewers, that is, we

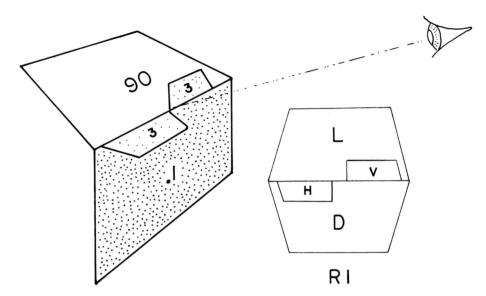

16-12   Changing gray scale with dimensiional cues. This experiment involves a configuration of tabs that have the same gray intensity but change from black to white, depending upon viewing the cues as two- or three-dimensional figures. The upper panel has a relative reflectance of 90; the lower panel is 0.1; the tabs are 3. The tabs are set vertically *(V)* and horizontally *(H)*. When viewed with one eye the horizontal tab looks white and the vertical tab looks dark. Viewed with both eyes, the horizontal tab will appear dark and the vertical tab will appear light. With one eye, the spatial cues are two-dimensional; with both eyes, the spatial cues are three-dimensional.

always reference our visual experience to other things in the visual field. This provides a remarkable range of visual perception without imposing an extraordinary physiology on the visual system.

Many aspects of the visual system carry a symmetry of activity or anatomy. We could ask if this applies also to our perception of gray colors. Do we see things differently in the form of white-on-black versus black-on-white? Based on the results of some simple images and cellular-level measurements, we do not see black-on-white and white-on-black the same way [6, 9, 11, 13]. For example, a white object on a black background appears physically larger and brighter than the same object now black but placed on the same-intensity white background [11, 13]. And measurements at the cellular level also show the same sort of difference [15]. At the cellular level, the visual system seems to handle a wider range of colors when presented as black-on-white than white-on-black. These cellular measurements are shown in Figure 6-13. And this visual process seems to extend even to the "spot in a void" problem, where a white object set in a black "void" must go through very large changes in intensity to produce a change in the visual system [7].

Having now described these unconnected events, we now need to draw some general rules about vision and data transfer.

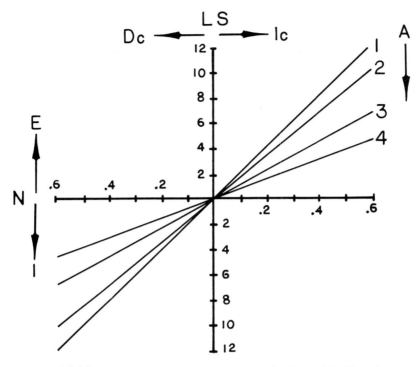

16-13 Changing Dynamic Range of the Eye with Changing Presentation. Cells within the geniculate nucleus respond in a graded way to diffuse light flashes that are different from an adapted background level. The X-axis shows the relative amount of shift in light intensity (LS) in relative log units as the light increments *(IC)* and decrements *(DC)*. On the Y-axis is the firing rate for the geniculate neurons in impulses/second *(N)*, *E* follows excititory responses. I are inhibitory responses. Curves 1, 2, 3, and 4 represent decreasing adaptive luminances. the changing slopes on the curves show the decreasing response range of the eye with dimmer adapting light levels. The dynamic range of the eye improves with brighter adaptive background levels. From Poggio, G.F.: Central Neural Mechanisms in Vision, in *Medical Physiology,* V.B. Mountcastle Ed., The C.V. Mosby Company, St. Louis, 1974; replotted from data by Jacobs, G.H.: Effects of Adaptation on the Lateral Geniculate Response to Light Increment and Decrement, J. Opt. Soc. Am. 55 (1965) 1535.

Preferred Modes of Data Transfer

One of the early applications of preferred data transfer involved the smoothing of digital images to decrease the high spatial-frequency aliasing. Some monitors offer a focus adjustment that can improve the harsh-appearing images produced by some uncorrected scan converters. Most scan converters, however, have employed a digital technique to smooth out the image and prevent the high frequencies from interfering with the information contained in the lower spatial frequencies.

Still, the adjacency principle on static images applies, indicating a need to recognize that the apparent gray color for any echo signal is a function of the surrounding signals. And gray-scale information can disappear in an image that creates cues suggesting a three-dimensional image with changing illumination rather than color. Masking out portions of the surrounding image can often change the apparent gray intensities dramatically.

Images in which we seek to draw information on boundaries and architecture might be better presented white-on-black. The subjectively larger boundaries and shallower contrast sensing can make overall architecture more apparent. On the other hand, textural information is conveyed in a major way through the gray scale of an image. Here a black-on-white image can offer the best chance of seeing the small changes in color that provide information on subtle tissue qualities. In this mode, the relative sensitivity of the eye can be improved by increasing the background intensity within the capabilities of the display monitor.

But along with appreciating the processes within the visual system is a need to minimize machine design limitations that would limit the capabilities of the visual system. Gray-scale images with 8 or 16 grays offer so many chances for subjective gray-scale contouring that they cannot be fully trusted. At least 32 or more grays are needed to show the real variations in gray across an image, as well as to handle the variations among signal levels without the risk of subjective contouring. Indeed, those relationships have been well known by those dealing with pulse code modulation of images prior to 1966 [16].

Conclusion

The eye is not an absolute intensity sensor. It is, rather, a contrast sensor and handles unreferenced intensity information poorly. To return to questions asked at the beginning of this chapter: Can the eye see more than 10 shades of gray? Yes, but the eye cannot measure these gray intensities in an absolute sense. Each apparent gray level will be a function of its surrounding intensities and where it appears on the retina. Measurement of absolute signal levels requires stable post-processing that can help the sonographer define like echo signals in the image and thereby determine the presence of unlike echo signals associated with anatomy and disease. How many shades of gray can the eye see? If we depend upon the smallest discriminable step within the functional range of the retina (normalized for a given background intensity), some experimental numbers appear as: 35 for background intensities less than 10^{-4} cd/m^2 about 185 steps for intermediate levels; and perhaps 1,000 for intensities near 5×10^4 cd/m^2 [11]. For the typical video display, it may be in the range of 100. Thus, a digital display carrying only 16 gray levels hardly matches the functional range of the eye.

When does the video inverse switch become valuable? It begins with a balanced video system that does not change intensity values of grays when the display mode changes from white-on-black to black-on-white. Images look different black-on-white and vice versa, each containing the same information but presenting it to the visual system differently. A look at an intensity-reversed image can often alter the appearance of image elements enough to form a confirmation or a denial of suspicious patterns. White-on-black should be used for boundary information and black-on-white for textural information. It is important not to limit one mode over the other. Whereas using both modes will not hide information, using only one increases the possibility of the user missing information.

We often think we can see motion in an absolute sense, but, clearly, we cannot. This raises doubts about using real-time images as accurate evaluations of dynamic structures like the heart. Complex motion appears even more complex and often incompletely in a complex signal mix. The degree to which this poses a problem in a real-time image will become evident when less-subjective motion analyzers evaluate the real-time image.

In the end, it appears that we see a great deal. But like other senses, we are often guided by what we expect to see rather than by what is really present. We still see what we look for, and look for what we know.

References

1. Werblin, F.S. January 1973. The control of sensitivity in the retina. Scientific American 228:71–79.
2. Hess, E.H. November 1975. The role of pupil size in communications. Scientific American 233:110–119.
3. Brown, J.L., and C.G. Mueller. 1965. Brightness discrimination and brightness contrast. In Vision and visual perception, ed. C.H. Graham. New York: John Wiley & Sons.
4. Barlow, H.B., and W.R. Levick. 1965. The mechanisms of directionally selective units in rabbit's retina. J Physiol 178:477–504.
5. Hubel, D.H., and T.N. Wiesel. 1962. Receptive fields, binocular interaction and functional architecture in the cat's visual cortex. J Physiol:106–154.
6. Gilchrist, A.L. March 1979. The perception of surface blacks and whites. Scientific American 240:112–124.
7. Land, E.H. December 1977. The retinex theory of color vision. Scientific American 237:108–128.
8. Sekuler, R., and E. Levinson. January 1977. The perception of moving targets. Scientific American 236:60–73.
9. Graham, C.H. 1965. Some fundamental data. In Vision and visual perception, ed. C.H. Graham. New York: John Wiley & Sons.
10. Campbell, F.W., and L. Maffei. November 1974. Contrast and spatial frequency. Scientific American 231:106–114.
11. LeGrand, Y. 1968. Luminance difference thresholds. Chap. 11 in Light, color, and vision. London: Chapman Hall, 1968.
12. Ophir, J. and N.F. Maklad. April 1979. Digital scan converters in diagnostic ultrasound imaging. Proc IEEE 67:654–664.

13. Hering, E. 1964. Outlines of a theory of light sense. Chapter 5, Cambridge: Harvard University Press.
14. Gogel, W.C. May 1978. The adjacency principle in visual perception. Scientific American 238:126–139.
15. Mountcastle, V.B. 1968. Medical physiology, vol. 2, 1613, 12th ed. Saint Louis: C.V. Mosby Co.
16. Mayo, J.S. March 1966. Pulse code modulation. Scientific American 218:103–108.
17. Bloom, W. and D.W. Fawcett. 1968. A textbook of histology, 776. Philadelphia: W.B. Saunders Co.

Chapter 17

Making Real Time Work for You

A look in any of the current buyers guides on diagnostic ultrasound shows a wide array of real-time sonographs on the market. Some move the ultrasound beam mechanically, others move the beam electronically, and still others combine both techniques. Despite the variations in beam movement, however, real time uses a common set of principles to achieve the uniform objective of moving the ultrasound beam automatically and presenting to the sonographer a constantly refreshed ultrasound image.

In the hands of an experienced sonographer, real time appears fast and therefore easy. Experience shows, however, that real time is not easy. It simply shifts the information required of the sonographer into another domain. Instead of requiring the user to be adept at physically scanning with the transducer, real time calls for well-developed imaging in order to correctly place the real-time scanhead and quickly evaluate the image contents. Real time *is* fast, but when improperly handled, fast can mean missed information, poorly adjusted TGCs, inappropriate preprocessing, unused postprocessing, and incomplete imaging information. The sonographer operating a real-time machine must, among other things, be able to adjust the machine according to the tissue presentations, scan all of the organs presented, and provide a complete set of pictures for the attending physician.

This chapter endeavors to provide users with an organized approach to the application of real-time sonography, while also conveying the notion that the concepts of good and fast are not necessarily mutually exclusive.

The Real Limitations of Real Time

One of the first and more obvious needs of real-time systems is a larger signal-to-noise ratio than exists in the typical B-scanner. The B-scanner has the ability to select the largest signal presented for any location on the display, often obtained over several pulse-listen cycles. In contrast, the real-time machine must acquire information from a single pulse-listen cycle for any line of sight in the image. To overcome this signal-to-noise ratio limitation, many real-time sonographs use a higher transmitted power than that in an equivalent B-scanner.

The frame rate in a real-time sonograph is limited by the round-trip time of the ultrasound within the tissues. This relationship involves a compromise among parameters such as the frame rate, the number of lines within a frame, and the depth of the display. Because of the trade-offs inherent in the compromise, the real-time image is not infinitely flexible. Many sonographs use different weightings among these parameters to obtain different functional goals. For example, high-resolution images of the abdomen often forgo frame rate. On the other hand, high frame rates are needed to portray heart motion in echocardiography, and therefore, use fewer lines to make an image.

Along with limited frame rates and short display depths, the field of view of a real-time device is not as large as that in the B-scanner. The small field of view in real time results from the fixed angle the beam is allowed to scan through, and the inability of the machine to show more than the current scanning area at any one time. By contrast, the lower pulse-repetition frequency and larger memory of the static B-scanner permit compound scanning and large fields of view.

Because the real-time scanning plane is free to move in any direction in space, the image is not referenced to any particular position on the body, as is often the case with the static B-scanner. This positional freedom for the transducer and the scanning sequence represents a basic problem in real-time scanning. A common question in the reading room is: "Where am I looking?" To help solve this problem, many real-time systems provide annotation of the image either through single-key "call-ups" on the screen along with the final image or through audio annotation on a videotape during the examination. Some even use a scanning arm like the static B-scanner.

The scanning angle in a real-time device is fixed; therefore, a single transducer position seldom includes all the boundaries of an organ or lesion, especially if the area of interest is comparatively large. Complete examinations often mean moving the transducer in a dynamic way to provide a complete presentation of the patient to the sonographer and sonologist. To a newcomer, this freedom of real-time imaging can create unusual and often unexpected difficulties.

Once the limitations of real time are understood, the sonographer can construct a framework of problems to solve. As described below, most of these limitations can be overcome by applying a consistent examination protocol.

Imaging Goals for Real Time

The operating objectives of a real-time system are the same as those for the B-scanner: To image the interior of the body and determine size, shape, position, texture, and, in addition, the dynamics of the internal organs. Sonographic activities that distort any aspect of this information can ultimately defeat the attainment of reliable imaging results. The section following discusses each of these elements in more detail.

Determining Size

Determining the size of an organ requires an image large enough to include the lesion and the organ under investigation. A look at many of the single-pass scans for the static B-scanner shows that a field of view on the order of 15 cm to 25 cm is typical and consistent with the largest fields of view found in many real-time systems.

Determining Shape

Determining shape requires a depiction of the organ or lesion boundaries. The quality of any real-time depiction should be such that depicted boundaries can be separated into smooth or rough. This will also require changing the acoustical window to permit several different views of the lesion.

Determining Position

The position of an organ or lesion is ultimately based on knowing the position of the transducer beam in space. Normally, structures are located with respect to external anatomy or in relation to internal structures that are readily identified during the examination. Any single image may not be understandable without landmarks within the image and indications on the film or records of the actual position of the transducer. The freedom of the transducer that is the essence of real time, however, makes external landmarks all but useless, forcing the user to rely totally on the internal landmarks.

Depicting Texture

Depicting the ultrasound image texture well enough to separate visually many organs and lesions requires a wide input dynamic range for the sonograph and more than 16 gray levels at the display. Few real-time systems exceed 16 gray levels, and most depend heavily on variable preprocessing to display texture adequately. The displayed texture is also influenced by the sampling rate of the digital scan converter within the sonograph. Accurate portrayal of textural information permits a dissection among slightly different tissues within the same organ as well as the recognition of differences among organs in the image.

Depicting Motion

A single-element M-mode sonograph can have a high pulse-repetition frequency, allowing an accurate portrayal of rapid motion. Depicting the dynamics of an organ in real time requires a frame rate high enough to sample adequately the motion that is involved. Trade-offs, as noted earlier, determine the applications of many real-time machines. For example, echocardiography needs rapid frame rates to depict valve motion, whereas abdominal scanning can succeed with much lower frame rates.

Having identified imaging goals of size, shape, position, texture and dynamics, let us now examine how to use the sonograph to attain each of them.

Organizing Transducer Movement

The first requirement is to understand the scan plane relative to the physical dimensions and architecture of the real-time scanhead. All scanhead movement can be thought of in terms of moving and positioning this scan plane. There are four major ways to move the scan plane. Each movement should be performed separately in the beginning; then all the movements can be integrated into rapid combinations when manual positioning skills improve.

Before discussing each of these types of movement, it should be pointed out that knowing where the scan plane is positioned both in space and within the body requires a scanning protocol that keeps the positional information delivered to the sonologist in the correct order. Such a protocol not only shortens the time required for delivery of information to the sonologist, but also speeds up the total examination time by providing additional assurances that the examination is complete.

The first type of motion is called *angling the scan plane*. This motion basically angles the scan plane from a constant position on the surface of the body. The motion can be achieved by gently rocking the transducer on the surface of the body and sweeping the scan plane through a large sector, as shown in Figure 17-1.

The second form of scan plane motion involves *rotating the scan plane* about a central axis. This motion can be depicted by visualizing a central axis that passes down through the shape of the scan as well as through the center of the transducer scanhead assembly. The operator simply rotates the scanning plane about this axis, as shown in Figure 17-2.

The third form of motion requires moving the *scanning pattern within the scanning plane* in a linear fashion, as shown in Figure 17-3. In a linear array, this requires sliding the array over the surface of the body along the axis of the array. A sector scanner, on the other hand, is slid along the skin, holding the direction and angle constant, with only the contact surface moving in a linear fashion over the surface of the body.

The fourth type of motion requires *angling the scanning segment within the scan plane*. This maneuver is much easier to perform with a sector scanner than with a linear array. The motion requires the sonographer to rotate the scanning segment within the scan plane but without moving the contact point on the surface of the body, as shown in Figure 17-4. Normally, the large dimensions of the linear array make this motion prohibitive.

Although these movements are easy to do, each depends on an understanding of the presented anatomy; thus the normal anatomy should be kept in mind for each movement.

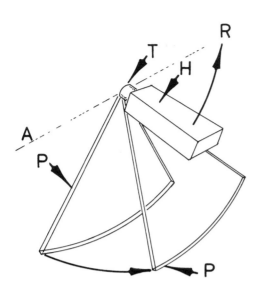

17-1 Rotating the scan plane perpendicular to the plane. The first rotating motion of a real-time scan head is in a plane perpendicular to the scan plane P. T is the transducer; H is the scan-head housing; R is the direction of rotation; A is the axis of rotation.

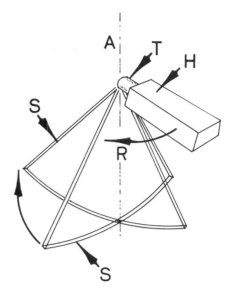

17-2 Rotating the scan plane about an in-plane axis. The second rotating motion of a real-time scan head is about an axis A, within the scan plane S. T is the transducer; H is the scan-head housing; R is the direction of rotation.

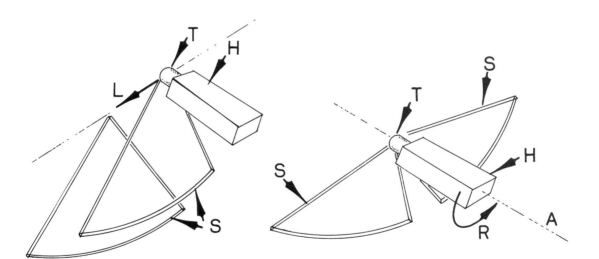

17-3 Linear displacement of the scan plane. The third form of scan-plane movement is a linear displacement that introduces no rotating motion. L is the linear motion line; T is the transducer; H is the scan head housing; S is the scan plane.

17-4 Rotating the scan plane about the scan-head central axis. The fourth form of scan-plane motion is to rotate the scan plane about the scan-head central axis. S is the scan plane; T is the transducer; H is the scan-head housing; A is the axis of rotation; R is the direction of rotation.

A Real-Time Examination Protocol

The purpose of any examination protocol is to help ensure that all the desired information is obtained during an examination. Without a well-established procedural pattern, the surprises offered by some presentations can easily divert the sonographer's attention from the task at hand. A carefully considered protocol, on the other hand, can enable all the needed data to be acquired, while still affording additional time to examine carefully any unusual presentations.

As an example of an effective real-time protocol, an upper-abdominal real-time examination is described below.

Before picking up the transducer, the user must be able to answer the following questions: What is the exam? What is the clinical question? and Why is it being asked? The answers to these questions come from the exam request form, the patient history, the results of previous tests, and the results of any previous ultrasound exams.

We will separate the protocol into two parts: first, the survey, and, second, the specific scans for detailed imaging information.

The Survey

Regardless of the final scanning sequence, the survey routine is the same for every patient. The survey begins with a survey scanhead, if one is available. The survey scanhead is usually a medium-frequency, medium-focus transducer system, providing penetration over the entire field of view. In performing the survey, we will use the same image-quality elements as in the static B-scanner (see Chapter 19).

A proper examination sequence takes on extra importance when the exam is being videotaped. A poorly sequenced examination on a videotape is almost impossible to interpret later. Voice-over explanations, along with a running commentary on the tape and image labels, are essential to determine where any single image is located in the abdomen.

The survey begins in the midline, in the true midsagittal plane. We set the TGC for the transducer and change the system response (transmitter power or system gain) for adequate penetration over the field of view.

The first observation to make is the size and position, both internal and external, of the left lobe of the liver. It may be a good idea to mark the lower edge of the liver on the patient's skin with a water-soluble pen. With no scan-arm references to come back to, the mark provides a good external reference.

We continue the survey by first moving to the patient's right, always keeping parallel to the sagittal plane. This enables a regular view of organ size, the relationships among organs, and the dynamics of each organ and great vessels. After surveying right, we begin at the midline and survey left, again maintaining the scan plane parallel with the sagittal plane. The result is a complete survey of the whole upper abdomen.

The next step is to change the scanning plane transversely to the sagittal plane and resurvey the upper abdomen. In these scans, we look in detail for:

1. The size of organs and vessels.
2. The angle of the boundaries.
3. The shape of organs and vessels.
4. The relationships among organs.
5. The positions of organs and boundaries relative to internal landmarks and to the external mark on the skin for specific scans that will follow. We will have to watch the patient's breathing through the exam, which can displace organs and lesions through the breathing cycle.
6. The changes in texture, such as the spatial separation of texture dots and the amplitude of textural components; and localized changes in attenuation rate to form enhancement or shadowing.
7. Artifacts common to real time and specific to this patient.
8. Any specific organ and vessel dynamics.

The survey provides more than a calibration of organ size, shape, and position, however. It offers a good mental three-dimensional image of the organs and their positions among one another, and sets the stage for the specific scans that follow.

Regardless of the scanning techniques used, we must always be aware of where the scanning plane is pointing and what anatomy we should see at that angle. If we fail to see the expected anatomy, the immediate question should be: Why not?

From the survey, we try to draw a specific set of conclusions or data about the patient that in turn suggest objectives for the next level of scanning. Before proceeding to scan for specifics, the following questions should be answered:

1. What specifics are to be scanned in more detail?
2. What transducer changes, if any, are needed?
3. What new patient positions are needed?
4. What new transducer scanning angles are needed?

Having determined the answers to these questions, we are now ready to scan the patient for specific imaging.

Scanning for Specifics

In scanning for specifics, a general real-time protocol should be kept in mind. First, scanning for specifics without landmarks can yield disappointing results when the images are later examined. Few things can grow as cold as real-time images without references. Therefore, the solution is to scan so as to have one or more internal references always within the image. These references can include structures such as the aorta, the inferior vena cava, the superior mesenteric artery, the superior mesenteric vein, portal veins, and the diaphragm. We also need to keep any anatomical references on a common base; thus, the patient's head or right-hand side always appears on the image left.

Second, in the heat of scanning, it is easy to forget the elements of image quality that help ensure that all the possible clinical information appears in the image. The goal is to illustrate the clinical problem through imaging. Each imaging sequence provides information on anatomy, which is what we are looking at; physiology, which includes the organ and vessel dynamics; and pathology, which relates to the presence of lesions and the textures they produce. Are we seeing what we think we see? The answer can come only by testing the image.

Some real-time sonographs also have "selectable" or variable postprocessing similar to the B-scanners with larger scan converters. The postprocessing techniques discussed in Chapter 14 deliver the same capabilities to the real-time sonograph as they do to the B-scanner. Thus, we can also test the image with postprocessing.

We test the texturing process by observing changes in transmission with small changes in scanning angle. By slowly rocking the transducer, enhancement and shadowing can be examined in detail, yielding information about the tissues that cause these changes in attenuation. The transducer should be rocked gently, so as not to change the echogenicity of the tissue beneath the transducer by compressing the tissue.

We test the dynamics of the organs and vessels at the highest frame rate possible, in order to prevent motion aliasing that might keep us from gathering information about tumor vascularization.

To help ensure maximum information from an image, a comfortable rule to keep in mind is: Never scan at a rate faster than you can understand what you are seeing. Such a simple rule seems almost a cliché, but it is worth reemphasizing for real time because real time is fast and thus invites scanning at a rate that exceeds our ability to comprehend.

With this general protocol for specific real-time scanning in mind, following are some hints on scanning specific organs.

Pancreas   If the pancreas is one of the organs being scanned, then it should be scanned first before any breathing maneuvers introduce air into the stomach and gut. If air is already in the stomach, the gas can be displaced by having the patient drink a glass or two of water. This will permit a clear view of the pancreas. With water in the stomach, it is easy to show the papilla of Vater and the common bile duct. Here, the speed of real time permits a thorough examination while the acoustical window is present.

Gall Bladder   The flexibility of the real-time scan head and the visual qualities of real time combine to make studies of the gall bladder even more informative. We can roll the patient while scanning to observe the movement of gallstones or sludge. With this maneuver, we can learn a great deal about the condition of the bile by watching how fast things move in the gall bladder.

It is important to show all the borders at 90°, in order to provide an accurate measurement of wall thickness. The 90° position will minimize the beam-width artifacts that are common to most real-time systems.

Liver   The liver provides one of the best settings to view the changes in texture resulting from tumors. But here, real time adds a dimension not available to the B-scanner. For example, a large tumor with a necrotic center can look like an abscess. However, a tumor of that size will have vessels feeding it that can impart a motion to the tumor. This motion is often observable in the real-time image. Also, we still look for motion of major vessels such as the hepatic veins and structures like the porta hepatis.

Kidney   With real time, it is easy to show the entire length of the renal artery and renal vein, and these vessels should be included in every renal examination. We need to stay at an angle 90° to the renal capsule in order to be sure to differentiate between retro- and intraperitoneal masses. And again, the flexibility of real time lets us stand the patient up to observe internal movements with leaning and tilting. The left kidney can be viewed through the spleen. A complete study requires imaging both kidneys.

Spleen   It is easy to show vessels and the diaphragm through the spleen, but it is also easy to forget the image conventions. These image conventions must be remembered in order to make the splenic images meaningful. Through the spleen, we have a view of the tail of the pancreas, which can sometimes be confused with food in the stomach. Here again, real time offers an observation not available to the B-scanner. Food in the stomach will move, distinguishing it from the more stable pancreatic tail.

The above example of an abdominal protocol not only provides the specifics of an abdominal examination but incorporates operating principles applicable to any ultrasound test. These principles are discussed in a broader overview of ultrasound image quality in Chapter 19.

Preprocessing and Image Enhancement

Most current real-time sonographs have 16 or fewer gray levels. This places a strong dependence upon the preprocessing to portray small- and medium-level signals. Depending upon the signal processing within the sonograph, the number of preprocessing curves that can be used effectively is usually limited to 2 or 3. Moreover, the signal mix among organs changes considerably, which suggests that some preprocessing curves are preferred for looking at specific organs. Handling these variations in echo-signal levels and mixes requires most real-time machines to have several preprocessing curves.

A variable preprocessing circuit changes the assignment of analog signal levels to the digital numbers that are finally stored within the scan converter memory. Because of constant image updating, preprocessing in a real-time system works rapidly to interrogate the signals and information in the image. As a result, the sonographer can quickly match a preprocessing curve to the needed task.

Preprocessing curves can be thought of as mechanisms to handle the assignment of small, medium, and large signals. In selecting a curve for an imaging job, we can thus study a preprocessing curve published by a manufacturer and decide whether small, medium, or large signals are preferentially enhanced. In the case of primary and secondary tumors, for example, we are often looking for alterations in the medium and small signals as well as changes in texture that indicate the presence of a tumor. Choosing the proper preprocessing enables us to match the range of signals presented for many of the lesions, both primary and secondary, with the available gray levels.

On the other hand, we use medium- and large-signal separation to improve obstetric exams and to measure biparietal diameters. Many of the signals within the obstetrics examination fall within the medium to high signal levels, and discriminating among structures within these signals requires a reassignment of the analog signals to the numbers stored in memory. The fetal cranium, for example, often produces very large echoes, especially at the soft-tissue–amniotic fluid interface. Separation of the outside from the inside of the cranium is often improved by providing a preprocessing signal separation for high amplitude signals.

Including Postprocessing in the Imaging Protocol

Real-time sonographs with more than 16 gray levels often provide variable postprocessing along with variable preprocessing. Unlike preprocessing, postprocessing assigns the stored numerical value in the random access memory to a video gray-level intensity. As in preprocessing, postprocessing can dramatically influence the image information content and overall image quality. A manual and automatic postprocessing capability in the sonograph offers the sonographer significant interrogating power. Some sonographs even let the sonographer design the gray-scale assignments. While keeping in mind the restrictions applicable to postprocessing protocols for B-scanner quantification (see Chapter 14), the sonographer can perform similar measurements to a limited degree with a real-time sonograph using 32 or more gray levels.

Some sonographs carry variable postprocessing curves on the front panel. These curves offer an opportunity to rapidly interrogate the image for visual separations among signals in the small-, medium- and large-signal ranges. The idea is to visually separate signals that appear very close together on the display. If we identify each of the curves in the postprocessing choices for the signal range being preferentially interrogated or enhanced, we can examine any suspected lesion in a manner that is consistent and reproducible.

Expectations in Real-Time Accuracy

Because the process of image production is basically the same in a real-time sonograph as in the static B-scanner, axial resolution and axial accuracy should not be affected just because the system is operating in real time. Thus, we expect the same axial resolution and range accuracy in a real-time sonograph as in a static B-scanner. A measured axial resolution greater than three wavelengths in either a B-scanner or a real-time sonograph indicates a defective machine (see Chapters 11 and 12).

On the other hand, the lateral movement of the ultrasound beam in real time is determined by the design of the machine, so lateral accuracy in depicting structures is a larger problem for real time than for the static B-scanner. Because it is not easy to change a real-time transducer to match the job at hand, we are often required to scan using a single transducer frequency and focal point for any number of scanning problems. As a result, we need to be acutely aware of the beam profile of the real-time sonograph. Often, by changing to different acoustic windows, the focal point can be placed over the region of interest. The beam width and signal processing will affect the overall accuracy of any lateral measurements, and knowing what the beam width is within the image will help guide any conclusions on lateral measurements.

Not all digital scan converters operate identically. For example, in some real-time systems, the individual lines of sight are loaded into the scan converter memory on a columnar basis, are read out horizontally and are then constructed into a sector image. If the synthesis process is not properly controlled within the machine, the image can be distorted as a result of poor image reconstruction. Examining the image carefully during quality assurance procedures can determine quickly if distortions are present and if the synthesis of the image follows the defined rules of the machine. A 90° sector, for example, should be tested to be 90° on the display. Testing the image production and overall machine performance are described in Chapter 12.

Real-time sonographs are as subject to scanning artifacts as are static B-scanners. As a result, scanning artifacts will influence image information content and accuracy in nearly the same manner as artifacts in the B-scanner. Reverberations, for example, may hide information in both cases, but the flexibility of a real-time scanhead often permits easy repositioning to remove many tissue-generated artifacts from the image.

Real-Time Designs and Applications

Whether or not to use a real-time system for a particular application depends upon four factors: 1) the scanning field design, which may be linear or sector; 2) the size of the scanning head that holds the transducers; 3) the gray-scale resolution within the scan converter; and 4) the frame rate capabilities of the sonograph. Each of these items is considered below.

Scanning Field Geometry and Its Use

The first deciding factor for a particular application of real time is the pattern of the scanning field. For example, linear arrays produce a rectangular field, in contrast to the pie-shaped fields of the sector scanner. On the other hand, the sector scanner does not produce a uniform field. As a result, without special signal processing, the sector portion close to the transducer may be so badly overwritten that near imaging can be difficult or, in some cases, impossible to carry out.

A special need in obstetrical scanning is to gain a view of the fetal head in order to measure the biparietal diameter. The linear array is one of the best ways to deal with this imaging problem, a solution well-accepted for this particular application.

On the other end of the spectrum, echocardiography uses sector scanners almost exclusively. Despite some successful applications of the linear array to echocardiography, it has not generally gained acceptance within the cardiology community. Echocardiography can certainly be carried out with a linear array, just as obstetric examinations can be performed with a sector scanner. However, the linear array and sector scanner are much better suited to obstetrics and echocardiography, respectively, and have found a niche in these areas.

In addition, sector scanners are used more often than linear arrays for upper-abdominal scanning. The narrow field in sector scanners close to the transducer provides an opportunity to circumvent some of the upper abdominal scanning problems, such as bowel gas and ribs. In general, linear arrays offer similar imaging capabilities, but may not be able to explore some of the tighter spots as well as the sector scanner.

Size of the Scan Head

The second deciding factor for real-time applications is the size of the scanning head. Large-sector scanning heads, for example, have limited use in echocardiography, but are useful in abdominal and obstetric scanning. Also, large linear arrays will have limited use in standard abdomens, but can be utilized in obstetrics examinations. Because of these inherent limitations in the physical characteristics of the real-time sonograph, many ultrasound departments have more than one type of real-time scanner. The division of labor for the ultrasound scanner within the department will depend upon the physical characteristics of the scan head and the characteristics of the imaging process.

Gray-Scale Resolution

Upper-abdominal scanning and often obstetrical scanning rely on an ability to visually discriminate among signals coming from subtle lesions. Thirty-two or more gray levels provide technology that can depict and discriminate among subtle tissue differences. In contrast, echocardiographers use the gray-scale information inherent to the real-time image much less than that of the abdominal scanner. As a result, the real-time echocardiograph can use 16 or even fewer gray levels successfully.

Real-Time Frame Rate

Any real-time sonograph is limited, of course, by the line density in each scanning frame, the depth of display, and the frame rate in a combination that fits within very specific limits. Real-time systems with high line densities used for detailed abdominal scanning are not useful in echocardiography, because the high line density produces a frame rate too low to visualize a moving heart. Echocardiography devices, in contrast, use about 100 lines of sight to make a given frame, and frame rates run from 18 frames per second to as high as 50 frames per second. The problem is clearly one of choosing the machine to fit the task.

Conclusion

The contemporary real-time sonograph offers a fast and effective means of examination. The automatic movement of the transducer beam, and the small size and light weight of the scan head provide freedom to move the transducer and the beam into new locations within the body. But with the freedom to move comes the risk of moving improperly. Improper movement can result in loss of information, loss of anatomical references, and missed information that would normally be found with a B-scanner. Lacking the discipline of the scan arm, a real-time system is best handled through use of an examination protocol that permits a rapid yet thorough examination. By understanding the trade-offs and limitations in design, as well as the design objectives, the sonographer can produce effective real-time images.

One of the more available ways to test the image contents is by using the variable or "selectable" preprocessing within the sonograph. Methods of successfully using preprocessing for the B-scanner were described in Chapter 15 and apply equally to real-time sonography.

Chapter 18

Artifacts We Should Know

Being able to recognize artifacts within an image and to separate these artifacts from anatomy or disease are essential sonographic skills. One way of understanding what artifacts look like in an image is to understand the mechanisms behind their production. This chapter discusses the fundamentals of artifact production and how to read artifacts in images. Wherever possible, it also endeavors to describe a means of removing the artifact from the image.

Defining the Artifact

Understanding artifacts and how they enter the image requires a clear comprehension of the events that make an ultrasonic image. For example, travel time within the tissue is represented as distance on the display. Consequently, artifacts that extend over time can appear to be structures within the image. The sonograph, in addition, assumes a linear path for ultrasound, and when the ultrasonic beam is bent from its normal path, the result is a displacement of echo signals within the image. Furthermore, the sonograph assumes that the ultrasonic beam is infinitely thin; as a result, wide beams introduce a common set of artifacts to the images. If the sonograph is a real-time machine, then along with image artifacts come distortions in the portrayal of motion.

Imaging artifacts fall into five categories, with an additional category for Doppler. Although the Doppler artifact has qualities different from those of imaging artifacts, it still represents an inaccurate depiction of events within the tissue.

Categories of Imaging Artifacts

The five types of artifacts that can be produced in the imaging process include: 1) displaying of nonstructural echo signals; 2) removal of real structural echo signals from the display; 3) displacement of echo signals on the display; 4) distortion of the echo signal; and 5) distortion of the organ dynamics on the display. Each of these is examined in turn.

Displaying of Nonstructural Echo Signals

Because the display of echo signals is on a time base, the sonograph shows time as distance. Thus, any time-dependent process in echo-signal events can appear as nonstructural echo signals extending over distance on the display. Because these echo signals do not represent real anatomical structures within the tissue, they are therefore artifacts.

One often-seen artifact is the formation of reverberations between the face of the transducer and a highly reflective interface close to the transducer. This process occurs when ultrasonic energy reflects repeatedly between the scanning transducer interface and a structure within the tissues. In the image, repeating echoes extend at regular intervals into the image as if they were from echo sources deeper within the tissue. This reverberation process is most often seen between the transducer face and a gas-bowel interface. It also appears at the anterior limits of fluid–soft tissue boundaries such as the gall bladder, at placenta–amniotic fluid interfaces, and at bladder wall–urine interfaces. These reverberations can produce what appear to be "fuzzy" structures in the anterior portion of a cystic structure or can produce a false physical extension of the placenta *in utero*. An example of this effect is shown in Figure 18-1. These reverberation artifacts can sometimes be removed by putting less gain on the TGC initial gain and delaying the TGC through the reverberation interface.

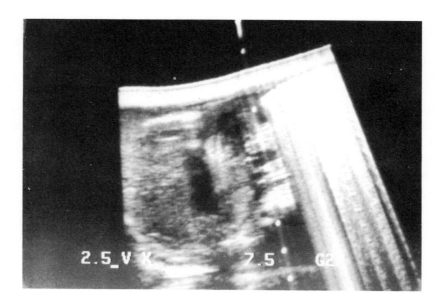

18-1   Reverberation between a transducer and a tissue interface. This patient has a strong reflecting interface close to the transducer, causing the reverberations that extend into the image. Note the repetitive intensity pattern of these reverberations.

In general, reverberations occur between any two highly reflective interfaces that are perpendicular to the direction of travel for the ultrasonic beam. These interfaces can include the transducer or other interfaces deeper within the body. On each reverberation, a small amount of the energy bouncing between the two interfaces leaks back to the transducer, producing a set of repeated signals. This sort of reverberation can often be identified because of the repetitive nature of the displayed signal and by noting that the echo signal vanishes when the beam is aimed away from perpendicular to the offending interfaces. This sort of artifact can appear after abdominal fat layers that have very reflective interfaces. The process is shown in Figure 18-2.

Echo signals that appear behind highly reflective interfaces, such as the peri-cardial-lung interface and the diaphragm-lung interface, are another example of reverberation. Distal to these structures is air-filled lung, which combines with the soft tissues to form an interface that is highly reflective. As a result, the tissue structures anterior to these reflecting interfaces appear again, posterior to the diaphragm or pericardium within the display. The reverberation process is shown in Figure 18-3; an example of the artifact is shown in Figure 18-4. These reverberations beyond the interface should not be confused with real structures.

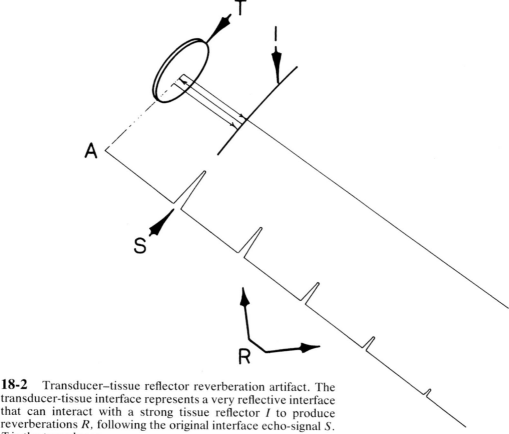

18-2 Transducer–tissue reflector reverberation artifact. The transducer-tissue interface represents a very reflective interface that can interact with a strong tissue reflector *I* to produce reverberations *R*, following the original interface echo-signal *S*. *T* is the transducer.

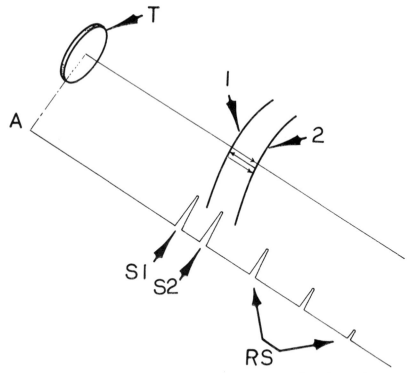

18-3 Deep-tissue reverberation artifact. Reverberation artifacts come from multiple reflections from very reflective interfaces, in this case, numbered 1 and 2. On the A-mode trace, *A,*
the original interface signals appear, *S1* and *S2.* The subsequent
reverberations appear as a multiple of the interface separation,
with a regular decrease in amplitude. *T* is the transducer.

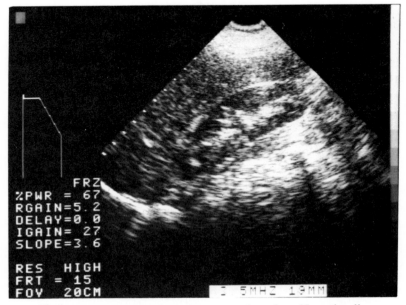

18-4 Example of a deep-tissue reverberation. Here the diaphram in the lower left portion of the image is forming a reverberation extruding downward from the diaphram.

Removal of Real Structural Echo Signals

The most frequent cause of real structural echo signals being removed is acoustical shadowing. Shadowing results from an inability of acoustical energy to penetrate beyond an interface or group of interfaces. As a consequence, deeper structures have either lower than normal echo signals or no echo signals, if the interfering structure interacts strongly. The reasons for the signal loss are either a highly attenuating or a very reflective interface or both. The loss can also result from structures that scatter ultrasound at a high rate. An example of acoustical shadowing is shown in Figure 18-5.

A second mechanism that can produce a loss of real structural echo signals results from using an elevated reject combined with viewing an interface off perpendicular. This is a common problem in real-time sonographs where the beam has a fixed angle of movement. An example of this information loss is shown in Figure 18-6. Real-time sonographs with a wide video dynamic range are often able to show an interface even though the reflection is not specular. Portraying the interface depends, then, upon the scattered echoes from the interface. This is frequently the case when using a real time sector scanner to view circular structures such as the gall bladder or the renal capsule.

Displacement of Echo Signals on the Display

Events can shift the echo signals on the display from their true orientation within the tissues. The most common source of this artifact is the beam width, which can move off-axis echo-signals onto an on-axis signal. Another source is a loss of echo-

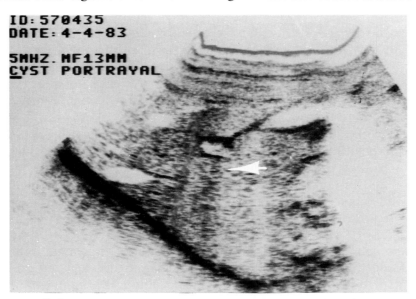

18-5   Shadowing from a higher-than-normal attenuator. A portion of the bile duct is casting a shadow in this image (arrow).

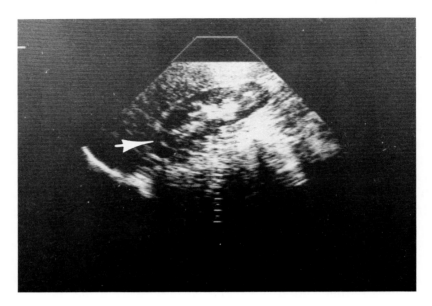

18-6 Signal dropout from reject function. The reject on this real-time sonograph is set too high, removing the smaller echo signals that portray the renal boundary (arrow).

signal registration because of poor signal processing or an inaccurate time base within the sonograph.

Regarding beam width, the beam produced by an ultrasound transducer is not infinitely thin. In addition, the diffraction characteristics of the transducer produce a set of side lobes that carry a significant amount of energy. The beam pattern from a transducer can have a major effect on the accurate positioning of echo sources on the display. The width of the beam also begins to affect the way in which echo sources are portrayed in the image. Chapter 7 points out that the beam width affects the lateral resolution of the system, as the beam width integrates information from all sources within its bounds onto the single display line of sight. Changing the sonograph gain or altering the output power can alter the effective beam width but runs the risk of removing desired information. Clearly, care must be taken in trying to remove this artifact. Along with the setup of the sonograph, the video dynamic range of the sonograph can also change the apparent beam width and thereby the appearance of the beam-width artifacts. The mechanism for beam width artifacts appears in Figure 18-7.

The techniques used within the sonograph signal processing can also affect the position of echo signals on the display. The tissue can play a role, as well, in this process, as regional changes in propagation velocity displace echo signals on the display.

A common source of registration problems is that of encoders on the scanning arm that do not register position properly. Scanning-arm registration can cause major artifacts in positioning the line of sight within a B-scan image. Along with registration is another source of artifacts in the image—known as B-mode jitter—that is due to an unstable referencing voltage that positions the line of sight within the scan converter memory. An example of this artifact is shown in Figure 18-8.

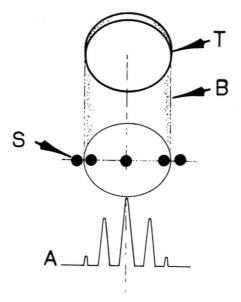

18-7 Beam-width artifact. As an echo source *S* enters the beam edge, the display shows a small echo signal. As the source reaches the center of the beam, the echo signal reaches a maximum. On a B-mode display, scanning a point source produces a line, not a point, with the line at least the beam width long.

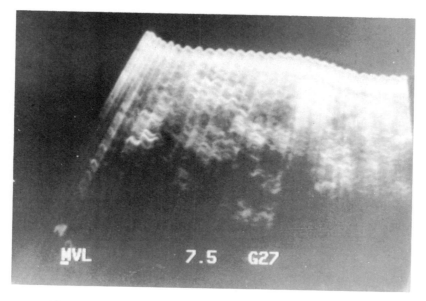

18-8 An example of B-mode jitter in a static B-scanner. When the scan arm encoding system fails to place the CRT trace on the display correctly, the trace "jitters" its position, producing distorted boundaries. This jitter produced a scaloped pattern for a linear scan.

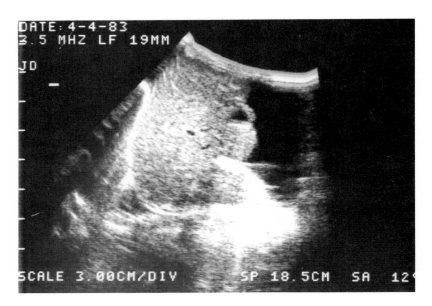

18-9   Increased echo-signal amplitudes with poor TGC adjust-ment. The band of echo-signals in the middle of the image come from placing the knee of the TGC right on the focusing of the transducer. The result is an improper portrayal of echo-signal amplitudes.

Distortion of the Echo Signal

Artifacts can enter the image with a poor depiction of echo amplitude. For example, a TGC slope set too high can produce a ''band'' of bright echo signals near the knee of the TGC curve. Signal processing within the sonograph can also alter the amplitude of the signals, with a nonlinear response to a linear TGC curve. An example of a TGC artifact is shown in Figure 18-9.

Removing this artifact may simply require resetting TGC, if that is the cause. Or, if the band results from the transducer or a nonlinear response, then changing transducers and realigning the sonograph are easy solutions.

A digital scan converter with 16 gray levels can produce another form of ampli-tude artifact called gray-scale contouring. This signal-processing artifact produces regions that flow together to form a common intensity. This can occur on the major signal dots, sometimes causing the so called ''blobby dots'' we often complain about. Contouring can also form ''structures'' within the image that are a result of dots flowing together on the same gray level, producing shapes and contours. An example of contouring is shown in Figure 18-10.

Another form of distortion is a shape distortion to the echo signal. This alteration comes from processes either within the tissue or the sonograph. For example, reflections added from ultrasonic beam side lobes can sum onto a major signal from an interface, extending the width of the echo signal on the display. This type of distortion can also occur at interfaces that intercept the beam at angles other than 90°. An example of this sort of axial-resolution distortion from beam width is shown in Figure 18-11 and is explained in detail in Chapter 7.

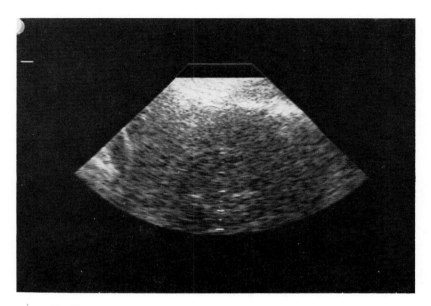

18-10   Gray-scale contouring with a limited gray-scale system. Because this system has too few gray levels available to show gray scale in the image, many of the smaller echo signals are all assigned the same gray level, making them run together and form contours.

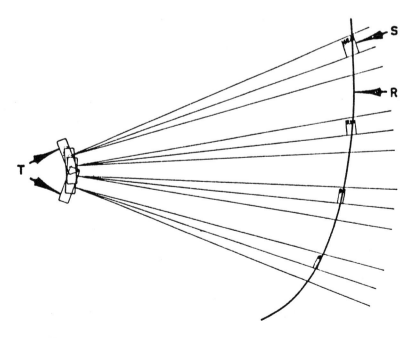

18-11   The integration of beam width onto axial resolution as an artifact. Intercepting a scattering interface at an angle will integrate the beam-width error onto the echo signal, causing a poorer axial resolution and poor portrayal of the interface. The artifact vanishes when scanning 90° to the interface.

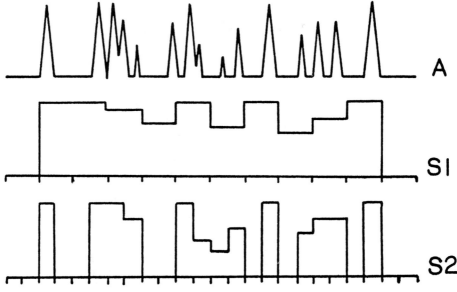

18-12   Digital sampling artifact. The rate of digital sampling in a digital scan converter can greatly influence the appearance of B-mode texture. A low sample rate, as shown in *S1*, hides the detail of the original trace, *A*. Increasing the sample rate, *S2*, improves the reproduction of the original.

Shape distortion can also result from digital scan converters that fail to sample the line of sight often enough to show the true signal mix. This is a common problem found in real-time systems that have limited sampling rates and small digital scan converters. We can test for this artifact by comparing the sample rate (depth of field in millimeters per the number of samples per line of sight) with the effective wavelength of the center operating frequency of the transducer. Sampling the center operating frequency means a sample every half wavelength.

This artifact is not really in the sonographer's power to remove; it resides in machine design. The mechanism for this artifact appears in Figure 18-12.

Distortion of Organ Dynamics

The basic means of image formation in a real-time sonograph involves scanning an ultrasound beam in space and producing an image from the collected echo signals. The finite time required to collect the information means that motion within the tissues is sampled and not shown continuously. Basic communications theory indicates that motion must be sampled at twice its highest frequency component in order to be accurately reproduced. This limitation sets up the possibility that motion aliasing will occur when a real-time frame rate is too low. This sort of artifact can be easily seen in real-time images of pregnancy close to term when the fetal heart rate is high and the large field of view causes a low frame rate. The heart motion is distorted under these conditions. Although detailed information about the motion of fetal heart valves is lost in this situation, an indication that the heart is moving will not be lost.

One of the more interesting artifacts produced by a real-time system is a process called "ring around." This is almost identical to a reverberation process in which echo signals that enter the transducer were actually transmitted much earlier in the frame formation. The result is a floating, almost beating artifact in the real-time image and a somewhat blurred structure in a frozen image. The artifact appears as an echo signal on a pulse-listen cycle later than the transmitted energy. The time delay results from a long travel time through the tissues. The artifact is most apparent when high frame rates are coupled with high transmitted power or when there is high system gain along with highly reflecting interfaces in the scanning field. Positioning the transducer will alter the position of the artifact, according to some of the rules of reverberation. An alternative is to change the frame rate. The artifact will often move out of the image field with either a higher or lower frame rate.

Nonlinear transducer motion in a mechanical scan head is a primary source of artifacts in mechanical real-time sonographs. Often the connection between the driving motor and the transducers is a belt or variable drive system, permitting the transducer to move independently of the motor under the right circumstances. The uncoupled motion produces wavy images and distorted perceptions of motion. The appearance of motion-dependent artifacts within a real-time image can be quickly detected on a tissue-equivalent phantom or other fixed-signal source that displays the inappropriate motion present in the system.

Each individual element of a phased array functions as an independent diffracting aperture. A linear array of elements, combined to make a scanhead as either a linear array or phased array, forms grating lobes, which appear largest when the beam is pointed away from the central array axis. These grating-lobe elements can cause "paradoxical" motion on the display, especially at the boundaries of the image sector for the phased array. The presence of such paradoxical motion can be examined by moving the scan head over a set of fixed echo sources such as a phantom or AIUM Test Object. This motion artifact is usually unsuspected until demonstrated with a phantom.

Artifacts in Doppler Processing

The echo-signal image produced by a Doppler ultrasound system is a spectral analysis with frequency on the Y-axis, time on the X-axis, and amplitudes of frequency components on the intensity or Z-axis. The ability to produce artifacts in this display is usually connected with the events within the tissue, especially in pulsed Doppler systems. Within the Doppler information display, we are interested in the form of the frequency changes over time, the number of frequency components present at any one time, and the direction of flow. The most sensitive portion of this display format in regard to artifacts derives from the increase in frequency components due to an interaction between the architecture of the blood flow and the sample volume size. Spectral broadening of this type is discussed in detail in Chapter 8, on Doppler systems.

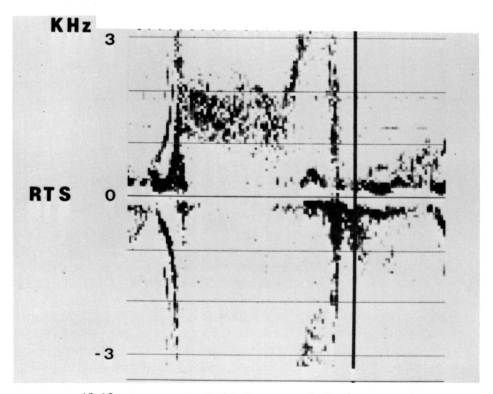

18-13   An example of high frequency aliasing in a spectral display. This spectral display of flow through a stenotic mitral valve shows a displacement of very high frequency Doppler signals (arrow) that exceeded the Nyquist limit.

Another form of distortion that is unique to pulsed Doppler systems is the process of Doppler frequency aliasing. This form of distortion occurs because the pulsed Doppler system is sample-rate limited by the pulse-repetition frequency. As a result, Doppler frequencies exceeding one-half the pulse-repetition frequency cannot be accurately shown, but are aliased into lower frequencies or different directions. An example of such aliasing is shown in Figure 18-13.

Another form of artifact present in some of the directional Doppler systems is a "ghost" of signals in a direction opposite that of the primary signal. This occurs when the signal level into the directional separating circuits is too high. This ghosting process is most frequently found in pulsed Doppler systems using a quadrature phase detector to separate signals into direction.

Conclusion

One of the most impressive capabilities of an experienced sonographer is the ability to separate the components of an image into real echo signals and artifacts. This skill comes from experience and an awareness of what to look for in an image. By knowing the classes and sources of these artifacts, as described in this chapter, the sonographer is able to separate artifacts from real image in less time and with more accuracy.

Chapter 19

Elements of Image Quality

Anyone who has attended a national ultrasound meeting or has compared the various ultrasound machines on the market is inevitably drawn into a consideration of the elements of image quality. Considering the range of imaging results, it is easy to feel that no real basis for image quality exists. Although any two sonograph operators may seek the same information, the resulting data may appear in a variety of ways in the image. Often, too, what we think of as image quality is absent. Just what is image quality? This chapter discusses the fundamentals of image quality, of what to look for and measure to maximize the amount of diagnostic information contained in an image. The elements we discuss will also be useful in evaluating the images of others, as well as in contributing to a quality assurance program both for real time and static B-scanning images.

Before identifying the elements of image quality, however, we must discard the long-held views that image quality is subjective, that producing diagnostic ultrasound images is an art form only, and that the information contained in the image is independent of any of the signal-processing techniques within the sonograph. In fact, image quality is a product both of signal processing within the sonograph, which supplies resolution, and the skills of the sonographer, who supplies definition to the images. When the sonograph ultimately changed to the digital scan converter, it made numerical determination of the elements of image quality possible. Thus, image quality is not subjective; it is objective, with measurable and determinable elements logically displaying the methods of signal processing within the sonograph and the operator's skills in setting up and using the sonograph.

Image Information Goals

Our investigation of the elements of image quality begins with a delineation of image information goals, from which we can generalize the qualities of an image that must be present. These goals will extend to the decision-making stages of diagnostic ultrasound, stages that are summarized in what we call a "decision tree" that shows the visual information used to determine the presence of a mass and its character. (The decision tree is discussed more later in the chapter.) By blending image information goals and the elements of the imaging decision tree, the elements of image quality become evident.

Our first goal is to gain information about size, shape, position, texture, and dynamics of organs, structures, and lesions within the body. This is, in fact, the overall aim of ultrasound procedures in general, and is repeated often in this book. The design of sonographic equipment, the signal processing within the equipment, and the display of information, all are geared to attaining specific objectives in this general imaging goal.

A determination of size provides information such as fetal gestational age, vessel enlargement, and the progress of tumor growth. A determination of shape provides, for example, evidence of tumor involvement with normal tissue and of anatomical distortions attendant with disease. A determination of position can aid, for example, in a biopsy; or provide a surgeon with evidence of what to expect at surgery; or determine if a placenta is obstructing a delivery. A display of texture assists in identifying similar tissues or helps separate normal from abnormal tissues and one organ from another. A display of motion can show a fetus to be alive, for example; or demonstrate pathologies of the heart; or separate a tumor from an abscess. Some or all of these capabilities can vanish with poor image quality.

Decisions in Ultrasonic Imaging

Described below are problems associated with imaging abdominal masses, problems chosen because they are characteristic of imaging difficulties in nearly all ultrasound applications. In the current application, five decision elements are used to determine the size, location, and organ of origin for a particular mass [1]. These

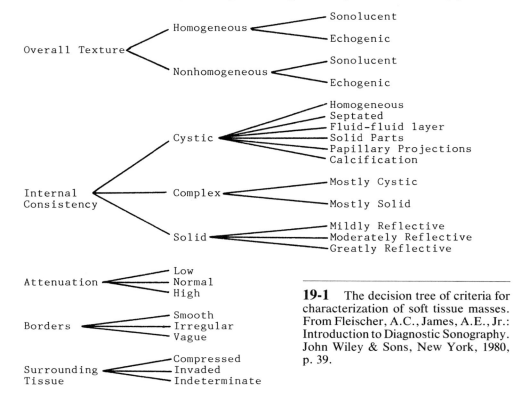

19-1   The decision tree of criteria for characterization of soft tissue masses. From Fleischer, A.C., James, A.E., Jr.: Introduction to Diagnostic Sonography. John Wiley & Sons, New York, 1980, p. 39.

decisions form the main trunk of the imaging decision tree. The entire sequence appears in Figure 19-1.

A look at Figure 19-1 shows that progression through this particular decision tree is predicated not only upon an ability to portray the texture of a mass as different from that of surrounding tissue, but upon the ability to depict the internal organization of a mass. At the same time, the borders of the mass must be defined, in addition to the character of its interface with the surrounding tissue.

To deliver the information needed to make the decisions shown in Figure 19-1, images must exhibit at least 12 elements of image-quality. As stated earlier, these elements apply to both static and real-time imaging.

Elements of Image Quality

Each of the 12 elements of image quality is described below, along with a visual example of each.

Ray Formation is Uniform

In a static B-scanner, the formation of a single-pass or compound scan depends as much upon the sonographer's skill in moving the ultrasound transducer over the surface of the body and sweeping the beam through the interior of the body as upon the signal-processing and image-forming capabilities of the sonograph. Also, the textural quality of an image depends upon an even distribution of ultrasonic energy. The first evaluation of an image, then, is the ray formation both along the ray and its lateral distribution over the image—in other words, both axially and laterally over the image. Whether a static B-scanning image or a real-time image, the rays must be correctly and evenly positioned in space; they must not change in consistency or intensity from one to the other; all lines of sight should be present; and pixels with real signals should be filled in the image.

An example of good and bad ray formation appears in Figure 19-2.

Like Tissues Look Alike

If the sonograph TGC is properly set up and the signal processing within the sonograph is working correctly, like tissues should look alike throughout the image, with similar texture and gray-scale intensities. This requirement extends rigorously over the region of compensation for the TGC. For example, liver should look like liver both close to the transducer as well as more deeply into the tissue, despite the changes in echo signals that result from frequency-dependent attenuation and alterations in system gain and signal mix. The test for this criterion is to look for adjacent tissues that have similar textural qualities and that appear alike in the image. A uniform liver texture appears in Figure 19-3.

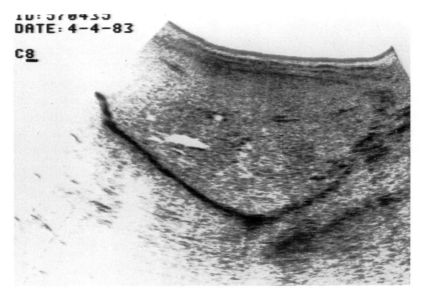

19-2   Part A

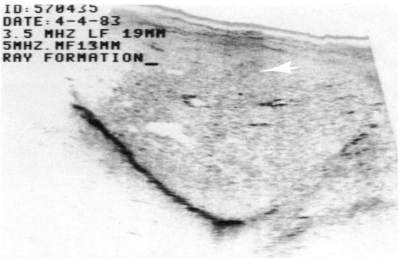

19-2   Part B

19-2   Looking at ray formation of the sonograph. Part A: Uniform ray formation, both axially and laterally, produced by a smooth, even movement of the transducer. Part B: An uneven movement of the transducer has produced a more intense region in the center of the scan (arrow). Bad ray formation can also result from electronic failures in the sonograph.

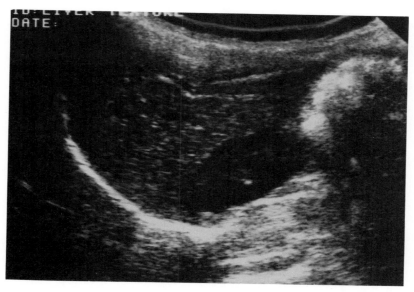

19-3   Part A

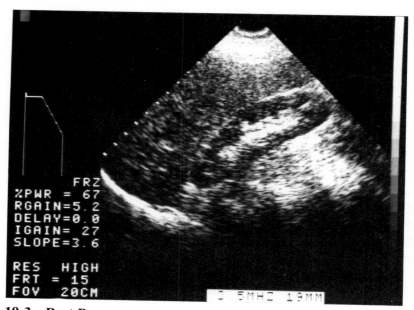

19-3   Part B

19-3   Like tissues should look alike. Part A: Like tissue looks alike in the image, both close to the transducer and more distant. The texture of the kidney looks quite different from the liver in this image. Part B: Real-time scan of liver and kidney. Like tissue looks alike and different for each organ.

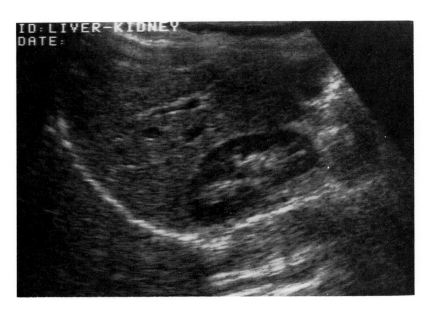

19-4 Unlike tissues should look different. This scan shows clear differences between the textures of liver and kidney that must appear to separate organs from one another and lesions from normal tissues.

Unlike Tissues Look Different

Unlike tissues with different distributions of scattering bodies and different reflectivities should appear to be different within the image. Each tissue carries its own internal anatomy, and these macro- and micro-variations in anatomy should interact with ultrasound in distinct ways, producing discernible modifications in texture within the image. Failure of unlike tissues to look different can produce situations where anatomy and architecture are lost in a diffuse pattern of scattering echoes. On the other hand, when unlike tissues do appear distinct from one another, masses with characteristics similar to but different from surrounding normal tissue will be evident within the image, and organs such as the liver and pancreas can be differentiated readily. Clearly recognizable differences between the liver and kidney are shown in Figure 19-4.

Full Scan-Converter Dynamic Range is Used

With the sonograph, signals are processed and assigned gray levels through preprocessing and postprocessing, both functions assuming that a full dynamic range of signals is present during the assignments. Failure to use the full dynamic range within a digital scan converter permits progressive digital error in the conversion of the analog signals into digital signals that are stored in memory. Images should "write to white," in other words, should use the full dynamic range of the display to prevent digital error, and should utilize fully both preprocessing and postprocessing functions.

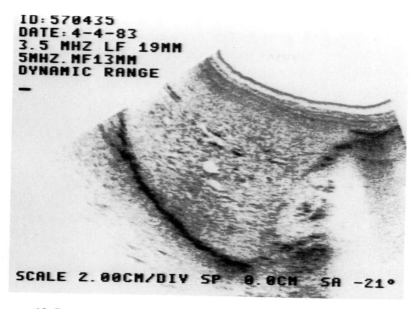

ID:570435
DATE:4-4-83
3.5 MHZ LF 19MM
5MHZ. MF13MM
DYNAMIC RANGE

SCALE 2.00CM/DIV SP 0.0CM SA −21°

19-5 Writing over the full display dynamic range. Using the digital scan converter to its full potential requires using the full display dynamic range for the echo signals. This scan is using the full dynamic range of the scan converter and display.

An example of using the full writing capabilities and ''writing to white'' appears in Figure 19-5.

Dot Size is Correct

The free-standing dots forming an image should be three wavelengths or less in length and should not vary greatly with amplitude (a tearing quality on large amplitudes). This physical criterion for dot size results from the length of time needed to stop and start the transducer vibration in order to separate signals in a gray-scale environment (see Chapter 3). Signal processing that produces dots greater than three wavelengths for single echo signals indicates malfunction within the sonograph, owing either to design or to the need for an adjustment. Usually, a poor dot formation will be accompanied by inadequate axial resolution. The most frequent violation of this criterion produces the so-called blobby dots that can destroy the gray-scale qualities of an otherwise fine image.

An example of good dot formation appears in Figure 19-6.

Cystic Structures Look Cystic

Cystic structures represent masses filled with materials that usually have uniform acoustical impedances. If a system is unable to portray echo-free cysts, then more-complex structures that include septations, multifluid layers, or solid components

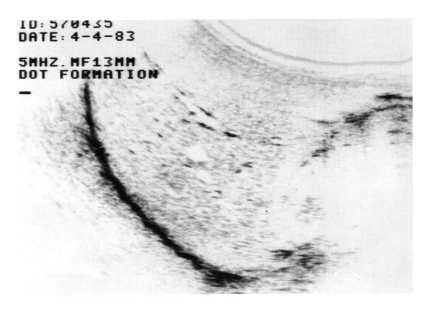

19-6   Image dot formation. Poorly aligned or poorly set up sonographers will produce dots larger than three wavelengths. This sonograph shows good dot formation and a consistent texture as a result.

may not be distinguished from truly cystic structures. A uniform distribution of acoustical impedance in a cystic structure should provide an echo-free image of the structure, while solid structures should still look solid.

Figure 19-7 shows both properly and poorly portrayed cystic structures.

Solid Structures Look Solid

Solid structures with a wide range of acoustical impedances should produce a continuous texture of echo signals on the display. Failure to produce textural information commensurate with nonhomogeneous structures is often the result of poor signal processing within the sonograph, or sometimes a consequence of using reject improperly to make the image. For example, the liver is a continuous set of scattering bodies, both on a micro and macro level. The imaging goal is to depict a solid tissue with numerous echo-sources *as such,* while cystic structures should still appear cystic.

Examples of good and bad portrayals of solids are shown in Figure 19-8.

Low Attenuators Show Acoustical Enhancement

Masses with low attenuation rates will make echosignals posterior to the mass look brighter within the image. If the TGC is correctly set within the sonograph, these increases in echo-signal level will indicate a low attenuating mass, and not a poorly set TGC. At the same time, an incorrectly set TGC or improper internal

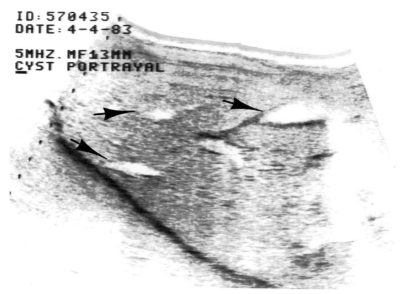

19-7   Part A

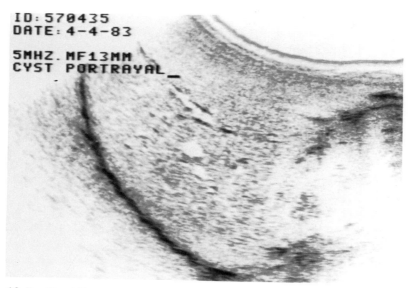

19-7   Part B

19-7   Cysts should look cystic. Part A: Most cystic structures
are fluid filled, with low internal attenuation rates. A good portrayal of cystic structures permits determination of complex
structures when they appear. This is a good portrayal of cystic
structures (arrow). Part B: This scan shows a partially filled cyst
because of the beam width integrating echo signals into the cyst.

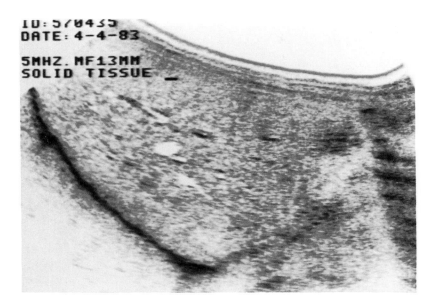

19-8   Part A

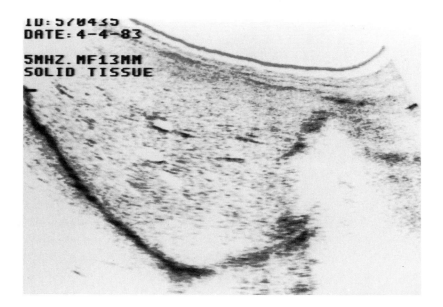

19-8   Part B

19-8   Solid tissues should show a solid mix of signals. Part A: A solid tissue with many echo sources should appear as a continuous set of echo signals. Part B: Failing to portray the full echo-signal mix produces incomplete images of solid tissues.

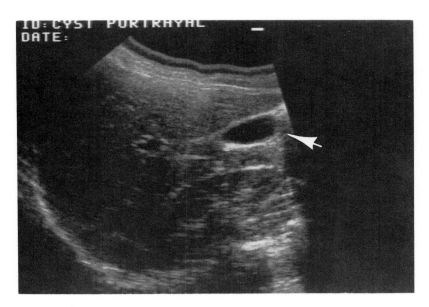

19-9   Low attenuating materials should show enhancement. Low attenuating materials such as the fluid in this gall bladder (arrow) produce acoustical enhancement. Enhancement is an indication of lower-than-expected attenuation rate inside a structure.

signal processing can hide this low-attenuator enhancement, removing information about the nature of the mass relative to the surrounding tissues. Clearly, low attenuating structures should produce visible acoustical enhancement in the image.

Acoustical enhancement is evident in Figure 19-9.

High Attenuators Show Shadowing

In contrast to the masses and structures with low attenuation, masses with higher-than-normal attenuation rates or unusually high reflectivity should produce various degrees of acoustical shadowing over posterior structures. Shadowing is undeniable evidence that ultrasound failed to penetrate well to the structures posterior to the mass. A shadow may result from two processes: 1) a higher-than-normal reflectivity, and 2) a higher-than-normal attenuation rate within the mass. Either process indicates an unusual interaction between the ultrasound and tissue. Shadowing is evident in Figure 19-10.

Boundaries of Organs and Structures Are Visible

Our imaging goals require a clear determination of the size, shape, and position of a mass within the body. To reach these goals requires organ boundaries and internal structures to be clearly displayed within the image. The ability to separate one organ from another or one vascular system from another hinges on more than the depiction of boundaries through specular reflections. Single-pass scanning in the

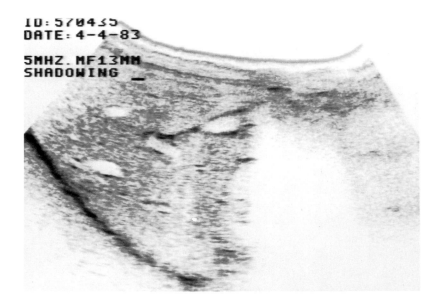

ID: 570435
DATE: 4-4-83

5MHZ. MF13MM
SHADOWING

19-10 High attenuators should produce shadows. Many tissues cause a greater-than-expected decrease in beam energy. The bile duct in this image is causing a greater-than-expected decrease in beam energy, causing a shadow. Shadowing is an indication of higher-than-expected energy loss in the beam, which can give information about tissue characteristics.

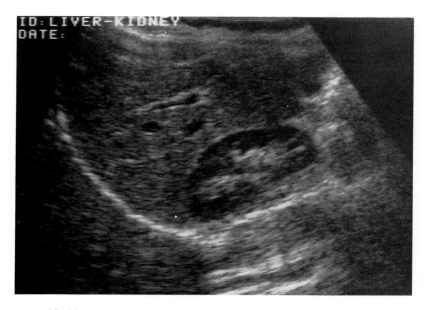

ID: LIVER-KIDNEY
DATE:

19-11 Clearly defined organ boundaries. In this image, the kidney boundary is defined with both specular and scattering echo signals. Good boundary definition helps determine the position of organs that may be displaced from normal locations and helps to locate organ-specific lesions.

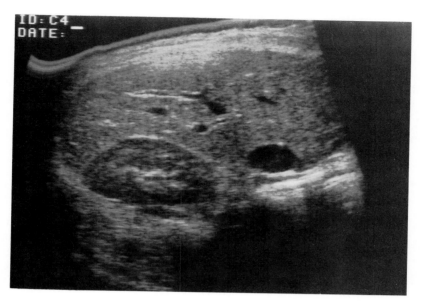

19-12   Good spatial accuracy supports assessment of size, shape, and position. This scan includes a complex set of structures, whose portrayal depends directly on the spatial accuracy of the sonograph.

static B-scanner and the fixed-angle scanning of the real-time sonograph require boundary depiction using scattering processes rather than specular reflections. Whether by specular reflection or by scattering, however, boundaries of organs, masses, and vascular structures need to be plainly visible within the image and sharp on both sides.

An example of good boundary definition appears in Figure 19-11.

Spatial Accuracy is Adequate

A properly running sonograph will accurately depict organ and lesion anatomy. For example, round structures should appear round, not square; elliptical fetal heads are not circular or radially bent; and lateral measurements are accurate. The correct determination of organ mass and position relies upon a clear depiction of lateral structures. Moreover, accuracy of timing within the sonograph determines both the ability to measure size and to place the position of the mass within the body accurately in the image. This particular image-quality element is more easily determined by the operating sonographer than by an outside evaluator, although gross distortions can be quickly picked up in a moving real-time image (see Chapter 12).

An example of good spatial accuracy appears in Figure 19-12.

Motion Depiction is Accurate

A static B-scanner has only limited capability to depict motion. A real-time son-ograph, however, can depict movement within the body with an accuracy that corresponds to the frame rate of the sonograph. The frame rate of the sonograph must, in the end, match the motion depicted. For example, frame rates less than about 30 frames per second are inadequate to depict motion in the heart. On the other hand, such frame rates are useful for scanning the abdomen.

Conclusion

Despite our community attempts to make image quality subjective, we can still draw out a number of objective image elements that let us judge the image on its ability to deliver information. The information we seek comes from the problems we are trying to solve. Thus, trying to characterize a mass forms a set of connected data that define what an ultrasound image must be able to deliver, and ultimately, what the sonograph and songrapher must be able to do.

The twelve elements of image quality tell us what to look for in an image that can make the image clinically valuable. They are, however just pieces of the imaging process. It is the pattern of the elements working together that can keep an image from ever reaching film or make it a source of pride. Knowing what to look for is a starting point, for we see what we look for and look for what we know.

Yet, an image can pass an inspection for the image quality elements and still fail to be a useful tool in making clinical decisions. Overlaying the elements of image quality are two major influences: image unity and context.

Unity refers to the wholeness or completeness of the image. An image is complete when we know the scanning plane location because key landmarks are present; when crucial information about a lesion is present to permit characterization; when we can express size, shape, position, and texture of a mass or lesion; when we have a context to evaluate the tissue-ultrasound interaction.

Ultrasound images abound with information, but it is all relative, for the sonograph uses only the time of arrival and echo-signal amplitude to make the image. Thus, to appreciate the texture of a mass, the image must also hold normal tissue; enhancement and shadowing can be seen only with normal echo-signal amplitudes in the image. A context means including the benchmarks for comparison in an image.

It is the twelve elements of image quality, surrounded by image unity and context that can keep an image esthetically pleasing and clinically useful.

References

1. Fleischer, A., and A.E. James. 1980.
   Introduction to diagnostic sonography,
   39. New York: John Wiley & Sons.

Chapter 20

Thinking Through the Study: an Organized Approach

Our final application of the previous chapters' scientific and clinical information on ultrasound involves "thinking through the study," an approach that is as much an attitude as a process. As an attitude, thinking through the study implies a framework of thinking that lends an organized approach to scanning, and thus permits recognition of changes within the image. As a process, thinking through the study involves the formation of a "thought model" of events that contribute to image formation. The model becomes a central tool in understanding the formation of an image and, thereby, interpreting the final results. Within the model are parts of the tissue-ultrasound interaction, such as: the production of ultrasound, the propagation of ultrasound in the tissue, the formation of echoes, and the arrival of ultrasound back to the transducer. Also contained in the model are signal-processing events within the sonograph that influence the amplitude, shape, and position of the echo signals on the display. These events include, for example: setting the TGC, picking the right transducer for the job, the type of preprocessing used within the sonograph, the use of postprocessing within the sonograph, and the method of placing signals into and taking them out of a digital scan converter. The thought model further includes an understanding of the behavior of disease within the body. For example, we expect fluid-filled structures to appear homogeneous; we expect solid masses that are heterogeneous to present a texture; and we use the known anatomy of the body to detect the presence of masses and to determine their involvement in normal tissue.

As both a thought pattern and a behavior, then, thinking through the study keeps established imaging information goals foremost in the mind of the examiner. Thinking through the study divides naturally into five activity segments that correspond to the normal sequence of an examination. Each of these segments is examined in turn below.

Before the Patient Arrives

Long before the patient arrives, we need to know that the sonograph is working properly in order to eliminate it from suspicion should the imaging not proceed well. We can verify the machine's functioning with the aid of a thorough, regular quality assurance program for each sonograph, whether static B-scanner or real time. An effective quality assurance program for each type of sonograph was discussed in detail in Chapters 11 and 12, using both the AIUM Test Object and a tissue-equivalent phantom. And a readily available phantom can be used to quickly eliminate or verify the possibility of a sudden failure in the sonograph should patient imaging be abnormally difficult. A highly attenuating patient can be shown to be truly so when a spot check with the phantom shows the sonograph to have adequate sensitivity and texture portrayal.

Each patient comes to the ultrasound department with a clinical question to be answered. The sonographer must first find out from the patient's record and examination request form what the patient's clinical question really is. First, we must determine whether or not the question—or any portion of it—can even be answered with ultrasound. Without knowing the clinical question to be answered, the examiner begins the study blind. And without a purpose to the examination, it is easy to be lured away from both diagnostic and imaging goals.

Within any general clinical question are a set of subquestions that help define the direction of the examination and the specific pieces of information that we seek with the sonograph. For example, the simple request to determine fetal age implies a second set of questions concerning the fetal size for dates, fetal viability, and any suggested growth-pattern abnormalities. The answers to these questions will come from a survey scan followed by specific techniques to derive the clinical information.

The Survey as Starting Point

With a specific set of clinical questions in mind, the examination begins with a survey of the region or organs being considered. The first prerequisite is to choose a transducer that can do the job. A good initial selection is a medium-frequency transducer with a medium (6-cm) focal-point position and long focal zone. The frequency must be low enough, however, to reach the deeper portions of the body during the survey scans. We set the TGC for the transducer, assuming a normal patient with normal tissue attenuation (see Chapter 13). Deviations from these settings required to image the patient will yield information about general tissue conditions of the patient.

The first scan with the sonograph yields a substantial amount of information. In fact, no single scan thereafter provides as much data about the patient and the setup of the sonograph. Consider the start of an upper abdominal survey examination as an example. The first scan is a longitudinal, midline, single-pass scan.

From this single image comes the following information: the size and position of the left lobe of the liver; the position of major landmarks including the great vessels, usually the aorta, and sometimes the inferior vena cava; the amount of gas within the stomach and the gut that can interfere with the examination; the location of the pancreas, often displaying the body and sometimes the head of the pancreas; an indication of the angle needed to visualize the pancreas well; visual evidence that the TGC is set up properly for the soft-tissue attenuation rate and transducer focusing; and immediate evidence of any unique qualities in the patient's anatomy such as skin thickness or fat distribution. This scan should be carried out slowly with an eye to image formation and to the clues within the image that tell us about the above-listed information.

From this first scan, we fix the position of major vascular landmarks and readjust the TGC if obviously needed, using the techniques discussed in Chapter 13. Continuing the survey, we watch the image formation, testing each image according to the elements of image quality (see Chapter 18). In each scan, we look for organ boundaries such as the boundaries that define the liver and pancreas, and regions of mutual organ contact such as the liver–right kidney interface. We look for textures that help define each of the organs. We look also for transmission qualities unique to the organs within this particular patient. (Transmission qualities appear as acoustical enhancement and shadowing that represent major ultrasound-tissue interactions.)

From the first longitudinal scan, the upper abdominal examination continues in a fixed investigative format, covering all of the organs in the region of interest in a series of compound or single-pass scans. Throughout the survey, we assay for texture and transmission changes that indicate the need for specific scans later in the examination. Often the survey raises new questions that will be answered in the subsequent specific examination techniques. And in Chapters 14 and 15 are protocols for interrogating the presentations using postprocessing and preprocessing.

Throughout the survey, we look for artifacts that alter the image information content, and for ways of avoiding these artifacts to produce images we can trust. (Chapter 18 provided a detailed discussion of artifacts, their sources and how to remove them from the image.) We also evaluate each image according to elements of image quality to make sure we include all the diagnostic information. When the image falls outside acceptable limits (discussed in Chapter 19 on image quality and Chapter 18 on artifacts), it is an easy decision to erase the image and begin again.

We should, moreover, anticipate what anatomy will be in the next scan, based on the anatomic information gathered from all the previous scans. As the scanning moves through a region, each image should contain an identifiable landmark that offers an "anatomical" annotation to the image. For example, major landmarks in the upper abdomen are the aorta, the inferior vena cava, the superior mesenteric artery, the superior mesenteric vein, and the diaphragm. Including one or more of these landmarks within an image and using standard display conventions provide evidence of the scanning plane position and scanning window for each image.

Each image should, in addition, be labeled and annotated for later review. The annotation should relate directly to the anatomical landmarks within each image.

The inclusion of established landmarks and the addition of printed annotation will keep the image as fresh to the reviewer as when first made by the sonographer.

Boundaries help define whether a mass resides within an organ or its adnexal organs. Obviously, boundary definition requires a clear depiction of the boundaries, which can be best achieved by placing the ultrasound beam 90° to the boundary. A flexible static B-scanner arm and a skilled sonographer in combination can provide a clear depiction of boundaries by reading the boundary orientation in the image *during* image formation and staying perpendicular to the boundary throughout the scan. These requirements also apply when using a real-time sonograph. The benefits of remaining perpendicular to boundaries in terms of both axial and lateral resolution were described in detail in Chapter 3 on transducers and Chapter 7 on real-time systems.

A survey is based on examining a single organ for disease, but many organs come in pairs, and in this case, both organs and adnexal organs should be included in the exam. For example, a suspected mass in one kidney may also appear in the other kidney, and may extend into adrenal tissue. A renal survey, then, should include both kidneys and both adrenals. We should rigidly follow a standard scanning sequence in order to image the complete organ volume. Examples of such a sequence are available in many of the available texts on diagnostic ultrasound [1, 2, 3].

The organ survey represents a critical, primary step in the application of diagnostic ultrasound. If we miss a mass in the survey portion of the examination, we will not be looking for it during the specific scanning later in the sequence. To make sure we are not neglecting important information in the survey, the investigating routine must be carefully followed, looking at each image in great detail.

Finishing the Examination

Finishing the examination involves an accurate determination of size, shape, position, texture, and dynamics of the lesion or lesions in order to answer the preliminary clinical questions as well as any new questions raised by the survey. The survey may offer evidence of focal disease (for example, stones in the gall bladder), in which case, continuing the specific examination will require only a limited amount of scanning with different sorts of transducers. If the survey demonstrates distributed disease or multifocal disease, however, defining the extent of normal tissue involvement will require scanning with a number of different transducers. The purpose is to answer all of the questions presented by the earlier survey.

As with the survey scan, the first step in carrying out a specific scan to obtain particular information is to choose the right transducer. This necessitates matching the imaging requirements and the transducer characteristics. In general, we seek the best axial and lateral resolution possible in order to make measurements of organ or lesion size, shape, position, and textural qualities. Lesions close to the surface of the body can be examined with high-frequency, short focus transducers. Chapter 9 emphasized the importance of placing the focal point of the transducer in front of or behind a particular type of lesion. And Chapter 13, on TGC, provided a protocol to ensure that the TGC is set for the scanning task. Moving to specific transducers for a specific task also reduces the opportunity for artifacts. Lesions more distant from the transducer, such as posterior metastatic lesions in the liver or a subphrenic abscess, will require long-focus transducers with a frequency defined by the attenuation rate of the patient's tissue. The expected resolution of the transducer can be determined through the procedures discussed in Chapter 3—for example, by calculating the HMBW and the effective depth of focus. And a quality assurance program such as that described in Chapters 11 and 12 gives some clues to the performance we can expect from the transducer-sonograph combination.

As in the patient survey, all of the boundaries of a lesion or affected organ must be clearly defined in any specialized scans. Boundary definition provides accurate sizing for the lesion and helps show the shape and type of boundary possessed by the mass. In addition, boundary definition begins to identify the organ of origin for the mass. For example, a retroperitoneal mass can appear to be part of a kidney until an outline of the renal capsule shows the mass to be outside the kidney. In such scans, we need to hold closely to the 90° position to the boundaries. This may require new positions for the patient, such as an oblique position to examine the kidney. A lesion often exhibits texture changes and attenuation rates different from the normal surrounding tissue. The task in this extended procedure is to determine the reasons for any observed changes away from normal both in transmission—which involves shadowing and enhancement—and texture. For example, some tissues such as uterine fibroids have a high attenuation rate because of increased scattering processes. These structures cause shadowing without the high specular reflections attendant with large changes in acoustic impedance. It is this combination of shadowing without specular reflections that indicates shadowing from scattering and not reflection. In addition, some tissues have variations in acoustical impedance so small that they appear cystic but show very little or no acoustical enhancement, usually attributed to structures truly cystic. These tissue-ultrasound interactions were discussed in detail in Chapter 9, dealing with the tissue effects on ultrasound.

As we move through the specialized imaging from different angles, using different acoustical windows and different transducers, we need to label and annotate the image with later viewing in mind. As in the survey scan, landmarks should be kept clearly in the image to prevent later confusion about the position of the scan plane or the particular acoustical window in use. This requirement grows in importance when scanning from unusual patient positions to more clearly delineate a mass. It also plays a major role in the applications of real-time sonography as detailed in Chapter 17.

Many lesions are surgically removed or biopsied. To aid the surgeon, we can provide positional information for specific surgical examinations. For example, renal surgery is seldom carried out from the anterior abdominal wall, rather it usually occurs through lateral and dorsal incisions. Providing information about mass position from the surgeon's point of view can tell the surgeon what to expect to see on the way to the mass.

Before The Patient Leaves

During the examination, the sonographer, the patient, and the sonograph form an interactive set of three independent systems. The result is a level of intimacy between sonographer and machine and between sonographer and patient not found in other forms of diagnostic information-gathering. This intimacy often provides impressions to the sonographer that can later be valuable additions to a diagnostic decision. These impressions are provided by the sonographer, whether or not the sonographer reads the final images for a diagnosis. The sonographer should write down impressions based on the imaging information and any experiments carried out during the examination.

Before the patient leaves, we need to be sure that all the questions formed at the beginning of the examination and resulting from the survey and specific scanning techniques are answered. A conscious forming of the questions in the beginning, followed by a methodical attempt to answer them, brings all the available scientific knowledge and clinical observations to bear on obtaining the answers. Just as we do not begin the examination until we understand what the questions are, we do not finish the examination until all the clinical questions *are* answered to the best of our ability.

An easy trap to fall into in reporting ultrasound examinations is to state the obvious: for example, a well-jaundiced patient is reported to have "enlarged bile ducts." On the other hand, citing the reason for the enlarged bile ducts is valuable. The sonographer needs to use his or her knowledge of disease and lesions to explain and test the reasons for the various presentations in the examination. Large bile ducts means an obstruction of the bile system. The real question is: Where is the obstruction located and what is its nature?

We should report the results of an examination as if this were the only information available. In other words, in arriving at an ultrasound-based conclusion, we scan to survey, scan the particular applications, and perform the necessary experiments to arrive at information that can stand alone without additional imaging. This does not discount the use of other clinical and imaging data to solve the question originally posed to the physician. But scanning for the "final word" encourages a completeness in the ultrasound examination that might otherwise be absent.

Reading the Images

The patient is gone, and we are now left with the images prepared during the examination and any additional history provided by the patient's record. Now the rigid survey format and the flexible special scanning techniques, along with the annotation, both anatomical and verbal, make the remaining information readable and useful. Given a rigid survey format, anyone reading the images knows both the sequence of images produced and the examination sequence. Reading the images requires repeating the sequence of the examination as if we were repeating the examination physically. Within the image, we look for the basic elements of image quality discussed in Chapter 19 that will let us examine, test, and trust the image contents. A carefully laid out labeling protocol and an anatomical annotation that includes landmarks helps to maintain a realistic perspective on the examination and the tissue-ultrasound interactions recorded in the images.

Conclusion

These are the basic elements, then, of thinking through the study. We prepare for the patient to arrive by ensuring that the machine is working properly; that we clearly understand the question being asked; and that we formulate the ultrasonic questions specific to the examination. We use the survey to gather the basic relationships and indications that will be examined in more detail in the study protocol. The survey is the starting point for this protocol, and even from the first scan comes a flow of information about the patient to guide us to the next stage in the protocol. We finish the examination with detailed scans using transducers geared for the job, not only in frequency, but in size and focal-point position. Before the patient leaves, we compile all the individual pieces of information, including written impressions, and prepare a report that states the reasons behind the obvious presentations.

In the end, both the sonographer and the sonologist must read the images. Through reliance on the survey format and careful annotation, reading the image becomes a direct extension of our organized approach to thinking through the study.

References

1. Shirley, I.M., et al. 1978. A user's guide to diagnostic ultrasound. Baltimore: University Park Press.
2. Fleischer, A.C., and A.E. James. 1980. Introduction to diagnostic sonography. New York: John Wiley & Sons.
3. Bartrum, R.J., and H.C. Crow. 1977. Gray-scale ultrasound: A manual for physicians and technicians. Philadelphia: W.B. Saunders Co.

Index